Reshaping Nursing Practice Through Cross-Border Partnerships

Athina Patelarou
https://orcid.org/0000-0002-0300-0650
Hellenic Mediterranean University. Greece

Alexandros Argyriadis
https://orcid.org/0000-0001-5754-4787
Hellenic Mediterranean University, Greece

Evridiki Patelarou
Hellenic Mediterranean University, Greece

IGI Global
Scientific Publishing
Publishing Tomorrow's Research Today

Vice President of Editorial	Melissa Wagner
Director of Acquisitions	Mikaela Felty
Director of Book Development	Jocelynn Hessler
Production Manager	Mike Brehm
Cover Design	Jose Rosado

Published in the United States of America by
IGI Global Scientific Publishing
701 East Chocolate Avenue
Hershey, PA, 17033, USA
Tel: 717-533-8845 | Fax: 717-533-7115
Website: https://www.igi-global.com E-mail: cust@igi-global.com

Library of Congress Cataloging-in-Publication Data

LCCN: 2025950951 (CIP Data Pending)
ISBN13: 979-8-3373-5931-1
Isbn13Softcover: 979-8-3373-5932-8
EISBN13: 979-8-3373-5933-5

British Cataloguing in Publication Data
A Cataloguing in Publication record for this book is available from the British Library.

Table of Contents

Detailed Table of Contents

nursing curricula is essential to prepare culturally competent nurses for a globally connected healthcare environment.

Barbara Kegl, Faculty of Health Sciences, University of Maribor, Slovenia
Petra Klanjsek, Faculty of Health Sciences, University of Maribor, Slovenia

International mobility of nursing students and faculty is crucial for building global competencies, cultural awareness, and adaptability. Programs such as Erasmus+, Fulbright, and bilateral agreements expose participants to diverse healthcare systems and foster intercultural skills that improve patient care. Beyond cultural and professional outcomes, ergonomics (physical, cognitive, and psychosocial) also plays an important role. A literature review will assess evidence on benefits, barriers, and best practices. Findings show mobility strengthens cultural sensitivity, critical thinking, and academic creativity, while driving institutional innovation through partnerships and curriculum development. Yet financial limits, rigid curricula, language barriers, and accreditation gaps restrict access and equity. To maximize impact, programs must reduce barriers, ensure inclusivity, and prepare participants.

R. Velmurugan, Karpagam Academy of Higher Education, Coimbatore, India
R. Bhuvaneswari, Dr. Mahalingam College of Engineering and Technology, Pollachi, India
Maksud A. Madraswale, Presidency University, Bangalore, India
S. Senthilkumar, Skyline University, Nigeria

The globalization of healthcare underscores the importance of faculty and student mobility in nursing education, defined as movement across institutional and cultural boundaries to enhance learning, practice, and research. Such mobility fosters knowledge exchange, skill development, and cultural competence, vital for a globalized healthcare environment. Students gain adaptability and cross-cultural awareness, while faculty benefit from exposure to diverse pedagogies and research methods. Despite challenges such as financial, institutional, and cultural barriers, mobility strengthens professional growth, curriculum innovation, and global partnerships. It enhances clinical competence, research collaboration, and global health outcomes. With supportive policies, funding, and technology-enabled exchanges, mobility can develop a culturally competent, innovative, and globally engaged nursing workforce.

Falls in people over the age of 65 is the most important factor of geriatric injuries leading to serious conditions, to increased death rates and serious socio-economic consequences. Hip fractures due to fall is an increased phenomenon, which quite regularly leads to secondary falls within six months after surgery, with all consequences that follows. Therefore, it is quite crucial to enhance the best treatment procedure for managing hip fracture after a fall, eliminating the incidence of further falls and improving the quality of patient's life. The multicomponent nature of geriatric hip fracture care demands a paradigm of a healthcare pathway from traditional single medical approaches to comprehensive multidisciplinary models. It is proved by various researchers that this phenomenon is being managed better by a multidisciplinary team, therefore it is quite crucial to design hip fracture rehabilitation plan and fall prevention strategies, based on cross border healthcare partnerships. This would ensure to implement strong and common healthcare policies in elderly care. Successful implementation strategies addressing these barriers typically include interprofessional education and team-building, communication protocols, and data-driven quality improvement with transparent outcome reporting. The role of advanced practice nurses and specialized care coordinators has emerged as crucial in recent studies. These professionals play a binding role in multidisciplinary teams together, ensuring that assessment findings translate into actionable care plans, facilitating communication across specialties and care transitions, and providing continuity for patients' healthcare plan in complex healthcare systems. The evidence increasingly suggests that dedicated orthogeriatric coordinators in multidisciplinary teams are not optional enhancements but rather essential substitute for high-quality hip fracture care.

In this chapter the author considers Social Capital Theory of Pierre Bourdieu, the Connected theory of Nicholas Christakis and James Fowler in order to help in finding out how social capital (that is - nurses, all social network of close relatives, friends, even followers in social media) matters in the process of passing through illness/ surgery smoothly and recover faster. Also, the Theory of Social Capital as Functional

Social Structure by James Coleman and a new approach to social capital of Robert Putnam are being considered by the author as constituent parts of contemporary approach to social capital.

This chapter examines how patient safety is integrated into nursing education by synthesizing international competency frameworks and their corresponding measurement instruments. It reviews general frameworks—the National Patient Safety Education Framework (NPSEF), the World Health Organization's Patient Safety Curriculum Guide, the Canadian Safety Competencies Framework, and EUNetPaS—and nursing-specific models including Quality and Safety Education for Nurses (QSEN) and the Patient Safety Competency Frameworks ($PSCF^a$, $PSCF^b$). The chapter maps core domains (teamwork, communication, human and system factors, risk management, and safety culture) to curricular design and clinical learning, and evaluates widely used tools (e.g., H-PEPSS, PaSNEQ, SAQ, HSOPS-NS, JCAT-NE) for their structure, validity, and applicability across various settings. The synthesis demonstrates how structured frameworks and validated instruments enable benchmarking, identify gaps, and advance a sustained culture of safety in nursing education and practice.

Creativity is considered one of the most complex human competences/abilities or behaviors. As sociologists, we consider creativity as a considerable factor in humanity's welfare, in terms of sense of fulfilment and happiness. We believe that social well-being, going hand in hand with the creative realization of one's purpose, is a two-way process. So, there are two factors that influence the enrichment of life: firstly, the state and conditions for creativity, which determines the feeling of inner satisfaction, and; secondly, the individual realization of one's own destiny and the socialization of an inner 'gift', i.e. abilities and talent. In this chapter we dive into the basic definitions of creativity and its theories, social conditions and beneficial, as well as hindering factors.The authors consider the ability of being creative as one of the main mental health conditions factors, as well as the opportunity to contact with art in all the ways during time of being disabled in the hospital as beneficial

Foreword

Modern nursing is transforming at a pace never witnessed before. Countries now face a wide range of complex public health challenges, including shifting demographics, widening health disparities, the impacts of climate change, environmental degradation, international migration, and persistent inequities in access to care. In this context, nurses stand at the core of health systems, serving not only as providers of direct care but also as educators, coordinators, innovators, and advocates for population health. Yet the realities they confront increasingly transcend traditional professional categories, institutional boundaries, and geographic limitations. For this reason, our ability to build meaningful, equitable, and enduring cross-border collaborations will be essential to the future of nursing, perhaps more than ever before.

The edited volume Reshaping Nursing Practice Through Cross-Border Partnerships offers a timely, insightful, and forward-looking contribution to this global conversation. The editors Athina Patelarou, Alexandros Argyriadis, and Evridiki Patelarou, bring together an exceptional group of scholars, practitioners, and educators whose work collectively demonstrates how international collaboration can strengthen nursing education, workforce development, clinical practice, and evidence-based decision-making across diverse health systems.

As an environmental health scientist, I am particularly encouraged by the attention given to how cross-border cooperation enhances our capacity to address emerging environmental and climatic risks. Nurses are often the first to observe shifts in health patterns among vulnerable populations such as children, older adults, migrants, and individuals living in underserved or environmentally stressed regions. When these insights are shared internationally, they become even more powerful facilitating comparative analyses, early identification of shared threats, and the dissemination of best practices. The chapters in this volume offer concrete examples of how such partnerships can support community-based health interventions, resilience, and preparedness.

This book arrives at a moment when global health challenges demand collective solutions. It provides an inspiring roadmap for institutions, policymakers, nursing leaders, and students seeking to expand their impact through collaboration. I am confident that this volume will make a meaningful contribution to contemporary discussions on nursing practice and will stimulate new models of international cooperation that advance environmental sustainability and health equity.

I extend my sincere congratulations to the editors for their vision and dedication, and I commend all contributors for their commitment to advancing the future of nursing. I hope the ideas presented here will foster new partnerships, spark innovation, and deepen our shared understanding of the vital role nurses play in shaping healthier, more resilient, and more just societies worldwide.

Petros Koutrakis
Harvard T.H. Chan School of Public Health, USA

Preface

The Laboratory of Evidence-Based Healthcare, Education and Clinical Protocols of the Hellenic Mediterranean University initiated the publication of this collective volume with the aim of fostering concrete collaboration among members of its wider network. The overarching objective was to promote international, interdisciplinary cooperation with faculty from universities around the world and to facilitate the translation of theoretical knowledge into clinical practice. The volume *Reshaping Nursing Practice Through Cross-Border Partnerships* emerges at a pivotal moment in global healthcare, when the boundaries between nations, disciplines, and professional identities are becoming increasingly fluid. Contemporary health systems face unprecedented demands—ranging from demographic shifts and the rising burden of chronic diseases to environmental challenges, transnational mobility, and widening inequalities in access to care. In this rapidly evolving landscape, nursing stands as one of the most dynamic forces capable of bridging divides and strengthening the resilience, equity, and sustainability of global health.

The chapters collected in this book reflect the diversity, creativity, and interdisciplinary nature of modern nursing practice. They also highlight a shared understanding: that meaningful progress in nursing can no longer occur within isolated systems. Instead, it is through international dialogue, collaborative learning, mobility programs, and the integration of multiple perspectives that nursing education and practice can aspire to meet the complexity of today's public health needs.

The first chapters explore cross-border partnerships as a catalyst for addressing structural vulnerabilities in insular and coastal populations. These contributions illuminate how international cooperation helps to reduce mental health inequities, promote environmental resilience, and strengthen local systems through comparative knowledge and shared methodologies. Subsequent chapters examine academic mobility as a transformative component of nursing education. Through European, Asian, and intercontinental perspectives, the book sheds light on how student and faculty mobility enhances cultural competence, broadens clinical experience, and enables institutions to co-create responsive curricula and innovative teaching strategies.

Equally important are the contributions addressing the intersections of nursing with social issues such as dating violence, creativity, and the sociocultural dimensions of mental wellbeing. These chapters emphasize that nursing is not simply a clinical profession; it is deeply embedded within social systems, relational networks, and evolving cultural landscapes. By engaging with these dimensions from an international standpoint, the book underscores the role of nurses as agents of change, advocates for vulnerable populations, and leaders in public health transformation.

Several chapters highlight how interdisciplinary teams, particularly in areas such as geriatric hip fracture rehabilitation and patient safety, reflect a shift toward collaborative, evidence-informed, and team-based models of care. The expertise presented demonstrates how interprofessional practice improves outcomes, strengthens communication, and enhances patient-centered approaches across borders.

The latter part of the book turns toward technological innovation and digital collaboration, essential elements of modern nursing. Whether through technology-enhanced mobility, integrated instructional design, or interdisciplinary partnerships with engineering and informatics, these chapters illustrate how digital tools can expand international cooperation and open new pathways for knowledge exchange. They also reflect the importance of preparing future nurses to navigate a technologically enriched global environment.

Taken as a whole, this volume aims to offer not only theoretical insights but also practical pathways for educators, practitioners, policymakers, and students who aspire to advance nursing through global partnerships. It highlights the power of collective learning, mutual respect, and transnational solidarity in shaping a more equitable healthy future.

We hope that this book will serve as an impetus for deeper collaboration, inspire new academic and clinical initiatives, and reinforce nursing's central role in building healthier and more resilient societies worldwide.

CHAPTER OVERVIEW

Chapter 1. Bridging the Shorelines: International Collaboration for Mental Health Equity in Insular and Coastal Areas examines how ecological vulnerability, systemic inequities, and cultural identity interact to shape mental health in insular and coastal regions. It aims to develop an integrative framework, the Shoreline Mental Health Equity Model (SMHEM), that links community resilience, cross border collaboration, and ethical governance. Using an interdisciplinary synthesis of empirical research, policy analysis, and case studies from Mediterranean and Caribbean contexts (2020–2025), the chapter adopts a qualitative meta,analytic approach informed by ecological systems theory and trauma,informed care principles. Findings reveal that mental health disparities in coastal populations stem from structural fragility, workforce shortages, and policy invisibility rather than geographic isolation alone.

Chapter 2. Role of Mobility in Advancing Nursing Education, Opportunities and Constraints examines the role of mobility in advancing nursing education within an increasingly globalized world. It discusses how physical, virtual, and institutional mobility foster intercultural competence, professional development, and ethical awareness among nursing students and educators. While mobility enhances curriculum internationalization and global collaboration, persistent inequalities in access, funding, and accreditation limit its inclusivity. The chapter argues for sustainable and ethical mobility frameworks that balance individual growth with global health equity. Integrating flexible and reflective mobility experiences into nursing curricula is essential to prepare culturally competent nurses for a globally connected healthcare environment.

Chapter 3. International Mobility in Nursing Education: Opportunities, Challenges, and Implications. International mobility of nursing students and faculty is crucial for building global competencies, cultural awareness, and adaptability. Programs such as Erasmus+, Fulbright, and bilateral agreements expose participants to diverse healthcare systems and foster intercultural skills that improve patient care. Beyond cultural and professional outcomes, ergonomics (physical, cognitive, and psychosocial) also plays an important role. A literature review will assess evidence on benefits, barriers, and best practices. Findings show mobility strengthens cultural sensitivity, critical thinking, and academic creativity, while driving institutional innovation through partnerships and curriculum development. Yet financial limits, rigid curricula, language barriers, and accreditation gaps restrict access and equity. To maximize impact, programs must reduce barriers, ensure inclusivity, and prepare participants.

Chapter 4. Faculty and Student Mobility in Nursing: Opportunities, Barriers, and Impacts. The globalization of healthcare underscores the importance of faculty and student mobility in nursing education, defined as movement across institutional and cultural boundaries to enhance learning, practice, and research. Such mobility fosters knowledge exchange, skill development, and cultural competence, vital for a globalized healthcare environment. Students gain adaptability and cross-cultural awareness, while faculty benefit from exposure to diverse pedagogies and research methods. Despite challenges such as financial, institutional, and cultural barriers, mobility strengthens professional growth, curriculum innovation, and global partnerships. It enhances clinical competence, research collaboration, and global health outcomes. With supportive policies, funding, and technology-enabled exchanges, mobility can develop a culturally competent, innovative, and globally engaged nursing workforce.

Chapter 5. Interdisciplinary Team in Geriatric Hip Fracture Care: A Clinical Rehabilitation Model. Falls in people over the age of 65 is the most important factor of geriatric injuries leading to serious conditions, to increased death rates and serious socio-economic consequences. Hip fractures due to fall is an increased phenomenon, which quite regularly leads to secondary falls within six months after surgery, with all consequences that follows. Therefore, it is quite crucial to enhance the best treatment procedure for managing hip fracture after a fall, eliminating the incidence of further falls and improving the quality of patient's life. The role of advanced practice nurses and specialized care coordinators has emerged as crucial in recent studies. These professionals play a binding role in multidisciplinary teams together, ensuring that assessment findings translate into actionable care plans, facilitating communication across specialties and care transitions, and providing continuity for patients' healthcare plan in complex healthcare systems.

Chapter 6. Social Capital of the Patient and Its Influence on the Mental Well-Being and Quick Recovery considers Social Capital Theory of Pierre Bourdieu, the Connected theory of Nicholas Christakis and James Fowler in order to help in finding out how social capital (that is - nurses, all social network of close relatives, friends, even followers in social media) matters in the process of passing through illness/surgery smoothly and recover faster. Also, the Theory of Social Capital as Functional Social Structure by James Coleman and a new approach to social capital of Robert Putnam are being considered by the author as constituent parts of contemporary approach to social capital.

Chapter 7. Patient Safety in Health Professions Education: Educational Frameworks and Evaluation of Patient Safety in Nursing examines how patient safety is integrated into nursing education by synthesizing international competency frameworks and their corresponding measurement instruments. It reviews general frameworks—the National Patient Safety Education Framework (NPSEF), the World Health Organization's Patient Safety Curriculum Guide, the Canadian Safety Competencies Framework, and EUNetPaS—and nursing-specific models including Quality and Safety Education for Nurses (QSEN) and the Patient Safety Competency Frameworks (PSCFa, PSCFb). The chapter maps core domains (teamwork, communication, human and system factors, risk management, and safety culture) to curricular design and clinical learning, and evaluates widely used tools (e.g., H-PEPSS, PaSNEQ, SAQ, HSOPS-NS, JCAT-NE) for their structure, validity, and applicability across various settings. The synthesis demonstrates how structured frameworks and validated instruments enable benchmarking, identify gaps, and advance a sustained culture of safety in nursing education and practice.

Chapter 8. Creativity as a sociological Category and a Factor of Mental Health consider the ability of being creative as one of the main mental health conditions factors, as well as the opportunity to contact with art in all the ways during time of being disabled in the hospital as beneficial factor for mental health. The authors consider that environment can be supportive to creativity and suppressive and that each organization (hospitals included) can help the creative potential to unfold, creating a proper environment – the authors call them socially harmonious (laminar, favorable) conditions for creativity, or suppress it by social rules and norms, we call them socialization unfavorable (conflict, turbulent) factors of creativity.

Chapter 9. Global Health Literacy and Nursing's Role in Health Promotion Across Borders. Global health literacy represents a fundamental pillar in promoting equitable health outcomes, reducing disease burden, and fostering informed decision-making across diverse populations. At its core, health literacy encompasses the ability of individuals and communities to access, comprehend, evaluate, and utilize health-related information to make informed decisions regarding their physical, mental, and social well-being. In an increasingly interconnected world, where health challenges transcend national boundaries, understanding global health literacy is crucial not only for individual empowerment but also for shaping resilient healthcare systems and sustainable public health strategies. Despite its recognized importance, global health literacy is unevenly distributed, reflecting and perpetuating existing socio-economic disparities. Populations in low- and middle-income countries (LMICs), marginalized communities, and vulnerable demographic groups.

Chapter 10. An Interdisciplinary Partnership of Nursing Education and Instructional Technology in Türkiye explores the significance of interdisciplinary study in the fields of nursing education and educational technology, with a particular emphasis on the integration of blended learning methodologies within nursing education. The chapter covers the role of nursing education in healthcare, the Turkish nursing education system, the legal and institutional framework of nursing education, the philosophy of nursing education and blended learning, the impact of paradigms on nursing education and blended learning, the role of educational technology in nursing education, the characteristics of nursing education. The necessity for an interdisciplinary partnership between nursing education and instructional technology is underscored. The authors posit that the integration of blended learning is conducive to effective learning and teaching opportunities across a wide range of disciplines in higher education, including nursing education. An interdisciplinary approach is considered essential for designing effective learning experiences in nursing education.

Athina Patelarou

Hellenic Mediterranean University. Greece

Alexandros Argyriadis

Hellenic Mediterranean University. Greece

Evridiki Patelarou
Hellenic Mediterranean University. Greece

Chapter 1
Bridging the Shorelines:
International Collaboration for Mental Health Equity in Insular and Coastal Areas

Agathi Argyriadi
American University in Dubai, UAE

Athina Patelarou
https://orcid.org/0000-0002-0300-0650
Hellenic Mediterranean University, Greece

Louiza Ioannidou
https://orcid.org/0000-0002-5320-1581
European University Cyprus, Cyprus

Evridiki Patelarou
Hellenic Mediterranean University, Greece

Efrosyni Kleanthous
Philips University, Cyprus

Alexandros Argyriadis
https://orcid.org/0000-0001-5754-4787
Hellenic Mediterranean University, Greece

ABSTRACT

This chapter examines how ecological vulnerability, systemic inequities, and cultural identity interact to shape mental health in insular and coastal regions. It aims to develop an integrative framework, the Shoreline Mental Health Equity Model (SMHEM), that links community resilience, cross border collaboration, and ethical governance. Using an interdisciplinary synthesis of empirical research, policy analysis, and case studies from Mediterranean and Caribbean contexts (2020–2025), the chapter adopts a qualitative meta,analytic approach informed by ecological systems theory and trauma,informed care principles. Findings reveal that mental health disparities in coastal populations stem from structural fragility, workforce shortages, and policy invisibility rather than geographic isolation alone.

DOI: 10.4018/979-8-3373-5931-1.ch001

INTRODUCTION

Insular and coastal regions sit at the intersection of environmental exposure, structural constraints, and cultural attachment, producing a distinct psychosocial terrain in which place operates as a determinant of health. The Intergovernmental Panel on Climate Change identifies small island and low,lying coastal zones as "hotspots of compounded risk," where climatic hazards (e.g., sea,level rise, storm surges, heat extremes) overlap with limited adaptive capacity (Intergovernmental Panel on Climate Change, 2022). In these settings, recurring shocks translate into cumulative distress, with anxiety, depressive symptoms, and post,traumatic stress reported following repeated disaster exposure and slow,onset environmental degradation (Coffey et al., 2021; Comtesse et al., 2021).

Environmental precariousness amplifies a collective sense of uncertainty. Qualitative and survey evidence links climate related worry with functional impairments in daily life among exposed populations, especially youth, while also noting heterogeneity in responses and the potential for constructive engagement (Clayton, 2020; Coffey et al., 2021). Importantly, the psychosocial burden is not limited to acute events. Slow transformations of seascapes and livelihoods can elicit enduring forms of ecological grief—an affective response to environmental loss that challenges belonging and meaning (Cunsolo & Ellis, 2018; Comtesse et al., 2021). For islands whose identities are inseparable from the sea, such losses reverberate across family rituals, intergenerational knowledge, and community cohesion.

Structural constraints compound these stressors. Many insular systems rely on small health workforces, costly supply chains, and fragile transport, which impede timely access to mental health care (World Health Organization, 2023). The Mental Health Atlas documents persistent service gaps worldwide and uneven progress toward parity for mental health in national plans, with resourcing deficits particularly salient in smaller states (World Health Organization, 2024). While the expansion of digital health during the COVID,19 era created new options for remote counseling and telepsychiatry, a "connectivity divide" persists across Small Island Developing States (SIDS): limited broadband, affordability barriers, and uneven digital skills restrict both care delivery and social participation that sustains wellbeing (United Nations Development Programme, 2024a, 2024b). Thus, geographic remoteness and digital exclusion often reinforce each other.

Economic volatility further shapes psychosocial risk. Tourism,dependent islands and coastal communities experience seasonal cycles and vulnerability to global shocks, with employment insecurity associated with stress, family conflict, and reduced help,seeking (United Nations Development Programme, 2024a). Demographic dynamics can intensify isolation: out,migration of young adults leaves aging residents with thinner support networks, elevating loneliness and undermining informal care—well,recognized predictors of poorer mental and physical health in later life (Intergovernmental Panel on Climate Change, 2022). These conditions frequently remain under,measured because routine mental health surveillance in small jurisdictions is sparse, limiting evidence,informed planning (World Health Organization, 2024).

Vulnerability is also intersectional. Gender, disability, age, and indigeneity modulate exposure and access to protection. Post,disaster assessments repeatedly show disproportionate risks for women and girls (including gender,based violence and economic precarity), barriers for persons with disabilities (from inaccessible evacuation to communication gaps), and heightened climate worry among youth (Intergovernmental Panel on Climate Change, 2022; World Health Organizaion, 2024). Intersectional framings suggest that risk multiplies across social positions, implying that generic psychosocial support is insufficient without accessibility, protection, and participation safeguards.

Against this backdrop, resilience should be understood relationally—as the capacity of communities, services, and institutions to reorganize under stress while preserving meaning and connection. Evidence,informed pathways include integrating mental health into climate adaptation and disaster,risk frameworks; scaling stepped,care and community,based psychosocial support; and investing in digital inclusion as a health enabler rather than a standalone technology agenda (Intergovernmental Panel on Climate Change, 2022; United Nations Development Programme, 2024a, United Nations Development Programme, 2024b; World Health Organization, 2024). Equally vital is knowledge co,production with island communities to ensure cultural resonance and to correct data invisibility that has historically marginalized small and peripheral places in national policy conversations (Intergovernmental Panel on Climate Change, 2022).

In sum, insular and coastal mental health is shaped by the convergence of environmental change, structural constraints, and cultural attachment. Addressing inequities requires moving beyond incident, focused care toward systemic strategies that pair service expansion with digital and social infrastructure, while recognizing ecological grief and climate anxiety as legitimate, heterogeneous responses to a transforming world (Clayton, 2020; Coffey et al., 2021; Comtesse et al., 2021; Intergovernmental Panel on Climate Change, 2022; World Health Organization, 2024; United Nations Development Programme, 2024a; United Nations Development Programme, 2024b).

RESEARCH TRENDS, GAPS, AND THE RATIONALE FOR INNOVATION

Over the past decade, research on climate-related mental health has expanded rapidly, reflecting a broader recognition that ecological change produces psychological, social, and cultural repercussions. Global scholarship increasingly examines constructs such as *eco-anxiety*, *ecological grief*, and *climate-related distress*, situating them within environmental psychology, public health, and climate adaptation research. Several large-scale studies—particularly those focused on youth and frontline communities—suggest that climate anxiety is becoming a widely distributed psychosocial phenomenon, with functional impacts on daily life, trust in institutions, and future orientation. Parallel qualitative work explores how communities interpret environmental loss through cultural narratives, spirituality, and intergenerational memory, thereby clarifying how meaning-making processes mediate distress. In insular and coastal settings, researchers have begun documenting the psychosocial effects of sea-level rise, erosion, livelihood transitions, and forced relocation, extending the conceptual vocabulary of climate-related emotional responses.

At the system level, another active research trend concerns the integration of mental health into disaster risk reduction, humanitarian response, and climate adaptation planning. Models of *psychosocial preparedness*, *stepped-care disaster support*, and *community-based resilience promotion* are increasingly prominent in the literature. Meanwhile, digital health scholarship has highlighted the potential of tele-mental health to address workforce shortages and geographical isolation. For island contexts, studies on digital inclusion and the "connectivity divide" have become central to understanding how digitalization intersects with mental health equity. Together, these bodies of work reflect a transition from conceptual articulation of climate-related distress toward applied research on health-system adaptation and multi-sectoral resilience.

Despite this momentum, several gaps remain pronounced—particularly for insular and coastal settings. First, much of the global climate-and-mental-health literature centers on large countries, urban zones, or highly visible crisis contexts. Small islands, remote archipelagos, and low-lying coastal regions remain under-represented in empirical studies, in part due to small population sizes and chronic data scarcity. As noted in global assessments, mental-health surveillance is extremely limited in these jurisdictions, leading to structural invisibility in national datasets and international comparisons. Consequently, evidence-informed planning is constrained, and many assumptions about vulnerability, resilience, or intervention effectiveness are extrapolated from dissimilar contexts without adequate validation.

Second, while emotional constructs such as eco-anxiety and ecological grief are now widely discussed, research rarely examines how these emotions interact with structural determinants—such as remoteness, digital exclusion, governance capacity, tourism-dependent economies, or migration patterns. Insular and coastal communities experience climate stressors within an ecosystem of pre-existing constraints. Yet few studies adopt multi-scalar frameworks that simultaneously address environmental exposure, cultural identity, and system fragility. This gap leads to fragmented policymaking: psychosocial programs may be designed without consideration of digital infrastructure; adaptation plans may ignore emotional wellbeing; and health policies may overlook cultural belonging as a protective factor.

Third, limited attention has been given to *knowledge co-production* with island communities. Although policy frameworks increasingly emphasize participation and local ownership, research practices often lack mechanisms for integrating experiential, indigenous, or community-generated knowledge. This is particularly problematic in contexts where place attachment, ritual, and intergenerational memory are central to wellbeing. Without participatory methodology, interventions risk being culturally misaligned or perceived as externally imposed.

Fourth, despite the emergence of digital health solutions, very few studies examine digital mental-health equity specifically for SIDS and coastal communities. Most telehealth evidence is generated in high-income settings and assumes stable broadband, digital literacy, and affordable devices—conditions not transferable to many islands. The absence of research on digital inclusion as a foundational health enabler limits the potential of remote counseling, telepsychiatry, and online peer support to reduce inequities.

Fifth, the literature tends to address climate-related mental health either through a clinical lens (diagnosable disorders) or through a psychosocial/emotional lens (eco-anxiety, grief), with limited integration across the two. For insular contexts, distress may manifest in ways that do not align neatly with psychiatric categories; conversely, major depressive or anxiety disorders may be under-diagnosed due to stigma, remoteness, or service gaps. A comprehensive framework must therefore bridge clinical, psychosocial, cultural, and structural perspectives.

These gaps underpin the rationale for innovation. The present work advances the field by proposing a conceptual reframing—mental health in insular and coastal settings as an *ecological, relational, and systemic phenomenon.* This perspective positions shoreline mental health equity not as a subset of disaster response, but as a cross-sectoral agenda embedded in climate governance, digital development, public health, and community resilience. In contrast with incident-based or pathology-focused models, this chapter emphasizes four interconnected dimensions: (a) environmental change and place-based emotional responses; (b) structural constraints in service delivery and governance; (c) cultural narratives and collective identity; and (d) opportunities for cross-border collaboration and digital solidarity.

A further innovation lies in identifying and articulating the *Shoreline Mental Health Equity Model (SMHEM)* as a coherent framework for these dynamics. By situating mental health within ecological systems theory, trauma-informed care, and critical public health, the model integrates previously siloed domains—environmental distress, cultural belonging, governance capacity, and cross-regional networks. Its emphasis on relational resilience, co-production, and ethical solidarity offers a conceptual advance beyond deficit-oriented understandings of vulnerability.

Methodologically, this work also highlights the need for research that combines psychometric assessment, qualitative inquiry, geospatial data, and digital-inclusion indicators. Such multi-method approaches can reveal how climate hazards, infrastructural fragility, and cultural identity co-produce mental-health outcomes. In doing so, the chapter points toward new avenues for comparative research across islands, the development of culturally grounded psychosocial indicators, and the design of early-warning systems that incorporate emotional and community-cohesion metrics.

Finally, the usefulness of this contribution lies in its policy relevance. By framing mental-health equity as inseparable from climate adaptation, digital inclusion, and multisectoral governance, the chapter provides practical guidance for governments, NGOs, and international partners. It underscores that improving mental health in insular and coastal communities requires integrated strategies: strengthening primary care, embedding psychosocial support in adaptation plans, investing in connectivity, and cultivating participatory platforms where local knowledge shapes decision-making.

In sum, while research on climate-related mental health is growing, it has not yet adequately captured the layered vulnerabilities—and capacities for resilience—found in insular and coastal regions. This chapter addresses that gap by offering a holistic, justice-oriented, and collaboration-driven approach that aligns environmental realities with culturally resonant mental-health responses.

CLIMATE CHANGE, ECO ANXIETY, AND THE EROSION OF PLACE IDENTITY

Climate change has become not only a biophysical phenomenon but also a deeply psychological and cultural experience that reshapes the ways communities understand belonging, stability, and hope. For inhabitants of islands and low,lying coastal regions, the changing climate is lived intimately—felt in the loss of fishing grounds, the encroachment of the sea, and the disruption of ancestral ties to land. Within this lived transformation, *eco anxiety* and *ecological grief* have emerged as salient concepts capturing the emotional and existential weight of environmental change (Clayton, 2020; Coffey et al., 2021). Yet their manifestations are profoundly context,dependent: in small island settings, these emotions intertwine with collective memory and place attachment, magnifying their psychological and sociocultural implications.

Empirical research demonstrates that climate related psychological distress is widespread and multifaceted. A landmark survey of 10,000 young people across ten countries revealed that 59 percent felt "very" or "extremely" worried about climate change, and 45 percent reported that these feelings negatively affected their daily functioning (Hickman et al., 2021). Although global in scope, such findings resonate acutely in insular communities where climate impacts are immediate and tangible. Coastal erosion, saltwater intrusion, and more frequent storms not only threaten livelihoods but also destabilize collective identity. The environment, once perceived as a source of continuity, becomes a reminder of impermanence.

Psychological frameworks suggest that eco anxiety is not inherently pathological but reflects an adaptive moral response to real ecological threats (Clayton, 2020; Panu, 2020). However, when persistent and coupled with perceived helplessness, it may exacerbate symptoms of anxiety or depression. Comtesse et al. (2021) conceptualize this reaction along a continuum from constructive engagement to functional impairment, emphasizing the importance of contextual factors—social support, cultural meaning systems, and governance trust—that mediate its outcomes. In island and coastal areas, where collective efficacy is constrained by structural marginalization, this continuum often tilts toward distress.

The notion of *solastalgia*, coined by Albrecht (2005) and elaborated by Cunsolo and Ellis (2018), captures the psychic dislocation that arises when environmental degradation transforms a once,familiar home into an alien landscape. It differs from nostalgia in that the individual remains physically rooted while the environment itself changes beyond recognition. In small island contexts, where cultural identity and livelihood are inseparable from land and sea, solastalgia constitutes a collective form of mourning. Residents of Arctic, Pacific, and Mediterranean coasts describe feelings of sadness, anger, and disorientation when coastal landmarks disappear or traditional practices become untenable (Cunsolo et al., 2020). These affective responses embody what Head (2023) calls *climate related loss of sense of place*—a phenomenon that erodes community cohesion and weakens mental health resilience.

Such ecological grief challenges conventional mental health paradigms that privilege individual pathology over social meaning. Cunsolo and Ellis (2018) argue for recognizing environmental loss as a legitimate driver of grief, requiring culturally responsive interventions rather than mere clinical treatment. Community,based rituals—such as storytelling circles, remembrance ceremonies for lost landscapes, or intergenerational art projects—have been shown to facilitate collective healing (Middleton et al., 2020). These practices align with indigenous epistemologies that frame emotional well being as relational and place,based, suggesting that psychological adaptation to climate change involves re,anchoring identity within altered environments.

Young people in particular inhabit an anticipatory form of distress, oscillating between activism and despair. Hickman et al. (2021) highlight that many youth perceive governmental inaction as betrayal, linking eco anxiety to moral outrage and loss of trust in institutions. In small island nations such as Fiji and the Maldives, qualitative studies describe pervasive fear of displacement and intergenerational guilt about the planet's future (Gibson et al., 2022). This "temporal compression," wherein the future feels simultaneously urgent and foreclosed, disrupts developmental trajectories and contributes to what Ojala (2023) calls *existential climate anxiety*. Importantly, hope emerges not from denial but from collective agency—education, civic participation, and the visibility of adaptive practices that reaffirm efficacy.

Educational interventions that integrate climate science with emotional literacy have shown promise in mitigating helplessness. For example, the Australian "Resilient Futures" curriculum links ecological knowledge with reflective exercises on grief and gratitude, fostering balanced engagement rather than avoidance (Burke et al., 2018). Comparable programs in Mediterranean schools emphasize local environmental stewardship, enabling students to translate anxiety into community action. These approaches illustrate that youth eco anxiety can serve as a catalyst for resilience when institutions provide avenues for participation and dialogue.

Cultural context shapes how environmental change is interpreted and emotionally processed. In Polynesian and Micronesian worldviews, land (*fanua*) and ocean are extensions of identity, and displacement represents not only material loss but spiritual rupture (McNamara & Jackson, 2019). Similarly, Mediterranean coastal communities articulate belonging through family continuity and ancestral memory; the degradation of these spaces evokes feelings of betrayal toward past and future generations (Albrecht et al., 2021). These narratives underscore that climate related distress is culturally embedded and morally inflected.

Collective resilience arises when cultural frameworks are mobilized for adaptation. Community,led coastal restoration projects in the Philippines and post,wildfire cultural renewal in Greece demonstrate how shared labor and narrative reconstruction foster recovery and meaning,making. Integrating such practices into mental health policy aligns with the World Health Organization's (2023) emphasis on community engagement as a cornerstone of psychosocial support in climate,affected settings. Rather than treating culture as a barrier, these examples illustrate its capacity to transform grief into solidarity.

Recognizing eco anxiety and ecological grief as legitimate responses to environmental transformation carries significant policy implications. First, it expands the scope of climate adaptation beyond infrastructure to include mental health and psychosocial dimensions (Intergovernmental Panel on Climate Change, 2022). Second, it calls for the ethical inclusion of affected communities in decision,making—what Cunsolo et al. (2020) term *emotional governance*. Policies that marginalize local voices risk perpetuating secondary trauma by denying recognition to lived suffering. Third, integrating mental health literacy into education, disaster,response training, and environmental planning can normalize help,seeking and reduce stigma.

The moral dimension is particularly salient in insular contexts, where environmental justice intersects with cultural survival. Protecting mental well being thus becomes an act of ecological and social justice. As Head (2023) argues, addressing climate related distress requires both adaptation of environments and transformation of ethics: societies must learn to coexist with change while sustaining empathy across generations and species.

The Greek islands and Crete occupy a unique climatic and geographical position within the Eastern Mediterranean, combining elements of a temperate, semi-arid, and subtropical environment. Their climate is shaped by prolonged dry summers, variable winter precipitation, intense heat episodes, and increasing frequency of extreme events—all of which exert direct and indirect effects on population health. Unlike continental settings, island microclimates can shift rapidly due to sea–land interactions, creating localized vulnerabilities that interact with demographic, infrastructural, and socio-economic factors. As climate variability accelerates across the Mediterranean basin, these regions face a complex mix of emerging health risks, changing care needs, and structural pressures on health services.

The Greek islands and Crete experience some of the longest and hottest summers in Europe. Heatwaves have become increasingly frequent and persistent, with temperatures surpassing 40°C even in traditionally milder coastal areas. Prolonged heat exposure is strongly associated with dehydration, renal stress, heat exhaustion, cardiovascular strain, and excess mortality among the elderly, infants, and individuals with chronic diseases. The population age structure of many islands—characterized by high proportions of older residents due to youth out-migration—magnifies vulnerability. Older adults living alone, especially in mountainous villages or remote coastal settlements, may have reduced access to cooling resources, transportation, and immediate medical assistance.

Tourism intensifies heat-related risks. Large influxes of seasonal visitors can overwhelm local health facilities, increase emergency-department load, and create transient populations unfamiliar with local climatic extremes. Reports from island clinics often highlight spikes in cases of heatstroke, syncope, arrhythmias, and electrolyte imbalance during July and August, placing additional strain on already limited medical staff. Moreover, outdoor workers—such as those in agriculture, construction, and hospitality—experience cumulative heat stress across the summer months, contributing to absenteeism, occupational injuries, and reduced productivity.

Air quality in the Aegean and Crete is strongly influenced by Saharan dust episodes, which have intensified due to shifting atmospheric circulation. These dust plumes elevate concentrations of PM10 and PM2.5, exacerbating asthma, COPD symptoms, allergic rhinitis, and cardiovascular stress. Children, older adults, and individuals with chronic respiratory conditions are particularly sensitive. Primary care centers in Crete and the Cyclades report noticeable increases in respiratory consultations during dust intrusion events, often coinciding with emergency responses for asthmatic crises or acute bronchitis.

In addition, heat and stagnant air masses contribute to ozone formation, compounding respiratory risks. Seasonal variability means that health systems must maintain surge capacity for pollutant-related exacerbations while simultaneously addressing heat-related illnesses, creating overlapping seasonal burdens that require integrated monitoring and preparedness protocols.

Many Greek islands face chronic water scarcity due to limited freshwater resources, saline intrusion, and increasing evaporation rates. Water is often imported, desalinized, or rationed during peak tourist periods. This scarcity impacts health in several ways. Limited water availability reduces hygiene capacity, contributing to minor gastrointestinal infections, dermatological issues, and increased vulnerability during heatwaves. Salinity changes in local supplies may affect vulnerable individuals, including those with hypertension or kidney disease.

Seasonal increases in water-borne infections—such as gastroenteritis, norovirus, and salmonella—have been reported in island health centers, particularly when water demand surges and distribution networks are strained. Wastewater management systems in smaller islands can become overwhelmed during the tourism season, increasing the risk of contamination and vector breeding.

Climate warming has expanded the geographical range and seasonal activity of vectors such as mosquitoes, sandflies, and ticks. The Aegean islands and Crete have witnessed episodic occurrences of West Nile Virus, increased phlebotomine activity linked to leishmaniasis, and sporadic chikungunya or dengue risk alerts associated with Aedes albopictus expansion. Warmer winters and prolonged autumn periods create longer breeding seasons, while water scarcity leads many residents to store water in containers—ideal vector habitats.

Moreover, the movement of large tourist populations provides opportunities for disease introduction and dissemination. Health services must maintain surveillance capacity, public education, and rapid diagnostic access despite limited laboratory infrastructure on many islands.

Climate stressors exacerbate psychosocial challenges already present in insular settings. Extended heat, drought, wildfire exposure, and recurring dust storms contribute to irritability, sleep disturbances, anxiety, and a persistent background of climatic worry. Islanders whose livelihoods depend on fishing, agriculture, or tourism experience profound uncertainty tied to environmental variability. In Crete, olive cultivation and viticulture are increasingly affected by drought patterns and pest proliferation, creating economic insecurity that reverberates in family wellbeing.

Social isolation, common in rural and mountainous island villages, intensifies heat-related psychological strain. When combined with infrastructure disruptions—power outages, transportation delays, water rationing—these conditions heighten emotional distress and reduce resilience. For many communities, climate-related loss of landscape (e.g., erosion, wildfire scars) produces grief responses that mirror ecological grief described in global literature.

Health services across the Greek islands and Crete face longstanding structural challenges. Hospitals are unevenly distributed, with many islands relying solely on small health centres staffed by rotating physicians, limited nursing personnel, and restricted diagnostic capacity. Emergency evacuations by boat or air are often delayed by weather conditions—strong Meltemi winds, rough seas, or fog—creating critical delays in acute care.

Seasonal population surges during tourism months amplify demand for emergency, primary, and preventive services, while staffing levels remain constant or even reduced. Pharmacies, diagnostic labs, and mental-health services may operate with limited hours or face supply chain delays. Telemedicine initiatives have expanded since the COVID-19 pandemic, yet persistent digital gaps—poor signal in mountainous zones, limited broadband on smaller islands, affordability issues—restrict consistent implementation.

SYSTEMIC INEQUITIES IN MENTAL HEALTH ACCESS AND RESILIENCE BUILDING

Insular and coastal populations face not only the physical consequences of climate change but also the entrenched inequities of health and governance systems that shape their access to mental health care. Structural determinants—such as limited infrastructure, workforce shortages, fragmented governance, and social stigma—combine with environmental risks to create what the World Health Organization (2024) describes as a "layered inequity." These inequities are systemic rather than incidental: they reflect historical marginalization, policy neglect, and the uneven distribution of global resources. Addressing mental health resilience in these regions, therefore, requires an ecological understanding of health systems, one that recognizes how structural and social conditions co,produce vulnerability and recovery.

In many island and coastal states, health infrastructure is small in scale, heavily centralized, and often dependent on imports or external aid. The Mental Health Atlas 2024 reports that more than two,thirds of Small Island Developing States (SIDS) lack a stand,alone mental health policy or an operational action plan, while less than half allocate more than one percent of their health budget to mental health (World Health Organization, 2024). The consequences are immediate and measurable: limited psychiatric beds, scarce community services, and delayed crisis response. Geographic dispersion further compounds these deficits, as transportation and referral networks are frequently disrupted during extreme weather events. For residents of remote islands, continuity of care can depend on a single ferry route, a satellite connection, or the availability of one overstretched nurse.

This infrastructural fragility renders systems reactive rather than preventive. As Rehm et al. (2022) observe, small states tend to allocate resources toward hospital,based crisis management rather than community,based prevention, perpetuating cycles of acute care and relapse. When disasters strike, mental health services are among the first to collapse and the last to recover. The absence of stable financing mechanisms further limits sustainability, leaving local authorities dependent on international donors whose priorities may shift with global trends. These dynamics underscore the need for health,system resilience frameworks that integrate mental health planning into broader disaster,risk management and climate adaptation policies.

Human resources represent another persistent bottleneck. WHO (2024) data show a median of fewer than two psychiatrists per 100,000 inhabitants across SIDS, compared with over nine in high,income countries. Psychologists, psychiatric nurses, and social workers are similarly scarce, and training opportunities remain limited. Health professionals in small island systems frequently assume multiple roles—clinician, administrator, and crisis responder—without adequate supervision or support. Such multitasking, though necessary, increases burnout and turnover, further weakening service continuity.

Innovative capacity building approaches are emerging to address these deficits. The Pan American Health Organization (PAHO) has piloted tele,education networks connecting Caribbean mental health workers with regional training hubs, demonstrating significant improvements in clinical knowledge and perceived confidence (Pan American Health Organization, 2023). Similarly, Mediterranean collaborations—such as the partnership between the Hellenic Mediterranean University and Frederick University Cyprus—illustrate the value of joint curricula in community mental health literacy and trauma,informed care. These initiatives show that capacity building must be both technical and relational, nurturing professional networks that can sustain morale and knowledge exchange despite geographic isolation.

Governance deficits compound infrastructure and workforce challenges. In many coastal and insular systems, mental health remains peripheral to public,health strategy, and accountability mechanisms are underdeveloped. Few nations collect disaggregated data on mental health service use, and even fewer integrate such data into planning or budgeting processes. The absence of reliable indicators hampers both national and international efforts to evaluate progress toward Sustainable Development Goal (SDG) Target 3.4—reducing premature mortality through prevention and treatment of mental disorders. Without systematic data, inequities remain invisible.

Recent analyses by the United Nations Development Programme (2024) highlight digital data governance as a critical enabler of equity. Investments in interoperable health,information systems allow small jurisdictions to aggregate and visualize mental health indicators alongside climate and socioeconomic variables. Such integrative data ecosystems support early warning for psychosocial distress following environmental shocks and enable more transparent resource allocation. However, governance reform also entails ethical challenges: ensuring data sovereignty, protecting confidentiality in small populations, and involving communities in defining what constitutes meaningful evidence. Equity, in this sense, is inseparable from participation.

Beyond institutional constraints, cultural stigma remains one of the most pervasive barriers to mental health access. In many tight,knit island societies, concerns about confidentiality and social judgment discourage individuals from seeking care. Research in Caribbean and Mediterranean contexts indicates that mental illness is often interpreted through moral or spiritual frameworks, reinforcing shame and concealment (Wainberg et al., 2023). Stigma is particularly pronounced in small communities where anonymity is impossible, and gossip functions as a form of social regulation.

Combating stigma requires culturally embedded approaches that transform rather than confront local belief systems. WHO (2023) advocates for community,led "anti,stigma ecosystems" that combine public education, peer support, and lived,experience leadership. Such approaches have shown success in Malta's *Mind the Gap* initiative and in Bermuda's community "talking circles," where storytelling and dialogue reframe mental illness as a shared human experience (World Health Organization, 2023). By aligning psychosocial messaging with cultural idioms of care—family, faith, and collective responsibility—these programs demonstrate that destigmatization must resonate emotionally as well as cognitively (Chatzea et al., 2022).

Resilience, in this context, denotes more than psychological endurance; it is a systemic property of communities and institutions. WHO (2023, 2024) frameworks emphasize integration—embedding mental health services into primary care, education, and climate adaptation planning. The success of such integration depends on governance coherence and cross,sectoral collaboration. For example, embedding mental health professionals within community nursing and disaster,response teams in Cyprus and Crete has improved early identification of trauma and eco anxiety. Digital platforms can augment these networks, facilitating teleconsultation and continuous professional development even in geographically fragmented settings.

True resilience also demands ethical reflexivity. As Allen et al. (2023) argue, health systems must balance efficiency with equity, ensuring that rapid digitalization does not deepen disparities by privileging those with connectivity or literacy advantages. Therefore, resilience building must be participatory—anchored in local agency, guided by inclusive governance, and evaluated through the lived experiences of those most affected. In insular and coastal contexts, where the boundaries between environment, economy, and emotion blur, such integrative models offer the only sustainable pathway to mental health equity.

CROSS BORDER COLLABORATION AND THE FOUNDATIONS OF THE SHORELINE MENTAL HEALTH EQUITY MODEL (SMHEM)

Global health is increasingly shaped by interconnected crises—climate change, migration, pandemics, and resource scarcity—that transcend national boundaries. In such a context, the mental health of insular and coastal communities cannot be addressed through isolated national programs. These populations share ecological vulnerabilities, economic dependencies, and psychosocial stressors that call for regional and international solidarity. Cross border collaboration thus emerges not as an optional enhancement but as a structural necessity for equity and resilience. The Shoreline Mental Health Equity Model (SMHEM) is conceived as a framework for translating that necessity into coordinated action, linking local agency with global partnerships to strengthen mental health systems in geographically and politically peripheral regions.

The rationale for transnational collaboration in mental health is both pragmatic and ethical. Pragmatically, small systems face limited economies of scale and human resources, making collaboration a cost,effective means to share expertise, data, and infrastructure (World Health Organization, 2023). Ethically, it affirms the principle of *shared responsibility* enshrined in the Sustainable Development Goals, particularly SDG 3 (health and well being) and SDG 13 (climate action). The WHO's *Comprehensive Mental Health Action Plan 2023–2030* explicitly calls for "regional solidarity mechanisms" that support low,capacity states in governance, financing, and workforce development (World Health Organization, 2023). Within this paradigm, islands and coastal regions become laboratories for innovation, testing scalable models of digital care, culturally grounded prevention, and climate,informed psychosocial support.

Collaborative mechanisms can take diverse forms: bilateral partnerships between universities, regional mental health networks, or multi,stakeholder consortia integrating academia, NGOs, and local governments. The Pan American Health Organization's Caribbean Network, for example, coordinates telepsychiatry, training, and shared protocols among member states, demonstrating measurable improvements in continuity of care (Pan American Health Organization [PAHO], 2023). In the Mediterranean basin, cross border university alliances between Greece, Cyprus, and Malta have developed joint curricula on trauma,informed community nursing and mental health literacy (Argyriadi et al., 2025). These cases show that collaboration does more than transfer resources—it redefines power relations, enabling smaller systems to become co,creators of global knowledge.

The Shoreline Mental Health Equity Model (SMHEM) arises from an ecological and justice,oriented understanding of health. It synthesizes three theoretical traditions: (a) Ecological Systems Theory, which situates individual wellbeing within interdependent micro,, meso,, and macro,environments (Bronfenbrenner, 1979); (b) Trauma,Informed Care, emphasizing safety, trust, empowerment, and peer support as principles guiding psychosocial interventions (Substance Abuse and Mental Health Services Administration [SAMHSA], 2020); and (c) Critical Public Health, which foregrounds participation, equity, and the redistribution of resources as prerequisites for mental health justice (Baum et al., 2022). Together, these perspectives reposition mental health from a purely clinical concern to a *relational ecosystem* encompassing environment, culture, and governance.

Within the SMHEM, four interlocking dimensions provide operational scaffolding:

- Community,Driven Service Design: Local actors co,create strategies reflecting their cultural narratives, ensuring ownership and sustainability.
- Culturally Contextualized Care: Clinical interventions are adapted to indigenous and local epistemologies, recognizing the role of spirituality, family, and place in healing.
- Cross border Partnerships: Regional and international collaborations strengthen capacity and harmonize standards while respecting local autonomy.
- Policy Advocacy for Maritime Health Equity: Mental health is embedded within environmental, social, and economic policies that address the specific vulnerabilities of coastal populations.

These dimensions are not hierarchical but cyclical, reflecting the feedback loops characteristic of socioecological systems. The model thus aspires to be both conceptual and practical, a blueprint adaptable to diverse contexts without imposing uniformity.

A central tenet of the SMHEM is *knowledge co,production*: the collaborative generation of evidence and practice between researchers, practitioners, and community members. Traditional models of knowledge transfer often perpetuate asymmetry, with expertise flowing unidirectionally from high,income to low,capacity regions. Co,production challenges this hierarchy by valuing experiential and indigenous knowledge alongside academic science (Baum et al., 2022). In coastal contexts, fisher communities, local nurses, and teachers frequently possess intimate knowledge of psychosocial needs, disaster patterns, and culturally acceptable coping mechanisms. Integrating these insights into formal systems increases cultural relevance and service uptake.

Capacity building under the SMHEM emphasizes networked learning rather than static training. Tele,education programs and hybrid workshops allow dispersed professionals to maintain continuous learning communities. For example, the *Digital Health for Islands* initiative supported by the United Nations Development Programme (2024) demonstrates how online platforms can enable small states to access global expertise while contextualizing it locally. However, as Allen et al. (2023) caution, digitalization must be governed by equity principles—ensuring that technology enhances, rather than replaces, interpersonal and community,based care. Thus, co,production and capacity building must advance simultaneously: technology extends reach, while local knowledge ensures resonance.

Beyond service delivery, cross border collaboration operates through *global health diplomacy*—the negotiation of shared norms, resources, and accountability frameworks that influence national agendas. The concept underscores that health equity is inherently political. For coastal and insular states, diplomacy provides access to funding mechanisms and regional policy platforms otherwise dominated by larger economies. Within the European context, initiatives such as the *EU4Health Programme* and the *European Education Area* offer models for integrating mental health and environmental resilience into cross,national governance (European Commission, 2024).

Diplomatic engagement also shapes data governance. Collaborative research protocols that respect community ownership and privacy help balance the need for transparency with ethical stewardship. International organizations can facilitate standardized data collection across islands, enabling comparative analysis while protecting sovereignty. Such frameworks align with the WHO's (2023) recommendation for "solidarity,based monitoring" that treats data as a shared global good rather than a proprietary asset. By embedding ethical diplomacy into health governance, the SMHEM envisions a pluralistic global network where diverse regions contribute to, and benefit from, collective resilience.

The Mediterranean region offers an emerging example of how the SMHEM framework can function in practice. Cross border collaborations among Greek, Cypriot, and Maltese institutions have focused on eco anxiety and trauma recovery following wildfires, floods, and heatwaves. Joint projects led by community nursing departments combine psychosocial education with participatory workshops on mindfulness, storytelling, and ecological restoration (Argyriadi et al., 2025). Preliminary evaluations indicate reductions in reported anxiety and strengthened perceptions of social belonging, supporting the model's premise that local participation and cultural expression are central to resilience.

Equally significant are the policy ripple effects: health ministries have begun incorporating psychosocial indicators into disaster,preparedness protocols, while universities embed climate related mental health modules into public,health curricula. These developments exemplify how academic collaboration can influence systemic change. The Mediterranean cluster thus represents a microcosm of the SMHEM in action—linking localized interventions to regional governance and, through European networks, to global policy dialogues.

POLICY INTEGRATION, PRACTICE PATHWAYS, AND THE ETHICS OF COLLECTIVE RESILIENCE

The transition from analysis to action in insular and coastal mental health systems demands a coherent integration of policy, practice and ethics. This final section addresses how policy frameworks can institutionalize resilient mental health pathways, how practice can be aligned with culturally and environmentally informed ethics, and how collective resilience emerges as a normative goal for communities facing layered vulnerabilities.

Existing national adaptation strategies frequently exclude explicit references to mental health. For example, a global review found that only 42% of national climate adaptation policies mention mental health, and a mere 17% implement concrete adaptation actions targeting psychosocial outcomes. Embedding mental health considerations in adaptation policy means shifting from siloed disaster response to holistic anticipatory governance. Coastal and insular contexts magnify this need: policy must connect environmental risk, psychosocial vulnerability and health-system resilience. For instance, one empirical study of sea,level rise impacts on coastal communities documented heightened depression and anxiety linked to place,loss, reinforcing the imperative for policy that spans environment, health and social care. Integration involves cross,ministerial cooperation (environment, health, social welfare), budgeting for mental health infrastructure in climate,vulnerable zones, and monitoring tools that track psychosocial metrics alongside traditional adaptation indicators.

Operationalizing policy requires practice pathways that prioritize prevention, local engagement and equitable access. Preventive care involves training primary,care and community workers in psychological first aid post,environmental disasters, deploying tele,mental health platforms in remote islands, and expanding mobile outreach during prolonged climatic stress. Studies in coastal settings show that community-based mental health initiatives anchored in local traditions and ecological stewardship enhance participation and outcomes. Moreover, literature on nature-based solutions suggests that access to green and blue spaces fosters psychological restoration and sense of place, which is critical for resilience in coastal populations. Practice pathways must also adopt community co-production models, where residents participate in design, evaluation and governance of interventions to ensure cultural relevance and ownership.

The ethics of collective resilience in coastal mental health revolve around three interlinked principles: justice, participation and place,based rights. Justice demands that persons in remote, vulnerable regions receive equitable mental health resources despite logistical challenges inherent to geography. Participation ensures that communities are not passive recipients but active agents in shaping their future wellbeing. Place-based rights emphasize the cultural and environmental embeddedness of identity: when coastlines erode or ecosystems change, the loss is not only physical but moral and communal. The ethical framework laid out by Mishra, Han & Ramanathan (2025) argues that societal transformation for climate resilience must incorporate mental health objectives, promote social connection within frontline communities, and build long,term policy that prioritizes human wellbeing alongside ecological sustainability. In coastal zones, upholding these ethics means recognizing environmental grief as legitimate, designing inclusive governance mechanisms and aligning interventions with local narratives of home.

Accountability is central to whether policy integration and practice pathways translate into tangible improvements. Traditional metrics—such as number of beds, professional ratios or treatment uptake—fall short of capturing psychocultural and ecological dimensions of wellbeing. Newer frameworks propose psychosocial indicators (e.g., eco anxiety prevalence, sense of place disruption) and integrated dashboards linking climate and health data (Eissa et al., 2025). Monitoring must disaggregate by gender, age, disability and geography to reveal inequities. Furthermore, coastal jurisdictions must adopt participatory evaluation models, where community feedback informs service redesign. The ethical imperative is clear: "what gets measured gets managed"—and without meaningful metrics, justice and resilience remain aspirational.

CONCLUSIONS

Collective resilience in insular and coastal communities emerges when mental health systems, social networks and environmental stewardship converge. A "Shoreline Futures" approach entails: (a) strengthening ecological literacy and emotional literacy concurrently; (b) fostering cross,sectoral platforms that link local government, health services, environment agencies and civil society; (c) leveraging digital connectivity while safeguarding universality and affordability; and (d) institutionalizing feedback loops where communities refine adaptation strategies based on lived experience. A recent perspective article in *npj Climate Action* underscores that mental health inclusion accelerates climate resilience by promoting social cohesion and sustainable behavior change (Mishra et al., 2025). In practice, coastal mental health models should integrate community festivals, eco,restoration projects, peer,support groups and digital counseling platforms—moving from crisis response to continuous ecosystem of care.

REFERENCES

Albrecht, G., Askland, H. H., & Head, L. (2021). Solastalgia: Living with environmental change. In Head, L. (Ed.), *Refugia: Radical adaptation in a time of ecological crisis* (pp. 65–82). Routledge., DOI: 10.4324/9781003121425

Allen, J., Black, N., Clarke, A., & Dixon-Woods, M. (2023). What is system resilience? *BMJ (Clinical Research Ed.), 382*, e073696. DOI: 10.1136/bmj-2022-073696 PMID: 37402509

Argyriadi, A., Katsarou, D., Patelarou, A., Megari, K., Patelarou, E., Kotrotsiou, S., Giakoumidakis, K., Abdoola, S., Mantsos, E., Efthymiou, E., & Argyriadis, A. (2025). Digital Stress Scale (DSC): Development and Psychometric Validation of a Measure of Stress in the Digital Age. *International Journal of Environmental Research and Public Health, 22*(7), 1080. DOI: 10.3390/ijerph22071080 PMID: 40724147

Baum, F., Freeman, T., & Lawless, A. (2022). Why critical public health matters for health equity. *Social Science & Medicine, 307*, 115188. DOI: 10.1016/j.socscimed.2022.115188

Burke, S. E. L., Sanson, A. V., & Van Hoorn, J. (2018). The psychological effects of climate change on children. *Current Psychiatry Reports, 20*(5), 35. DOI: 10.1007/s11920-018-0896-9 PMID: 29637319

Chatzea, V. E., Mechili, E. A., Melidoniotis, E., Petrougaki, E., Nikiforidis, G., Argyriadis, A., & Sifaki-Pistolla, D. (2022). Recommendations for young researchers on how to better advance their scientific career: A systematic review. *Population Medicine, 4*(September), 1–17. DOI: 10.18332/popmed/152571

Clayton, S. (2020). Climate anxiety: Psychological responses to climate change. *Journal of Anxiety Disorders, 74*, 102263. DOI: 10.1016/j.janxdis.2020.102263 PMID: 32623280

Coffey, Y., Bhullar, N., Durkin, J., Islam, M. S., & Usher, K. (2021). Understanding eco-anxiety: A systematic scoping review of current literature and identified knowledge gaps. *The Journal of Climate Change and Health, 3*, 100047. DOI: 10.1016/j.joclim.2021.100047

Comtesse, H., Ertl, V., Hengst, S. M. C., Rosner, R., & Smid, G. E. (2021). Ecological grief as a response to environmental change: A mental health risk or functional response? *International Journal of Environmental Research and Public Health, 18*(2), 734. DOI: 10.3390/ijerph18020734 PMID: 33467018

Cunsolo, A., & Ellis, N. R. (2018). Ecological grief as a mental health response to climate change-related loss. *Nature Climate Change*, *8*(4), 275–281. DOI: 10.1038/s41558-018-0092-2

Cunsolo, A., Harper, S. L., Minor, K., Hayes, K., Williams, K. G., & Howard, C. (2020). Ecological grief and anxiety: The start of a healthy response to climate change? *The Lancet. Planetary Health*, *4*(7), e261–e263. DOI: 10.1016/S2542-5196(20)30144-3 PMID: 32681892

European Commission. (2024). *EU4Health Programme 2024–2027: Building stronger health systems in Europe.* https://health.ec.europa.eu/funding/eu4health-programme_en

Gibson, K. E., Barnett, J., Webber, M., & Friel, S. (2022). Environmental change and mental health: Understanding climate-related distress in the Pacific. *Nature Climate Change*, *12*(2), 146–155. DOI: 10.1038/s41558-021-01216-2

Head, L. (2023). Climate change and sense of place. *Progress in Human Geography*, *47*(1), 3–20. DOI: 10.1177/03091325221111910

Hickman, C., Marks, E., Pihkala, P., Clayton, S., Lewandowski, R. E., Mayall, E. E., Wray, B., Mellor, C., & van Susteren, L. (2021). Climate anxiety in children and young people and their beliefs about government responses to climate change: A global survey. *The Lancet. Planetary Health*, *5*(12), e863–e873. DOI: 10.1016/S2542-5196(21)00278-3 PMID: 34895496

Intergovernmental Panel on Climate Change. (2022). *Climate Change 2022: Impacts, adaptation and vulnerability* (WGII Sixth Assessment Report). https://www.ipcc.ch/report/ar6/wg2/

McNamara, K. E., & Jackson, G. (2019). Loss and damage: When adaptation is not enough. *Climate Policy*, *19*(6), 667–678. DOI: 10.1080/14693062.2019.1594967

Middleton, J., Cunsolo, A., Jones-Bailey, M., & Harper, S. L. (2020). Moving toward a framework for cultural climate grief. *Emotion, Space and Society*, *37*, 100738. DOI: 10.1016/j.emospa.2020.100738

Ojala, M. (2023). Hope and meaning in times of climate change: Promoting agency in young people. *Current Opinion in Psychology*, *49*, 101554. DOI: 10.1016/j.copsyc.2023.101554

Pan American Health Organization. (2023). *Caribbean Mental Health Network: Strengthening capacity through regional cooperation.* https://www.paho.org/en/topics/mental-health

Panu, P. (2020). Anxiety and the ecological crisis: An analysis of eco-anxiety and climate anxiety. *Sustainability (Basel)*, *12*(19), 7836. DOI: 10.3390/su12197836

Rehm, J., Shield, K. D., & Gmel, G. (2022). The contribution of mental and substance use disorders to global burden of disease. *The Lancet. Psychiatry*, *9*(2), 107–118. DOI: 10.1016/S2215-0366(21)00429-0 PMID: 35065719

United Nations Development Programme. (2024a). *Small Island Digital States: How digital can catalyse SIDS development.* https://www.undp.org/publications/small-island-digital-states-how-digital-can-catalyse-sids-development

United Nations Development Programme. (2024b). *How digital is transforming the lives of young people in Small Island Developing States.* https://www.undp.org/sites/g/files/zskgke326/files/2024-04/undp-how-digital-is-transforming-the-lives-of-young-people-in-small-island-developing-states-v2.pdf

Wainberg, M. L., Scorza, P., & Collins, P. Y. (2023). Cultural stigma and global mental health inequities. *World Psychiatry; Official Journal of the World Psychiatric Association (WPA)*, *22*(1), 1–9. DOI: 10.1002/wps.21029 PMID: 36640397

World Health Organization. (2023). *Comprehensive Mental Health Action Plan 2023–2030.* https://www.who.int/publications/i/item/9789240072244

World Health Organization. (2024). *Mental Health Atlas 2024.* https://www.who.int/publications/i/item/9789240114487

Chapter 2
Role of Mobility in Advancing Nursing Education:
Opportunities and Constraints

Ulrike Tscherne
https://orcid.org/0009-0008-9594-0228
Carinthia University of Applied Sciences, Austria

ABSTRACT

This chapter examines the role of mobility in advancing nursing education within an increasingly globalized world. It discusses how physical, virtual, and institutional mobility foster intercultural competence, professional development, and ethical awareness among nursing students and educators. While mobility enhances curriculum internationalization and global collaboration, persistent inequalities in access, funding, and accreditation limit its inclusivity. The chapter argues for sustainable and ethical mobility frameworks that balance individual growth with global health equity. Integrating flexible and reflective mobility experiences into nursing curricula is essential to prepare culturally competent nurses for a globally connected healthcare environment.

1 INTRODUCTION

Globalization and internationalization have profoundly reshaped the landscape of higher education, and nursing-rooted in care, ethics and applied science has not been immune to these transformations. Academic mobility has become a central strategy for fostering global citizenship, intercultural competence and transnational

DOI: 10.4018/979-8-3373-5931-1.ch002

collaboration among nursing students and educators (Dobrowolska et al., 2015; Kunaviktikul et al., 2019; Roy et al., 2019, 2019). The growing recognition that health and illness transcend borders underscores the need for a nursing workforce capable of delivering equitable and culturally sensitive care worldwide.

Mobility initiatives – ranging from structured exchange programs like Erasmus+ and Nordplus to short-term placements and virtual collaborations – allow nursing students to experience diverse healthcare systems, pedagogical models and socio-cultural contexts (Bjørnnes et al., 2024; Borrelli et al., 2022)

However, while these programs offer immense professional and personal benefits, they also expose persistent disparities in access, funding and recognition across global regions. The challenge for contemporary nursing education lies in ensuring that such mobility remains inclusive, ethical and sustainable.

Recent literature has shifted from descriptive accounts of mobility to empirical and theoretical analyses of its impact. Roy et al. (2019) and Johnston et al. (2022) emphasize that mobility can enhance learning outcomes, reflective capacity and employability, but these gains depend heavily on program design, duration and institutional support. Moreover, socio-political factors such as global inequalities and credential recognition systems continue to constrain the democratization of educational exchange (Bani et al., 2025; Ghimire & Neupane, 2025).

This chapter explores the role of mobility in advancing nursing education, critically examining its opportunities and constraints through a global lens. It integrates evidence from Europe, Asia, Australia and Latin America to articulate a comprehensive understanding of mobility's educational, ethical and policy dimensions.

2 BACKGROUND AND RATIONALE

Historically, the Bologna Process and the Lisbon Strategy transformed European higher education by promoting harmonization of degrees and mobility of students and staff. In nursing, this led to structural reforms aligning curricula, competency frameworks and assessment systems to facilitate cross-border exchanges. Lino et al. (2022) note that the Bologna architecture enabled not only physical mobility but also academic-professional mobility, supporting the mutual recognition of learning outcomes and qualifications across EU states (Dobrowolska et al., 2015; Lino et al., 2022)

However, harmonization has also revealed disparities in resources and readiness among institutions. While Western European universities embraced mobility as a pedagogical priority, Eastern and Southern European schools often faced resource shortages and uneven clinical training capacity. Restaino et al. (2020) social network analysis revealed a core-periphery dynamic in which certain nations – such as Spain,

Finland and the UK – dominate exchange networks, leaving peripheral countries underrepresented (Dobrowolska et al., 2015; Restaino et al., 2020). From a theoretical perspective, mobility aligns with experiential and transformative learning theories. Keogh and Russel-Roberts (2009) proposed that exposure to new healthcare environments compels students to re-examine professional values and assumptions. This reflective process fosters transformative learning, where experiences abroad reshape personal and professional identities. More recently, Heiberg et al. (2019) linked short-term mobility to intelligent kindness – a deepened empathy and moral sensitivity cultivated through global clinical encounters.

Collectively, these studies underscore that nursing mobility extends beyond skill transfer. It nurtures a holistic professional identity grounded in cultural humility, ethical reasoning and global awareness.

3 CONCEPTUAL FRAMEWORK

Mobility in nursing education can be conceptualized as a multidimensional process that facilitates the exchange of knowledge, skills and values across cultural and institutional boundaries. Within nursing mobility reflects both educational and professional imperatives. Educationally it promotes curricular innovation, intercultural learning and alignment with global standards. Professionally it supports the development of a flexible, competent workforce capable of responding to global health challenges (Dobrowolska et al., 2015).

This duality positions mobility not as an isolated phenomenon but as an integral element of nursing's evolution toward a global discipline. From a sociocultural perspective, mobility aligns with constructivist learning theory, emphasizing experiential learning and reflection. When students engage in international exchanges, they encounter unfamiliar healthcare-systems, communication styles and ethical frameworks. These encounters foster transformative learning, where assumptions are questioned and professional identities reshaped through cross-cultural engagement (Carvalho et al., 2016; Guedes et al., 2018).

In the policy domain, the Bologna Process and the ASEAN Mutual Recognition Agreements (MRAs) provide structural frameworks for facilitating academic degrees and transferable credits across Europe, enabling students and educators to move more freely between institutions (Dobrowolska et al., 2015) Similarly, the ASEAN MRAs on Nursing Services aim to enhance mutual recognition of credentials and promote regional collaboration (Kunaviktikul et al., 2019). Despite these frameworks, implementation remains uneven due to persistent disparities in curricula, licensing and institutional resources. A critical global nursing perspective underscores that mobility should advance not only personal and institutional benefits but also global health equity. Ethical mobility requires that international exchanges be mutually beneficial, respect local health system capacities and avoid exacerbating the "brain drain" from resource-limited settings (Ghimire & Neupane, 2025). Therefore, mobility policies must balance individual aspirations for global experience with collective responsibilities to sustain equitable healthcare delivery worldwide.

4 TYPOLOGIES OF MOBILITY IN NURSING EDUCATION

Mobility in nursing education manifests in several interconnected forms – physical mobility, virtual mobility and institutional or programmatic mobility. Each type contributes distinctively to professional development and international collaboration while posing unique challenges.

4.1 Physical Mobility

Physical mobility refers to the movement of students, educators or researchers across national or regional borders for the purpose of study, clinical placement or academic exchange. This traditional form remains the cornerstone of internationalization in nursing education. The Erasmus+ programme established by the European Commission in 1987, has been instrumental in promoting physical student exchanges. Within nursing, Erasmus experiences enable students to immerse themselves in different healthcare systems, thereby enhancing cultural awareness and professional adaptability (Tuncer Unver et al., 2021). Tuncer Unver et al. (2021) found that nurses who studied abroad during their undergraduate programs reported profound benefits across five thematic areas: adaptation, support systems, perceived differences, challenges and benefits. Participants emphasized increased self-confidence, linguistic competence and professional autonomy which later translated into enhanced employability and leadership skills.

However, physical mobility also entails significant constraints. Financial burdens, language barriers and limited recognition of foreign clinical placements often deter participation (Borrelli et al., 2022)Midwifery students across Europe, for instance, cited financial difficulties, family responsibilities and incompatibility between mobility periods and clinical requirements as major deterrents to participating in Erasmus placements (Borrelli et al., 2022). Similarly, Guedes et al. (2018) highlighted that Brazilian nursing students experienced logistical and emotional challenges during international placements, including homesickness and adaptation stress. Beyond individual experiences, physical mobility plays a broader role in harmonizing professional standards. Dobrowolska et al. (2015) observed that exposure to diverse clinical practice models through mobility fosters critical reflection on students' home systems and contributes to the standardization of nursing competencies across borders. Yet, complete harmonization remains elusive due to the heterogeneity of regulatory frameworks and healthcare contexts.

4.2 Virtual Mobility

With the digital transformation of education, virtual mobility has emerged as an inclusive and sustainable alternative to traditional exchange programs. Defined as the use of digital technologies to enable cross-border learning and collaboration without physical relocation, virtual mobility became especially significant during the COVID-19 pandemic, when travel restrictions halted most international exchanges. According to Borrelli et al. (2022) midwifery students demonstrated strong interest in short-term or hybrid forms of mobility that combine online collaboration with limited physical exchange. Students expressed preferences for interactive virtual tools – videos, peer discussions and online quizzes – that foster engagement and cultural exchange. Such models democratize access to international experiences by reducing costs, overcoming geographic constraints and accommodating students with caregiving or work responsibilities. Virtual mobility also aligns with sustainability and inclusivity principles. It supports equitable access for students from LMICs, where financial and visa-related barriers often prevent physical exchange (Ghimire & Neupane, 2025). Moreover, it facilitates long-term institutional partnerships, enabling continuous collaboration beyond the duration of physical placements. Nevertheless, virtual mobility is not a complete substitute for face-to-face intercultural immersion. The absence of embodied experiences – nonverbal communication, clinical practice in real-world settings and informal cultural interactions – may limit the depth of professional and cultural learning (Dobrowolska et al., 2015). Thus, the optimal approach may be blended mobility, integrating the flexibility of virtual platforms with the transformative power of physical engagement.

4.3 Institutional and Programmatic Mobility

Beyond individual mobility, institutional mobility involves transnational collaboration in curriculum design, joint degrees, research partnerships and faculty exchange. These initiatives create systemic change by embedding international perspectives within educational structures. The Southeast and East Asian Nursing Education and Research Network (SEANERN), described by Kunaviktikul et al. (2019) exemplifies institutional mobility aimed at aligning educational and research standards across ASEAN nations. SEANERN fosters joint research, faculty development and the exchange of best practices, thereby enhancing collective capacity and influencing national policy. Similarly, international visiting scholars' programs (IVS) serve as vehicles for faculty and doctoral-level exchange. Kung et al. (2025) demonstrated that such programs promote research collaboration, mentorship and curriculum innovation while cultivating global networks that extend beyond individual participants. Through IVS programs, nursing PhD students developed enhanced critical thinking, cross-cultural communication and academic writing skills-competencies that contribute to the internationalization of doctoral education.

Programmatic mobility also includes bridging and dual-degree programs, such as collaborative bachelor's or master's degrees between institutions in different countries. These programs facilitate credit transfer and mutual recognition of qualifications, directly supporting global employability of nurses. Yet, such collaborations often require substantial administrative coordination, resource investment and alignment of accreditation standards-factors that may limit their scalability in resource-constrained contexts (Ghimire & Neupane, 2025).

5 INTEGRATING MOBILITY INTO THE NURSING CURRICULUM

For mobility to effectively advance nursing education, it must be integrated into curricula as a pedagogical strategy rather than an extracurricular opportunity. This requires embedding intercultural learning objectives, ethical competencies and reflective practice within nursing education frameworks. Dobrowolska et al. (2015) and Tuncer Unver et al. (2021) emphasize that students derive maximum benefit when mobility experiences are connected to clearly defined learning outcomes – such as Evidence-based practice, communication and ethical reasoning. Likewise, Carvalho et al. (2016) found that international academic exchanges foster autonomy and broaden students' horizons when supported by structured mentorship and reflection mechanism.

Curricular integration also implies preparing students before, during and after mobility experiences. Pre-departure orientations enhance cultural competence and adaptability; ongoing supervision ensures learning continuity; and post-mobility debriefings promote reflection and reintegration of global insights into local practice. Furthermore, embedding virtual exchange components into standard courses can extend mobility benefits to all students, even those unable to travel. Collaborative online international learning (COIL) models – where students from different countries engage in shared projects – represent a promising approach to inclusivity and sustainability (Borrelli et al., 2022).

Ultimately, the conceptual framework of mobility in nursing education is grounded in interdependence: the recognition that local and global health challenges are interconnected and that nursing education must prepare professionals capable of navigating this complexity.

6 OPPORTUNITIES AND BENEFITS OF MOBILITY IN NURSING EDUCATION

Mobility in nursing education offers transformative opportunities that extend beyond academic achievement to encompass personal growth, professional competence and institutional innovation. Through exposure to diverse clinical settings, cultural contexts, and pedagogical approaches, students and faculty gain valuable perspectives that enrich both teaching and practice (Carvalho et al., 2016; Dobrowolska et al., 2015).

These benefits are particularly salient in a global health landscape marked by workforce shortages, technological change, and increasingly multicultural patient populations.

Empirical studies consistently highlight the ways in which mobility fosters academic excellence, intercultural competence, professional development, and research capacity. Furthermore, institutional participation in mobility initiatives contributes to the internationalization of curricula and the enhancement of nursing's social status as a globally engaged discipline (Kunaviktikul et al., 2019; Kung et al., 2025).

6.1 Academic and Professional Development

International experiences expand nursing students' clinical and cognitive skills by immersing them in health systems with differing structures, resources and patient populations. According to Dobrowolska et al. (2015) clinical placements abroad expose students to novel care protocols and ethical challenges, thereby encouraging critical reflection on their own practice environments. This process of comparative learning strengthens students' analytical and problem-solving capacities—core components of professional competence.

Similarly, Carvalho et al. (2016) found that academic mobility enables students to contextualize professional knowledge through firsthand encounters with diverse healthcare models. Participants in their Brazil-Portugal exchange described the experience as a catalyst for developing autonomy, decision-making, and adaptability—attributes essential for nursing leadership. These findings align with Kolb's experiential learning framework, suggesting that reflective engagement with unfamiliar clinical contexts transforms tacit knowledge into professional expertise.

Language acquisition represents another major benefit of educational mobility. Effective communication is fundamental to patient safety and interprofessional collaboration, and international exposure strengthens linguistic and interpersonal competencies. Studies of Erasmus participants revealed substantial improvement in English proficiency and intercultural communication skills, which subsequently enhanced graduates' employability and leadership potential (Tuncer Unver et al., 2021).

Beyond linguistic competence, cross-cultural communication experiences cultivate empathy and tolerance—key attributes of patient-centered care. Guedes et al. (2018) reported that Brazilian students participating in Science Without Borders programs developed heightened awareness of cultural differences in health beliefs, patient autonomy, and professional hierarchies. These insights translated into more holistic and culturally sensitive approaches upon their return.

6.2 Development of Global and Intercultural Competence

The acquisition of intercultural competence is central to nursing's global mission. As Borrelli et al. (2022) observed, intercultural sensitivity enables students to communicate effectively and ethically in multicultural clinical settings. Exposure to different norms surrounding childbirth, gender roles, and patient-family relationships deepens nurses' understanding of cultural determinants of health.

Erasmus and other exchange programs have been shown to nurture cultural humility—an awareness of one's own biases and a willingness to learn from others (Tuncer Unver et al., 2021). Participants frequently described their experiences as "life-changing," reflecting shifts in attitudes toward diversity, equality, and professional identity. Such outcomes support the International Confederation of Midwives' (ICM, 2019) call for a globally aware workforce capable of delivering equitable care across contexts.

Mobility also reinforces nursing's ethical and humanistic dimensions. Interaction with diverse health systems exposes students to varying interpretations of autonomy, justice, and care ethics. Dobrowolska et al. (2015) argue that this diversity fosters moral reasoning and critical engagement with professional values. When students witness disparities in access to care or resource allocation, they gain a broader appreciation of social justice as a nursing responsibility. Kung et al. (2025) found that doctoral-level mobility further strengthens ethical awareness through exposure to global research ethics, data protection standards, and culturally sensitive methodologies. Such experiences equip emerging nurse scholars to conduct responsible international research and to advocate for ethical collaboration in global health initiatives.

6.3 Research and Knowledge Exchange

Mobility fosters research collaboration by linking institutions and individuals across borders. The integrative review by Kung et al. (2025) demonstrated that international visiting-scholar programs enhance academic productivity and innovation among nursing PhD students. Participants developed advanced research design skills, improved critical analysis, and established long-term partnerships leading to joint publications and grant proposals.

At the regional level, SEANERN provides an example of how transnational networks can accelerate evidence-based practice (Kunaviktikul et al., 2019). By coordinating multicountry studies on nursing education and clinical competencies, SEANERN has facilitated comparative research that informs both national and regional policy. These collaborative structures help disseminate innovations such as simulation-based training, tele-nursing education, and culturally adapted patient-care models.

6.4 Employability and Career Advancement

International exposure often enhances graduates' career trajectories by signaling adaptability, cultural competence, and global citizenship. Studies across regions consistently associate participation in mobility programs with improved job prospects and professional recognition (Guedes et al., 2018; Tuncer Unver et al., 2021). Employers value candidates who demonstrate flexibility and an understanding of global health dynamics. Furthermore, mobility nurtures leadership potential. Students who navigate complex intercultural environments often acquire skills in negotiation, teamwork and problem-solving that prepare them for supervisory and managerial roles. Borrelli et al. (2022) reported that midwifery students viewed international experiences as stepping-stones toward leadership in maternal health policy and education.

At the doctoral level, international visiting-scholar programs foster academic career progression through mentorship and global networking (Kung et al., 2025). Participants frequently transitioned into international research collaborations or faculty positions, demonstrating the long-term professional dividends of academic mobility.

6.5 Institutional and Social Benefits

From an institutional perspective, mobility programs are powerful tools for curriculum internationalization and quality assurance. Dobrowolska et al. (2015) emphasized that transnational comparisons of clinical education promote standardization and the development of shared competency frameworks. Such harmonization aligns with global accreditation efforts led by organizations like the International Council of Nurses (ICN).

Kunaviktikul et al. (2019) observed that policy dialogue within SEANERN influenced national reforms in Thailand and neighboring countries, leading to curriculum upgrades and expanded research capacity. These systemic effects illustrate how mobility catalyzes educational modernization and regional integration.

Beyond academia, mobility initiatives contribute to strengthening global health systems by fostering cross-border collaboration and knowledge transfer. When returning nurses apply newly acquired skills, they enhance clinical standards, introduce innovative teaching methods, and participate in international public-health projects (Carvalho et al., 2016).

Moreover, equitable mobility supports the global distribution of nursing expertise. Ethical recruitment and mutual-recognition policies, as advocated by the WHO and ASEAN, help balance workforce shortages between high- and low-income countries (Kunaviktikul et al., 2019). In this way, mobility serves not only as a mechanism for individual advancement but also as a strategy for addressing global inequities in healthcare delivery.

6.6 Personal Transformation

Perhaps the most profound yet intangible benefit of mobility is personal transformation. Participants in multiple studies described increased self-awareness, independence and resilience (Carvalho et al., 2016; Guedes et al., 2018). Living and studying in a foreign culture requires adaptability and openness-qualities that translate into professional empathy and emotional intelligence. Tuncer Unver et al. (2021) found that nurses who studied abroad reported a stronger sense of global citizenship and professional identity. They perceived nursing not merely as a national vocation but as a universal commitment to human well-being. Such internalization of global ethics represents the ultimate educational outcome of mobility—an expansion of perspective that aligns personal growth with collective responsibility.

7 CONSTRAINTS AND CHALLENGES OF MOBILITY IN NURSING EDUCATION

While mobility in nursing education offers transformative opportunities, it also presents significant constraints and structural inequalities that can limit participation and impact. These constraints operate across multiple levels—individual, institutional, national, and global—reflecting the complex interplay between education systems, economic structures, and sociocultural contexts. Although international mobility programs are often framed as universally beneficial, evidence suggests that access remains uneven, with students from high-income countries and well-resourced institutions enjoying greater opportunities than those from low- and middle-income countries (LMICs) (Ghimire & Neupane, 2025; Kunaviktikul et al., 2019).

Moreover, issues such as financial cost, accreditation disparities, cultural adjustment, and ethical dilemmas complicate the implementation of equitable mobility frameworks.

This section critically examines these challenges, emphasizing the need for systemic reform to ensure that mobility contributes not only to individual growth but also to global health equity.

7.1 Structural and Financial Barriers

Financial cost is one of the most persistent obstacles to participation in international exchange. Tuition differences, travel expenses, and living costs abroad often exclude students without substantial financial support. Borrelli et al. (2022) found that midwifery students across four European countries identified financial difficulty as the primary deterrent to engaging in physical mobility. Despite Erasmus+ grants, many students perceived funding as insufficient to cover actual expenses, particularly in high-cost destinations. In LMICs, financial inequities are even more pronounced. Programs such as Brazil's Science Without Borders sought to democratize access to global education, but their discontinuation revealed the fragility of state-funded mobility (Guedes et al., 2018; Guskuma et al., 2016). Participants emphasized that while the program expanded horizons, its termination left a vacuum, highlighting the need for sustainable financial models. Dobrowolska et al. (2015) noted that even within Europe, disparities among higher education institutions (HEIs) affect students' access to high-quality placements. Differences in mentorship quality, clinical site availability, and supervision ratios create inconsistent learning experiences. These inequities undermine the harmonization goals of initiatives like the Bologna Process.

7.2 Policy and Regulatory Constraints

Variations in accreditation and licensure systems across countries pose major barriers to mobility. Ghimire and Neupane (2025) identified significant discrepancies between Nepal's four-year Bachelor of Science in Nursing and Australia's three-year Bachelor of Nursing programs. These differences in curriculum structure, clinical hours, and licensing examinations create hurdles for internationally educated nurses seeking recognition abroad.

Similarly, Kunaviktikul et al. (2019) observed that within the ASEAN region, inconsistent regulatory standards limit the full implementation of mutual recognition agreements. Despite regional efforts, countries maintain divergent competency frameworks and credentialing processes, preventing seamless professional mobility.

Without standardized accreditation and reciprocal recognition mechanisms, students risk having their qualifications undervalued or unrecognized. This lack of portability can lead to underemployment or "brain waste," where highly trained nurses are restricted to lower-level positions in destination countries (Ghimire & Neupane, 2025).

Curricular misalignment further complicates academic exchange. Dobrowolska et al. (2015) found that differences in course content, assessment criteria, and learning outcomes across European nursing programs made credit transfer challenging. Institutions often struggle to match local requirements with those of partner universities, resulting in incomplete credit recognition or extended study durations.

The absence of harmonized frameworks reduces student motivation to participate in mobility programs and discourages institutions from expanding partnerships. It also perpetuates regional disparities, as HEIs in high-income countries dominate the design of curricula and mobility policies, often imposing epistemological hierarchies that marginalize local knowledge systems.

7.3 Sociocultural and Linguistic Barriers

Language remains one of the most immediate challenges in international education. Although English dominates academic communication, proficiency levels vary significantly among nursing students. Tuncer Unver et al. (2021) reported that participants in Erasmus programs initially faced anxiety and communication barriers due to limited language skills, which affected their confidence in clinical settings. Language difficulties can compromise patient safety and learning outcomes during clinical placements, where nuanced communication is critical. Host institutions often underestimate the need for pre-departure language preparation or ongoing linguistic support. Consequently, students may experience frustration, social isolation, or limited engagement with local teams (Borrelli et al., 2022).

Cross-cultural adaptation presents another significant barrier. Guedes et al. (2018) and Carvalho et al. (2016) both noted that Brazilian nursing students abroad experienced culture shock, homesickness, and challenges in understanding local norms of communication and authority. Students often struggle to reconcile differing approaches to hierarchy, teamwork, and patient care.

These experiences, while potentially transformative, can also lead to psychological distress if insufficient support systems are in place. Dobrowolska et al. (2015) highlight that mentorship and structured reflection are essential for helping students integrate foreign experiences into their professional development. In the absence of such scaffolding, mobility may result in confusion or negative coping responses rather than growth.

Mobility opportunities are not equally accessible across social groups. In nursing - a profession historically dominated by women - gendered constraints such as caregiving responsibilities, safety concerns, and societal expectations often limit participation in international programs. Borrelli et al. (2022) observed that female midwifery students frequently cited family obligations as barriers to travel, reflecting broader gender inequalities in higher education mobility.

Socioeconomic status further compounds these disparities. Students from underrepresented or first-generation backgrounds may lack the financial or social capital to pursue international experiences (Ghimire & Neupane, 2025). Thus, mobility programs can inadvertently reproduce global inequities if they fail to address intersectional barriers.

7.4 Ethical and Political Considerations

The international migration of nurses, while addressing workforce shortages in high-income countries, often results in **brain drain** from LMICs. Ghimire and Neupane (2025) describe how bilateral recruitment agreements, such as those between Nepal and the United Kingdom, exacerbate the depletion of skilled personnel in source countries. This phenomenon undermines health system capacity and perpetuates inequities in global healthcare delivery.

Ethically, mobility policies must reconcile the rights of individual nurses to seek better opportunities with the collective need to sustain local healthcare systems. Sustainable solutions include bilateral agreements that ensure skill circulation rather than permanent loss, and reintegration programs that encourage returning professionals to share expertise. Mobility programs often reflect asymmetrical power relations between sending and receiving institutions. Partnerships dominated by Western universities may privilege Eurocentric knowledge and research paradigms, marginalizing indigenous or context-specific nursing perspectives (Kunaviktikul et al., 2019). Such epistemics inequities can manifest in curriculum design, research priorities and authorship representation. Ensuring equitable collaboration requires recognizing diverse epistemologies and fostering South-South partnerships that value local expertise as much as global standards.

Cross-cultural placements also raise concerns about ethical supervision and cultural competence. Students may inadvertently violate local norms or ethical standards due to inadequate preparation. Dobrowolska et al. (2015) called for international ethical guidelines to govern undergraduate clinical placements, ensuring that students act responsibly and that host communities benefit rather than bear risks. Similarly, Kung et al. (2025) emphasized that PhD-level visiting scholars must receive structured guidance on research ethics, data governance, and cultural sensitivity to avoid exploitative or culturally insensitive practices. Ethical frameworks thus form a cornerstone of responsible mobility.

7.5 Digital Divide and Limitations of Virtual Mobility

While virtual mobility offers inclusivity and sustainability, it also exposes a new dimension of inequality—the digital divide. Students and institutions in regions with limited internet access or digital infrastructure may be excluded from online exchange opportunities. Ghimire and Neupane (2025) noted that technological disparities between countries like Nepal and Australia hinder equitable participation in global online education initiatives.

Moreover, virtual platforms can reproduce linguistic hierarchies and accessibility barriers for students with disabilities or limited technological literacy. Without deliberate design for inclusivity, digital mobility risks becoming another form of exclusion rather than empowerment.

7.6 Institutional and Pedagogical Challenges

Integrating mobility into curricula requires significant pedagogical innovation and faculty engagement. However, resistance to change, limited training, and administrative burdens often constrain implementation. Faculty members may lack experience in intercultural pedagogy or virtual exchange methods, reducing the educational impact of mobility programs (Dobrowolska et al., 2015). In addition, the short-term nature of many exchanges limits long-term learning outcomes. Without structured reflection and follow-up students may fail to integrate international experiences into their ongoing practice or research. Carvalho et al. (2016) emphasize that sustainable mobility must include post-exchange evaluation and opportunities for continued engagement to maximize educational benefit.

8 INNOVATIVE MODELS AND FUTURE DIRECTIONS IN NURSING EDUCATION MOBILITY

In response to the constraints discussed earlier, nursing education systems worldwide have sought innovative strategies to make mobility more equitable, sustainable, and pedagogically meaningful. These emerging models reimagine mobility not merely as physical relocation but as a dynamic ecosystem of global engagement, encompassing digital collaboration, policy harmonization, and mutual capacity building.

The 21st-century vision of nursing mobility integrates the goals of educational excellence, workforce sustainability, and global health equity. This section examines key innovations—blended mobility, virtual collaboration networks, mutual-recognition frameworks, and global partnerships—that are redefining how nursing education advances across borders.

8.1 Blended and Flexible Models

Blended or hybrid mobility combines short-term physical experiences with long-term virtual collaboration. This approach emerged strongly after the COVID-19 pandemic, when institutions recognized the need for flexible and inclusive exchange models.

Borrelli et al. (2022) demonstrated that midwifery students across Europe expressed a preference for short-term placements supplemented by digital engagement—such as virtual discussions, shared assignments, and intercultural reflection sessions. These programs reduce cost barriers and accommodate students with caregiving or work commitments. Importantly, they sustain international engagement beyond the physical visit, transforming mobility into an ongoing learning process rather than a single event.

Hybrid mobility also fosters environmental sustainability by reducing the carbon footprint associated with long-term travel while maintaining essential interpersonal and clinical learning experiences. As universities pursue climate-conscious education, blended models align with global sustainability goals such as the UN Sustainable Development Goal (SDG) 13: Climate Action and SDG 4: Quality Education.

Short-term exchange programs—ranging from one-week study tours to one-month clinical immersions—represent another flexible model gaining traction. Dobrowolska et al. (2015) note that short-term placements allow students to experience alternative health systems without disrupting academic progression. These programs can be embedded within existing curricula and tailored to specific competencies, such as public health, palliative care, or community nursing.

Additionally, summer schools and global nursing camps provide cost-effective avenues for intercultural exposure. Through structured reflection, mentorship, and teamwork, these programs cultivate global citizenship and professional identity in a condensed yet impactful format.

8.2 Virtual Internationalization and Digital Collaboration

Virtual mobility has evolved from a pandemic necessity into a cornerstone of internationalization at home. COIL—Collaborative Online International Learning—enables students from different countries to engage in shared projects and virtual classrooms, fostering intercultural communication without physical travel (Borrelli et al., 2022). For instance, nursing faculties in Europe and Latin America have implemented COIL-based simulations where students jointly design care plans for hypothetical global health scenarios. Such digital exchanges promote teamwork, critical thinking, and cross-cultural awareness, echoing the experiential benefits of physical mobility.

To maximize inclusivity, COIL initiatives must address linguistic diversity, time-zone differences, and technological access. As Ghimire and Neupane (2025) caution, disparities in digital infrastructure can exclude students from low-resource regions. Hence, investment in digital literacy, broadband access, and multilingual platforms is crucial to ensuring equitable participation.

At the postgraduate level, virtual networks have revolutionized research collaboration. Kung et al. (2025) found that international visiting-scholar programs increasingly integrate virtual mentorship, enabling PhD students to participate in global projects remotely. These platforms facilitate joint publications, webinars, and peer review, thus democratizing academic exchange.

Moreover, digital repositories and open-access databases enhance the visibility of nursing research from underrepresented regions. By encouraging open science practices, institutions contribute to decolonizing knowledge production and fostering equitable research ecosystems.

8.3 Policy Harmonizations and Mutual Recognition

Harmonization of education and licensure standards remains pivotal to enabling sustained mobility. The Bologna Process in Europe and the ASEAN Mutual Recognition Agreements (MRAs) in Asia illustrate how regional cooperation can facilitate credit transfer and professional recognition.

Kunaviktikul et al. (2019) reported that SEANERN has played a vital role in aligning nursing competencies across Southeast Asia. Through shared research and curriculum mapping, SEANERN supports policy dialogue that bridges national gaps in regulation and accreditation. This approach exemplifies how regional frameworks can transform fragmented mobility into structured, policy-driven collaboration.

Global organizations such as the International Council of Nurses (ICN) and the World Health Organization (WHO) advocate for standardized credentialing systems that promote ethical recruitment and equitable workforce distribution. Ghimire and Neupane (2025) argue that transparent credentialing pathways would reduce bureaucratic barriers for internationally educated nurses while protecting local healthcare capacities.

Additionally, the development of micro-credential systems—short, competency-based certifications recognized across borders—represents an innovative solution. These digital credentials verify specific skills such as infection control, leadership, or telehealth, enabling mobility without full degree equivalence.

8.4 Equity and Inclusion in Mobility Programs

To make mobility genuinely transformative, inclusion must be embedded as a guiding principle. Borrelli et al. (2022) and Guedes et al. (2018) emphasize that female nursing students often face compounded barriers due to caregiving responsibilities and economic constraints. Institutions can address these disparities through flexible timelines, childcare support, and targeted scholarships.

Equally important is the diversification of mobility destinations. Historically, programs have concentrated on North America and Western Europe, reinforcing global hierarchies. Expanding South–South exchanges between Latin America, Africa, and Asia promotes mutual learning and contextual innovation while reducing dependency on Global North institutions (Kunaviktikul et al., 2019).

Ethical collaboration requires reciprocity and shared governance. Dobrowolska et al. (2015) and Kung et al. (2025) both call for mobility programs designed to benefit host and sending institutions equally. This involves joint curriculum development, equitable authorship in research, and transparent funding arrangements.

For example, capacity-building exchanges, where faculty from high-income countries co-teach or co-supervise in LMIC institutions, support local empowerment rather than talent extraction. Similarly, return programs that facilitate reintegration of graduates into home systems ensure that mobility outcomes contribute to national development.

Emerging discourse advocates for the decolonization of nursing education, emphasizing the need to challenge Eurocentric dominance in knowledge production. Kunaviktikul et al. (2019) and Ghimire and Neupane (2025) highlight that global mobility must respect local epistemologies and community-based care practices.

Integrating indigenous health perspectives, traditional healing knowledge, and culturally grounded pedagogy into mobility curricula ensures that global education remains contextually relevant and socially just. Reciprocal learning—where students from the Global North learn from Southern practices—can dismantle hierarchical narratives and foster genuine intercultural exchange.

8.5 Institutional Innovations and Leadership

Institutions that embed global perspectives into every aspect of their curricula—rather than relying solely on exchange programs—achieve more sustainable internationalization. Dobrowolska et al. (2015) suggest integrating global health modules, comparative ethics, and intercultural communication across courses.

Faculty development plays a critical role here. Through participation in visiting-scholar programs (Kung et al., 2025), educators acquire cross-cultural teaching competencies and global research skills. These faculty experiences trickle down into classrooms, enriching learning for students who may never travel abroad.

Furthermore, universities should collaborate in consortia that share best practices and resources. Networks like SEANERN and the European Federation of Nurse Educators demonstrate how collective governance strengthens regional influence and enhances quality assurance (Kunaviktikul et al., 2019).

9 FUTURE DIRECTIONS FOR GLOBAL NURSING MOBILITY

The future of mobility will be deeply intertwined with technology. Artificial intelligence, virtual reality, and simulation-based learning can replicate intercultural and clinical experiences in virtual environments. For example, virtual reality (VR) simulations can expose students to global health scenarios—such as managing epidemics or disaster response—within safe and controlled settings.

Kung et al. (2025) predict that PhD education will increasingly rely on virtual mentorship and AI-supported data analysis, democratizing access to global expertise. However, technological integration must remain inclusive, ensuring accessibility for institutions with limited infrastructure (Ghimire & Neupane, 2025). To sustain equitable mobility, global nursing organizations must integrate educational mobility into broader health workforce strategies. Aligning with the WHO Global Strategy on Human Resources for Health (2030), educational mobility should be guided by principles of ethical recruitment, skill circulation, and global solidarity.

Cross-border partnerships should prioritize mutual development, shared funding, and transparent monitoring. Data on student outcomes, retention, and reintegration can inform evidence-based policy, ensuring mobility programs yield measurable benefits for both individuals and health systems.

As climate change reshapes global priorities, nursing mobility must evolve to minimize environmental impact. Universities can adopt carbon offset programs, promote virtual collaboration, and design short-term, low-impact exchanges. By embedding environmental ethics into mobility design, institutions align nursing education with global sustainability imperatives (Borrelli et al., 2022).

10 IMPLICATIONS AND CONCLUSION

As nursing continues to evolve as a globally interconnected discipline, academic mobility has become a cornerstone of professional development, curricular innovation, and transnational collaboration. The preceding sections have demonstrated that mobility enriches nursing education through experiential learning, intercultural competence, and global research partnerships. Yet, these opportunities coexist with financial, structural, and ethical constraints that demand deliberate, equitable solutions.

The future of nursing education depends on the ability of policymakers, educators, and institutions to transform mobility from a privilege into a standard, accessible component of professional preparation. This concluding section synthesizes key insights, outlines practical implications for policy and curriculum design, and articulates a forward-looking vision for the role of mobility in advancing global nursing education.

10.1 Implications for Nursing Education Policy

Mobility must be institutionalized through coherent policy frameworks that ensure continuity, inclusivity, and quality assurance. Universities should embed internationalization objectives within their strategic plans, establishing dedicated offices for global engagement and partnerships (Greenleaf, n.d.). Policies should mandate equitable access by offering scholarships, stipends, and credit recognition mechanisms that enable all students—not just the affluent or well-connected—to participate.

Dobrowolska et al. (2015) recommend that international clinical placements be regulated by standardized guidelines addressing supervision, ethical conduct, and competency evaluation. Institutional policies must also prioritize reciprocal benefit by ensuring that host organizations and communities gain from visiting students' contributions, rather than serving merely as training grounds for outsiders.

At the national level, nursing councils and ministries of education should align curricula and accreditation systems with international standards to facilitate seamless mobility. Kunaviktikul et al. (2019) highlight the importance of regional cooperation through initiatives such as SEANERN and ASEAN MRAs, which harmonize competencies and facilitate mutual credential recognition.

National policies should also address ethical recruitment and workforce retention. Ghimire and Neupane (2025) argue that mobility frameworks must prevent brain drain by promoting skill circulation—where professionals return home with enhanced expertise to strengthen local systems. Governments can achieve this through bonded scholarships, reintegration programs, and bilateral agreements that balance workforce flows.

10.2 Implications for Curriculum Design

Curricula should integrate global and intercultural learning outcomes across all levels of nursing education. These competencies include cultural humility, ethical reasoning, communication across diversity, and understanding of global health systems (Borrelli et al., 2022; Tuncer Unver et al., 2021).

Embedding mobility as a pedagogical principle—rather than an optional activity—ensures that every student gains exposure to international perspectives. Virtual exchange modules, global health simulations, and collaborative online projects can provide accessible pathways for all learners.

Faculty must be equipped to facilitate intercultural learning through reflective pedagogy, mentorship, and continuous professional development. Faculty exchanges, such as international visiting scholar programs, strengthen teaching capacity and align classroom instruction with global standards (Kung et al., 2025). Reflection is the mechanism that transforms experience into learning. As Carvalho et al. (2016) and Guedes et al. (2018) demonstrated, structured reflection allows students to internalize the lessons of mobility, integrating cultural insights into their professional identities. Institutions should incorporate pre-departure orientation, ongoing supervision, and post-return debriefing into mobility curricula to maximize learning outcomes.

Assessment should evaluate not only technical skills but also intercultural competence and ethical awareness. Tools such as reflective journals, intercultural sensitivity scales, and group projects can provide multidimensional evidence of learning (Dobrowolska et al., 2015).

10.3 Implications for Research and Faculty Development

Mobility fosters research capacity and innovation by linking nursing scholars across continents. Institutions should actively support international research networks, co-authorship, and joint doctoral supervision. The integrative review by Kung et al. (2025) revealed that participation in visiting-scholar programs enhances research productivity and career advancement.

To ensure equity, research funding mechanisms should prioritize collaborative, cross-national projects that include institutions from the Global South. Open-access publishing and shared databases can further democratize knowledge dissemination, ensuring that research findings benefit the global nursing community.

10.4 Ethical and Equity Considerations

As global mobility expands, nursing education must prioritize ethical practices grounded in fairness, reciprocity, and respect for cultural contexts. Ethical guidelines should govern student placements, ensuring that communities are not exploited for learning purposes and that patient rights are upheld.

Dobrowolska et al. (2015) and Kung et al. (2025) advocate for codes of conduct that outline the responsibilities of both sending and host institutions. These codes should address issues of consent, supervision, and benefit-sharing, particularly in clinical or research contexts involving vulnerable populations. True internationalization is inclusive, not exclusive. Policies must actively dismantle economic, gendered, and linguistic barriers that limit participation. Programs should target underrepresented groups through scholarships, mentorship, and flexible delivery modes (Borrelli et al., 2022; Guedes et al., 2018).

Furthermore, decolonizing nursing education requires the recognition of diverse epistemologies and the promotion of South–South collaborations. As Kunaviktikul et al. (2019) and Ghimire and Neupane (2025) note, equitable partnerships that value local knowledge can rectify historical imbalances in global education.

11 THE FUTURE OF NURSING MOBILITY: A TRANSFORMATIVE VISION

The next decade will witness a convergence of global health challenges—pandemics, aging populations, migration crises, and climate change—that demand a highly mobile, culturally competent nursing workforce. Mobility must evolve from a privilege for the few to a strategic necessity for all.

Future nursing education should embrace:

- Technological integration through AI, virtual simulation, and digital collaboration (Kung et al., 2025).
- Ethical globalization, guided by WHO and ICN frameworks to ensure sustainable workforce distribution (Kunaviktikul et al., 2019).
- Interdisciplinary collaboration, connecting nursing with public health, technology, and policy studies.
- Environmental responsibility, promoting low-impact and blended exchange models (Borrelli et al., 2022).

Through these pathways, nursing mobility can become a transformative force that strengthens both education and global health systems.

12 CONCLUSION

Mobility has become an indispensable catalyst in advancing nursing education. It enables the exchange of knowledge, fosters intercultural understanding, and equips nurses with the competencies required to navigate a globalized world. Yet, mobility's transformative potential can only be realized when accessibility, ethics, and reciprocity are prioritized.

The studies reviewed—from European Erasmus programs to Asian and Latin American exchanges—demonstrate that mobility enriches not only individuals but entire systems of nursing education. When thoughtfully designed, it cultivates reflective practitioners, empowers educators, and strengthens global health solidarity.

The future lies in inclusive, equitable, and sustainable mobility frameworks that blend digital innovation with human connection. By embracing this vision, nursing education can lead the way in shaping a more compassionate, competent, and interconnected world.

REFERENCES

Bani, M., Zorzi, F., Russo, S., Del Greco, A., Ardenghi, S., Rampoldi, G., Putoto, G., Invernizzi, P., & Strepparava, M. G. (2025). International Mobility Experiences Among Italian Students: A Cross-Sectional Survey Comparing Motivations Towards High- Versus Low-Income Countries. *BMJ Open*, *15*(7), E093935. Https://Doi.Org/10.1136/Bmjopen-2024-093935. DOI: 10.1136/bmjopen-2024-093935 PMID: 40744513

Bjørnnes, A. K., Skaufel, H., Holmström Rising, M., Gädda, M., Nieminen, A.-L., Misvær, N., Bender Monggaard, M.-L., Greve Sørensen, K., Alondere, L., Butkuviene, A., & Torbjørnsen, A. (2024). Short-Term Student Exchange In Nursing Education: A Descriptive Pilot Study. *SAGE Open*, *14*(4), 21582440241299522. Https://Doi.Org/10.1177/21582440241299522. DOI: 10.1177/21582440241299522

Borrelli, S., Walker, L., Coolin, K., Fumagalli, S., Karema, A., Konstantinidis, S., Mets-Oja, S., Nespoli, A., Smit, A.-M., Van Oost, M., & Spiby, H. (2022). Midwifery Students' Perspectives Of Physical And Virtual Mobility Activities Including Preferences For E-Learning: A Cross-Sectional Survey. *Nurse Education Today*, *109*, 105214. Https://Doi.Org/10.1016/J.Nedt.2021.105214. DOI: 10.1016/j.nedt.2021.105214 PMID: 34799193

Carvalho, J., Backes, D., Lomba, M., & Colomé, J. (2016). International Academic Mobility: An Education Opportunity For Future Nurses. *Revista De Enfermagem Referência, Iv Série*(10), 59–68. Https://Doi.Org/10.12707/Riv16018

Dobrowolska, B., Mcgonagle, I., Jackson, C., Kane, R., Cabrera, E., Cooney-Miner, D., Di Cara, V., Pajnkihar, M., Prlić, N., Sigurdardottir, A. K., Kekuš, D., Wells, J., & Palese, A. (2015). Clinical Practice Models In Nursing Education: Implication For Students' Mobility. *International Nursing Review*, *62*(1), 36–46. Https://Doi .Org/10.1111/Inr.12162. DOI: 10.1111/inr.12162 PMID: 25559068

Ghimire, A., & Neupane, M. S. (2025). Navigating Global Mobility: A Comparative Study Of Nursing Education In Nepal And Australia. *International Journal of Nursing Education Scholarship*, *22*(1), 20240108. Https://Doi.Org/10.1515/Ijnes -2024-0108. DOI: 10.1515/ijnes-2024-0108 PMID: 40643086

Guedes, G. F., Da Cavalcante, I. M. S., & Püschel, V. A. D. A. (2018). Mobilidade Estudantil Internacional: A Experiência De Estudantes De Graduação Em Enfermagem [International Academic Mobility: The Experience Of Undergraduate Nursing Students]. *Revista da Escola de Enfermagem da USP*, *52*(0), E03358. Https://Doi.Org/ 10.1590/S1980-220x2017039403358. DOI: 10.1590/s1980-220x2017039403358

Guskuma, E. M., Dullius, A. A. D. S., La Godinho, M. S. C., Costa, M. S. T., & Terra, F. D. S. (2016). Mobilidade Acadêmica Internacional Na Formação Em Enfermagem: Relato De Experiência [International Academic Mobility In Nursing Education: An Experience Report]. *Revista Brasileira de Enfermagem*, *69*(5), 986–990. Https://Doi.Org/10.1590/0034-7167-2015-0128. DOI: 10.1590/0034-7167-2015-0128 PMID: 27783744

Kunaviktikul, W., Turale, S., Petrini, M. A., Tungpunkom, P., & Avant, K. C. (2019). Experiences From Southeast Asia On Nursing Education, Practice, Mobility And Influencing Policy. *International Nursing Review*, *66*(4), 474–481. Https://Doi.Org/10.1111/Inr.12556. DOI: 10.1111/inr.12556 PMID: 31606912

Kung, P.-J., Chang, Y.-C., & Chiu, C. A., Li, M., Fang, C.-J., & Reynolds, N. R. (2025). The Impact Of International Visiting Scholars Programmes On Nursing Phd Students: An Integrative Review. *Journal Of Advanced Nursing*. Advance Online Publication. Https://Doi.Org/10.1111/Jan.70116

Lino, M. M., Martini, J. G., & Barbieri-Figueiredo, M. D. C. (2022). Academic-Professional Mobility And Internationalization Of Nursing: Contributions Of The Bologna Process. *Texto & Contexto Enfermagem*, *31*, E20210319. Https://Doi.Org/10.1590/1980-265x-Tce-2021-0319en. DOI: 10.1590/1980-265x-tce-2021-0319pt

Restaino, M., Vitale, M. P., & Primerano, I. (2020). Analysing International Student Mobility Flows In Higher Education: A Comparative Study On European Countries. *Social Indicators Research*, *149*(3), 947–965. Https://Doi.Org/10.1007/S11205-020-02282-2. DOI: 10.1007/s11205-020-02282-2

Roy, A., Newman, A., Ellenberger, T., & Pyman, A. (2019). Outcomes Of International Student Mobility Programs: A Systematic Review And Agenda For Future Research. *Studies in Higher Education*, *44*(9), 1630–1644. Https://Doi.Org/10.1080/03075079.2018.1458222. DOI: 10.1080/03075079.2018.1458222

Tuncer Unver, G., Celebi Cakiroglu, O., Gungor Satilmis, I., & Harmanci Seren, A. K. (2021). The Experiences Of Nurses Who Studied Abroad With The Erasmus Program During Undergraduate Education: A Qualitative Study. *Nurse Education in Practice*, *51*, 102993. Https://Doi.Org/10.1016/J.Nepr.2021.102993. DOI: 10.1016/j.nepr.2021.102993 PMID: 33621924

Chapter 3
International Mobility in Nursing Education: Opportunities, Challenges, and Implications

Barbara Kegl
https://orcid.org/0000-0002-4749-4509
Faculty of Health Sciences, University of Maribor, Slovenia

Petra Klanjsek
https://orcid.org/0000-0003-3631-6691
Faculty of Health Sciences, University of Maribor, Slovenia

ABSTRACT

International mobility of nursing students and faculty is crucial for building global competencies, cultural awareness, and adaptability. Programs such as Erasmus+, Fulbright, and bilateral agreements expose participants to diverse healthcare systems and foster intercultural skills that improve patient care. Beyond cultural and professional outcomes, ergonomics (physical, cognitive, and psychosocial) also plays an important role. A literature review will assess evidence on benefits, barriers, and best practices. Findings show mobility strengthens cultural sensitivity, critical thinking, and academic creativity, while driving institutional innovation through partnerships and curriculum development. Yet financial limits, rigid curricula, language barriers, and accreditation gaps restrict access and equity. To maximize impact, programs must reduce barriers, ensure inclusivity, and prepare participants.

DOI: 10.4018/979-8-3373-5931-1.ch003

INTRODUCTION

In an increasingly interconnected world, international mobility in higher education has emerged as a key pillar of academic and professional development, particularly within healthcare-related disciplines such as nursing. Faculty and student mobility refers to the cross-border movement of academic staff and students for the purposes of education, training, teaching, and research. For nursing professionals, such experiences support professional growth by fostering adaptability, cultural sensitivity, and a deeper understanding of global health challenges. Moreover, international mobility promotes the dissemination of best practices in both nursing education and clinical care, encouraging innovation and the continuous improvement of standards (World Health Organizaion, 2016; Sailsman et al., 2021).

Global health challenges—such as pandemics, aging populations, and the rising prevalence of chronic diseases—have highlighted the need for a well-prepared and culturally competent nursing workforce (Adhikari & Smith, 2023; Sharplin et al., 2025). Participation in international mobility programs enables nursing students and educators to gain comprehensive experience with diverse healthcare settings and to engage in meaningful collaboration with international peers. These experiences contribute significantly to enhanced cultural sensitivity and the development of transcultural competencies, both of which are essential for providing patient-centered care in multicultural contexts. Exposure to multicultural environments fosters critical thinking, adaptability, and intercultural communication—skills that are increasingly vital for effective nursing practice within increasingly globalized healthcare systems (GalanLominchar et al., 2024; Perez-Encinas et al., 2023; Mackavey et al., 2024; University of Primorska, Faculty of Health Sciences, 2022).

Safe, efficient, and human-centered work is the foundation of professional excellence and patient safety; yet student and teacher mobility entails confronting unfamiliar equipment, facilities, documentation systems, and work norms — all of which are central concerns of ergonomics and human factors (Carayon et al., 2020). Empirical evidence further indicates that students who participate in structured international exchanges programs or collaborative learning initiatives, whether conducted in-person or virtually, exhibit statistically significant improvements in cultural intelligence and a deeper understanding of global health issues (GalanLominchar et al., 2024; Perez-Encinas et al., 2023; Mackavey et al., 2024; University of Primorska, Faculty of Health Sciences, 2022). International mobility programs —such as Erasmus+, the Fulbright Program, and various bilateral academic exchanges—are widely recognized as effective mechanisms for fostering global competencies among nursing students and faculty. According to the World Health Organization (2016), international exposure during nursing education enhances nurses' adaptability, leadership skills, and ability to function effectively within multicultural teams, all of which contribute to improved patient care outcomes. These programs not only broaden clinical and cultural perspectives but also cultivate essential professional qualities that equip nursing personnel to meet the demands of increasingly diverse healthcare environments (European Education and Culture Executive Agency, 2023; Forward Pathway, 2025; Morley & Cunningham, 2021; Perez-Encinas et al., 2023).

ADVANTAGES AND CHALLENGES OF NURSING FACULTY AND STUDENT MOBILITY

For nursing students, international mobility offers experiential learning opportunities that go beyond the confines of the traditional classroom. Exposure to diverse healthcare systems enables students to compare clinical practices, deepen their understanding of health disparities, and develop intercultural communication competencies (Ryan, 2011). In addition, participation in such mobility programs also contributes to personal growth, the formation of professional identity, and enhanced employability (Dobrowolska et al., 2015; de Wit, 2019).

From the perspective of nursing faculty, international mobility facilitates academic collaboration, supports curriculum development, and fosters transnational research partnerships. It also promotes the exchange of pedagogical innovations and dissemination of evidence-based practices across institutions (Green & Whitsed, 2015). Despite the well-documented benefits of international mobility, several significant barriers persist, several significant barriers continue to impede participation in such programs for nursing students and faculty. Commonly cited obstacles include financial constraints, limited institutional support, inflexible curricula, language barriers, and challenges related to visas or accreditation processes (Bjørnnes et al., 2025; European University Association, 2024; European University Foundation, 2022; Herath & Garbarino, 2023; Morley et al., 2018). Additionally, some nursing programs often face structural limitations on international clinical placements due to variations in licensure requirements and national healthcare regulations, which vary widely across countries (Knight, 2012). For instance, notable differences in educational curricula, duration of nursing programs, clinical practice requirements, and national licensure procedures represent substantial challenges to the international mobility of nurses and the mutual recognition of their professional qualifications (Ghimire & Neupane, 2025). These structural and systemic barriers tend to affect students from lower-income backgrounds and those enrolled in institutions located in low- and middle-income countries disproportionately, limiting their access to international mobility opportunities (Knight, 2012). Cultural challenges—such as adaptation difficulties and experiences of culture shock during international placements—underscore the importance of comprehensive preparatory support and structured post-exchange debriefing to optimize learning outcomes (Cunningham, 2020).

Concerns have also been raised about the potential for cultural misunderstandings or superficial engagement during short-term mobility experiences in nursing education. Without adequate preparation, both students and faculty may encounter difficulties integrating meaningfully into host environments, thereby limiting the transformative potential of the exchange (Green & Whitsed, 2015). To address these challenges, many mobility programs now incorporate structured pre-departure training, cultural competence workshops, and post-experience reflective debriefing sessions as integral components of program design (Sailsman et al., 2021). The impact of international mobility extends well beyond individual benefits, influencing institutional development and contributing to broader global health goals. At the institutional level, mobility fosters the internationalization of nursing education by promoting curriculum alignment with global standards, facilitating accreditation recognition, and supporting the development of joint degree programs. Participation in such programs enhances an institution's reputation, increases research productivity, and strengthens long-term international partnerships (de Wit, 2019).

METHODS

Following PRISMA guidelines, a descriptive method using systematic literature review was employed to gather and analyse relevant studies from the PubMed and CINAHL Ultimate. Figure 1. presents the PRISMA flowchart, illustrating the selection process of articles for this review. The search engines used the search strategies: ("nursing students" OR "nursing academic staff") AND ("mobility" OR "faculty mobility" OR "international exchange" OR "international educational exchange" OR "study abroad" OR "Erasmus") AND ("opportunities" OR "benefits" OR "impacts" OR "outcomes" OR "barriers" OR "challenges" OR "obstacles"). The literature searches were carried out on August 28, 2025.

The inclusion criteria required systematic reviews that focused on international mobility programs in nursing education, examining opportunities for professional development, associated challenges, and their implications for both faculty and students. The exclusion criteria included studies that were thematically irrelevant, as well as article types such as qualitative research, duplicates, editorials, protocols, and non-peer-reviewed contributions. The systematic literature review was limited to studies published in English, with no restrictions applied to the publication period. Included systematic review were assessed using the critical appraisal tool AMSTAR 2 for systematic reviews that include randomised or non-randomised studies of healthcare interventions (Shea et al., 2017). Each of the items from the checklists were judged with low risk of bias, some concerns or high risk of bias. Total scores were used to grade the methodological quality of each study. A synthesis of the selected studies was conducted using content analysis, following the approach of Elo and Kyngäs (2008).

RESULTS

As shown in Figure 1, 14 articles relevant to the research topic were identified through searches in the PubMed and CINHAL Ultimate databases. The search results were exported to the EndNote X21 software, and duplicated studies were removed using this software. Three articles were excluded as duplicates, and two were excluded based on the exclusion criteria. We analysed nine full-text articles, of which five were included in the systematic literature review.

Figure 1. Flow chart based on the PRISMA methodology

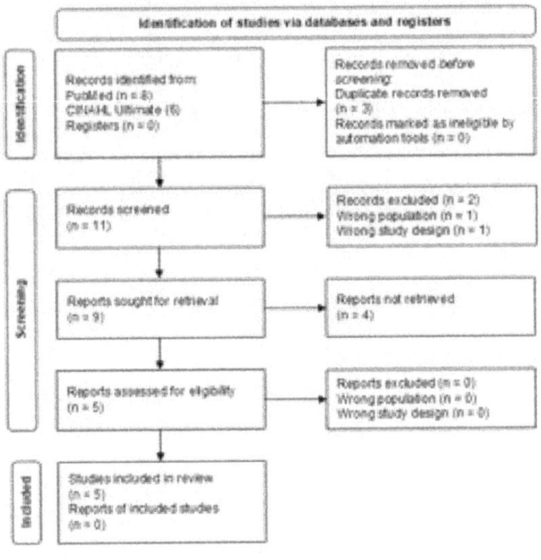

Table 1 summarizes the key characteristics of international mobility in nursing education, focusing on opportunities, challenges, and implications for faculty and students. Included study (Figure 2), methodological confidence is limited: three reviews were rated critically low (Mikkonen et al., 2016; Kulbok et al., 2012; Browne et al., 2015) and two low (Brown et al., 2016; Johnston et al., 2022). The deficiencies clustered in critical AMSTAR 2 domains, especially comprehensive searching (Item

4), reporting/justifying study exclusions (Item 7), and—most notably—assessment and use of study-level risk of bias (Items 9 & 13).

As shown in Figure 2, the overall, the quality of evidence was rated low to moderate across studies, indicating the need for more rigorous methodologies, standardized evaluations, and long-term outcome assessments (Browne et al., 2015; Brown et al., 2016; Johnston et al., 2022; Kulbok et al., 2012; Mikkonen et al., 2016).

Figure 2. Quality assessment with AMSTAR 2 tool (Shea et al., 2017), (AMSTAR, 2025)

Author (Year)	Quality of the Evidence																
	1	2	3	4	5	6	7	8	9	10	11	12	13	14	15	16	Overal rating
Browne et al. (2015)	?	-	+	?	-	-	-	+	-	-	N/A	N/A	-	-	N/A	-	Critically low
Brown et al. (2016)	?	-	+	?	-	-	+	+	+	-	N/A	N/A	?	-	N/A	-	Low
Johnston et al. (2022)	+	+	?	?	+	-	-	+	+	-	N/A	N/A	?	?	N/A	+	Low
Kulbo et al. (2012)	?	-	-	?	-	-	-	+	-	-	N/A	N/A	-	?	N/A	-	Critically low
Mikkonene et al. (2016)	?	-	+	?	+	-	-	+	+	-	N/A	N/A	-	-	N/A	+	Critically low

Legend: + = Yes; ? = Partial Yes; - = No; N/A = Not applicable; 1 – Did the research questions and inclusion criteria for the review include the components of PICO?; 2 – Did the report of the review contain an explicit statement that the review methods were established prior to the conduct of the review and did the report justify any significant deviations from the protocol?; 3 – Did the review authors explain their selection of the study designs for inclusion in the review?; 4 – Did the review authors use a comprehensive literature search strategy?; 5 – Did the review authors perform study selection in duplicate?; 6 – Did the review authors perform data extraction in duplicate?; 7 – Did the review authors provide a list of excluded studies and justify the exclusions?; 8 – Did the review authors describe the included studies in adequate detail?; 9 – Did the review authors use a satisfactory technique for assessing the risk of bias (RoB) in individual studies that were included in the review?; 10 – Did the review authors report on the sources of funding for the studies included in the review?; 11 – If meta-analysis was performed did the review authors use appropriate methods for statistical combination of results?; 12 – If meta-analysis was performed, did the review authors assess the potential impact of RoB in individual studies on the results of the meta-analysis or other evidence synthesis?; 13 – Did the review authors account for RoB in individual studies when interpreting/ discussing the results of the review?; 14 – Did the review authors provide a satisfactory explanation for, and discussion of, any heterogeneity observed in the results of the review?; 15 – If they performed quantitative synthesis did the review authors carry out an adequate investigation of publication bias (small study bias) and discuss its likely impact on the results of the review?

Table 1. Characteristics and Quality assessment of the included Systematic reviews

Author (Year)	Main findings	Quality of the Evidence			
Participants		**CL**	**L**	**M**	**H**
Browne et al. (2015)	Included eight studies on Australian undergraduate nursing students' international clinical placements (7 qualitative, 1 quantitative); placement length 8 days–5 weeks; most studies examined a single program. Thematic synthesis identified **five core outcome themes: Developing cultural awareness and competence:**	+			
	– International clinical placements improve cultural awareness, global perspectives, personal growth, and professional development. – Enablers: motivation to learn, financial support, role models, program feasibility. – Barriers: cost, limited language skills, family separation,				
	administrative difficulties. – Positive mentoring and integration with local students support mutual learning and reduce discrimination **Providing a Global Perspective on Health Care systems:** – International placements expose students to different cultures and health systems.				
	– Contrasts are most evident in developing countries. – Some view limited resources & high patient loads as barriers to "effective/Westernized" care. – Others recognize clinical principles can offset resource constraints. – Effective care relies on knowledge, sound practice, and				
	community education, not only equipment. **Translating theory into clinical practice:** – Clinical practicums help translate theory into practice. – ICPs enhance learning in child health, assessment, and nursing in disadvantaged settings. – Students report greater confidence, skills appreciation, and				
	cultural awareness. – Some evidence shows modest intellectual/attitudinal shifts, less than anticipated. – Knowledge transfer to local contexts after placements was limited. – Most significant changes were in perceptions of living				
	conditions and work habits. **Personal growth through reflection** (greater confidence, maturity, career influence) – Personal development is a key outcome of ICPs. – Motivations: travel, self-challenge, gaining experience, helping others.				
	– Helping others was often cored to nursing career choice. – Placements encouraged reflection on identity and career paths, including interest in aid work. – Experiences in low-resource settings led to reassessment of assumptions. – Students developed deeper appreciation of humanity, spirituality,				

continued on following page

Table 1. Continued

Author (Year)	Main findings	Quality of the Evidence			
Participants		**CL**	**L**	**M**	**H**
	and cultural care. – ICPs act as catalysts for personal growth and global nursing perspectives **Overcoming Apprehension to Successfully Meet the Challenge** (safety, language, communication), aided by reflection and support: – ICPs involve challenges in culturally and linguistically diverse care. – Pre-departure concerns: safety, professional competence, and not burdening host communities. – Anxieties decreased as placements progressed - importance of targeted pre-departure preparation. – Language barriers: use of interpreters, adapted strategies, language less problematic, acquired basic vocabulary quickly. – Despite barriers, students developed adaptive strategies, enhancing learning and cross-cultural competence.				
Brown et al. (2016)	Studies & participants: 10 studies (5 qualitative; 5 surveys), N = 1,489 healthcare students (pharmacy 489; physician-assistant 482; nursing 452; medical 66). Samples came mainly from North America and Europe. The same clusters of factors shape healthcare students' decisions to study abroad across professions and regions. **Factors that encourage participation:** – Desire to travel and to experience other cultures/health-care systems. – Enablers: Adequate, early information about opportunities (how to apply, timing, credit). – Strong predictors: Previous positive travel experience. – Role models and networks: knowing peers who went; faculty visibly involved in overseas projects. – Financial support (grants/bursaries) and feasible programme length (short, elective-style placements). – Choice of destination aligned with students' interests and language abilities; many prefer English-speaking (or linguistically familiar/easier) sites; safety and stability also considered. – Smaller role: faculty, family, and peer recommendations. **Factors that deter participation:** – Costs/finances and lack of bursaries. – Limited foreign-language skills. – Common barriers to studying abroad: Separation from family/friends; family responsibilities. – Institutional factors: Inadequate information/low institutional support (e.g., poor visibility of Erasmus-type options). – Concerns about personal safety/political situation in host countries; administrative burden/time to prepare. – Interest tends to be higher early in programmes and wanes later, partly due to workload/costs. **Recommendations:**		+		

continued on following page

Table 1. Continued

Author (Year)	Main findings	Quality of the Evidence			
Participants		**CL**	**L**	**M**	**H**
	– Provide clear information early, with named faculty "champions". – Offer/advertise funding, allow time for language preparation, and build partnerships in linguistically compatible sites. – Support social connection while abroad (e.g., planned communication with family) and teach coping strategies for family duties				
Johnston et al. (2022)	n = 56 primary studies (mostly qualitative; a few mixed/quantitative), English-language, 2010–2020. Participants mainly nursing students; very few midwifery-only studies. Destinations were largely low- or middle-income countries; most programs were short-term (≤4 weeks). Outcome themes: **Cultural learning** – Outcomes: global awareness, cultural competence, sensitivity, adaptation. – Students reported reduced bias, broader worldviews, and confidence with diverse populations. – Transformative experiences: understanding poverty, advocacy, language skills, cultural awareness. – Importance of collaboration with host communities for culturally acceptable care.		+		
	– Challenges: culture shock, ethical dilemmas, sustaining cultural learning post-return. **Personal growth** – Life skills: communication, confidence, flexibility, relationship-building. – Deeper transformations: worldview shifts, self-reflection, maturity. – Described as life-changing experiences, extending beyond				
	academic/professional development. **Professional development** – Enhanced nursing/midwifery skills, reflective practice, professional identity. – Cultural sensitivity shaped care approaches at home. – Influenced career goals, teamwork, leadership, and global professional outlook. Follow-up: Evidence is short-term—most outcomes measured within 6				
	months; very few studies followed students beyond 1–2 years. Measurement: Outcomes assessed heterogeneously; mainly reflections/interviews/journals. Few validated tools; little consistency across programs. Gaps/limits highlighted by authors: Scarcity of long-term outcomes, limited midwifery evidence, little on host community perspectives; variable program length/content; lack of robust evaluation frameworks.				

continued on following page

Table 1. Continued

Author (Year)	Main findings	Quality of the Evidence			
Participants		**CL**	**L**	**M**	**H**
Kulbok et al. (2012)	Review of 23 empirical studies (2003–2010); most conducted in the USA; truly two-way exchanges were rare. **Culture:** – *Cultural learning* – most frequently cited goal of international exchanges; Cultural differences central to the experience. – *Cultural competence* – both benefit and challenge. Depends on students' motivation and effort for adjustment and insight. – *Personal growth* – living abroad fostered self-development and understanding of multicultural care; often required unlearning misconceptions – *Motivation and effort* – crucial for successful cultural adjustment, insight, and effective functioning abroad. – *Personal growth* – living in another culture enhances self-development and understanding of multicultural care. – *Unlearning misconceptions* – students may need to revise or discard erroneous assumptions about host countries. **Global health:** – *Goal of global health learning* – students aim to understand healthcare systems, health problems, and nursing practices abroad. – *Knowledge diffusion* – exposure supports transfer of knowledge and skills between countries. – *Recognition of effective models* – students gain appreciation for efficient healthcare practices. – *Awareness of global health issues* – placements increase understanding of international health challenges. **Barriers to International Experiences:** – *Complexity of arrangements* – organizing and implementing international nursing experiences is often difficult. – *Stress of living abroad* – students reported high stress when living in foreign countries, particularly for extended periods. – *Cultural challenges* – cultural differences and complexities created obstacles in communication with host faculty and patients. – *Language barriers* – communication difficulties were intensified by limited foreign language proficiency. – *Financial issues* – lack of adequate funding was consistently highlighted as a significant problem. **Evidence gaps**: Very few long-term follow-ups; limited evaluation of clinical or patient outcomes; underrepresentation of low-income settings; nonstandard measures and largely descriptive reporting. **Conclusion**: International experiences are generally beneficial, but programs need more rigorous, standardized evaluation, more two-way partnerships, and stronger evidence on long-term and practice outcomes.	+			

continued on following page

Table 1. Continued

Author (Year)	Main findings	Quality of the Evidence			
Participants		**CL**	**L**	**M**	**H**
Mikkonen et al., 2016	Review of 5 studies. **Positive intercultural mentoring** is pivotal for international healthcare students' learning in clinical settings—it fosters reciprocal learning and reduces stress. When mentors lack time, skills, or support, learning quality declines. **The Positive Intercultural Mentor's Role:** – *Role of mentors* – supportive intercultural mentors were central to enhancing international clinical learning. – Intercultural mediation – mentors acted as mediators, helping students adapt, reducing stress, and fostering reciprocal learning. – *Reflection and dialogue* – identified as crucial for processing clinical experiences and exploring intercultural differences.	+			
	– *Impact on empathy* – intercultural sensitivity promoted empathy, with students articulating what it means to be "different." – Professional relevance – these insights shaped students' perspectives on future nurse–patient relationships **Encountering Lack of Knowledge, Skills and Time in Mentorship:** – *Need for dedicated mentors* – successful support of international students requires mentors who are well-prepared, skilled, and have sufficient time available. – *Practical challenges* – mentors often struggled with time constraints, limited teaching skills, and language barriers, making mentorship stressful and exhausting. – *Intercultural complications* – cultural differences complicated mentor–student relationships and created additional challenges. – *Institutional gaps* – mentors expressed dissatisfaction with insufficient institutional support and a lack of information about students' cultural backgrounds **The Student's Own Role in Learning**: – *Student's own role* – a decisive factor in clinical learning outcomes. – *Positive traits* – motivated, proactive, responsible, and open to feedback students adapted better, overcame language barriers, and maximized learning. – *Challenges for mentors* – students who were disengaged,				

continued on following page

Table 1. Continued

Author (Year)	Main findings	Quality of the Evidence			
Participants		CL	L	M	H
	unmotivated, or irregular in attendance were difficult to support. – *Key insight* – self-direction and commitment are essential for success in international placements **The Language Competence of Students:** – *Language competence* – identified as a decisive factor for success in international clinical placements. – *Strong skills* – verbal and written proficiency supported communication with patients/staff, accurate documentation, and positive mentor relationships. – *Weak skills* – inadequate proficiency led to barriers, isolation, and even clinical failure. – *Adaptive strategies* – students developed non-verbal				
	communication methods to support integration despite difficulties. **The Integration of International Students with Domestic Students in the Clinical Environment:** – *Integration* of international and domestic students is crucial for reciprocal learning and preventing discrimination. – *Challenges* – mentors reported cases of social isolation, rejection, and even bullying of international students linked to language barriers and cultural differences. – *Facilitating shared experiences* helps broaden global perspectives, strengthen social networks, and reduce isolation. – *Mentors' role* – pivotal in fostering inclusion and supporting positive intercultural learning environments.				

Legenda: H - High; M = Moderate; L = Low; CL = Critically Low; ICPs = International clinical placements.

Table 1 presents the characteristics and quality assessment of the included systematic reviews.

Browne et al. (2015) analyzed eight studies on Australian undergraduate nursing students' international clinical placements and identified five core themes: (1) **Developing cultural awareness and competence**: International clinical placements improve cultural awareness, global perspectives, personal growth, and professional development. The key factors enabling this were motivation to learn about other cultures, financial support, role models, and program feasibility, while barriers included cost, limited language skills, separation from family, and administrative difficulties. It was emphasized that positive intercultural mentoring and integration with local students are key to mutual learning and reducing discrimination. Overall, the quality of evidence was rated as low to moderate, highlighting the need for more robust methodologies and long-term evaluation of outcomes. (2) **Providing a Global Perspective on Health Care**: International clinical placements enable students to experience different cultures and health care systems, with contrasts most evident in placements in developing countries. While some students perceived limited resources and high patient loads as barriers to "effective" or "Westernized" care, others recognized that sound principles of practice can compensate for resource constraints. This understanding was illustrated by students in Tanzania and India, who emphasized that effective care depends not only on equipment and facilities but also on knowledge, sound clinical principles, and community education. (3) **Translation of Theory to Practice**: Undergraduate nursing programs integrate clinical practicum experiences to help students consolidate theoretical knowledge in real practice. Evidence suggests that international clinical placements (ICPs) support this progression, with students reporting valuable learning about child health, physical assessment, and the scope of nursing in disadvantaged settings. Placements highlighted students' appreciation of their own skills and the cultural dimensions of care. Students also reported increased confidence and perceived knowledge as placements progressed. However, some studies caution that actual intellectual and attitudinal shifts may be more modest than anticipated. It was found that the transfer of knowledge acquired during the internship to scenarios in the local community was limited, while minor changes were also reported in the attitudes of students who completed the internship, with the more significant changes being limited mainly to the perception of living conditions and work habits. (4) **Growing Personally Through Reflection**: Personal development is a central outcome of international clinical placements. Students reported motivations such as travel, self-challenge, gaining experience, and helping others, with many reflecting that their desire to help was integral to their decision to pursue nursing. Placements also fostered reflection on professional identity and future career pathways, including aspirations to work with international aid organizations. Confronting experiences in low-resource settings encouraged students to reassess their assumptions, leading to deeper appreciation of humanity, spirituality, and the cultural acceptability of care. Overall, ICPs were seen as catalysts for both personal growth and the development of global nursing perspectives. (5) **Overcoming Apprehension to Successfully Meet the Challenge**: International clinical placements present students with challenges that must be addressed to provide holistic care in culturally and linguistically diverse settings. Common concerns prior to departure included personal safety, professional competence, and the ability to contribute meaningfully without burdening host communities. These anxieties often diminished as placements progressed, suggesting the value of targeted pre-departure preparation. Language barriers were a consistent challenge, with students in Cambodia reporting reliance on interpreters and the need to adapt communication strategies for cultural compatibility. However, students in Thailand found language difficulties less severe than anticipated, noting that they quickly acquired essential vocabulary. Overall, while barriers were evident, students developed adaptive strategies that facilitated learning and strengthened cross-cultural competence. Brown et al. (2016), synthesizing ten studies with 1,489 healthcare students, highlighted factors that encourage participation in international exchanges (e.g., desire for cultural experience, financial support, role models, and alignment of destination with students' interests) as well as barriers (e.g., costs, limited language skills, separation from family, inadequate institutional support, and administrative burden).

Browne et al. (2016) identified **factors that encourage participation** and **factors that deter participation**. Most healthcare students expressed interest in studying abroad, motivated mainly by the desire to travel and experience different cultures and healthcare systems. Religious beliefs also influenced participation, with some students viewing overseas placements as opportunities to serve disadvantaged populations. Prior international experience and awareness of existing programs were strong predictors of interest. Faculty, family, and peer recommendations played a smaller role, though early access to information and supportive academic environments increased engagement. Furthermore, several barriers to studying abroad were consistently identified across studies. The most frequently reported deterrents included limited foreign language proficiency, separation from family and friends, and family responsibilities. Financial cost emerged as the most significant limiting factor, with student interest declining as anticipated expenses increased. Awareness and promotion of study abroad programmes also played a critical role: low participation was often linked to insufficient institutional support and limited knowledge of available funding. Evidence indicates that providing information early in training and increasing awareness of grants, such as Erasmus funding, can enhance students' confidence and willingness to participate.

Johnston et al. (2022) identified three outcome themes: (1) **Cultural Learning** encompassed outcomes related to global awareness, cultural competence, sensitivity, and adaptation to cultural differences and challenges. Students describing progression toward cultural competence, reduced bias, expanded worldviews, and increased confidence in working with diverse populations. Some studies highlighted transformative experiences, such as recognizing the complexities of poverty and developing advocacy skills, or gaining language skills, cultural awareness, and changed perspectives. Students also emphasized the importance of collaboration with host communities to ensure culturally acceptable practices and reported building meaningful relationships abroad. However, challenges such as culture shock, ethical dilemmas, and difficulty sustaining cultural learning upon return were also evident. (2) The theme of **Personal Growth** encompassed both the acquisition of life skills and deeper transformative change. Outcomes at the personal level, ranging from improved communication, confidence, flexibility, and relationship-building to profound shifts in worldview. Students frequently described their experiences as life-changing, with some stating they would "never be the same". Similar findings highlighted international placements as opportunities for personal transformation and maturation, providing students with skills and perspectives that extended beyond academic or professional development. (3) The theme of **Professional Development** encompassed outcomes related to the advancement of nursing and midwifery practice. International experiences were reported to enhance nursing skills, reflective practice, and professional identity. Reflection was emphasized as a key component of learning, while cultural sensitivity was identified as shaping students' approaches to care in their home settings. These experiences were regarded as transformative, influencing career goals, strengthening teamwork and leadership skills, and fostering a global professional outlook. Collectively, ICPs were found to expand competencies and inform future professional pathways.

Kulbok et al. (2012) found that **Cultural learning** was one of the most frequently cited goals of international exchanges, with all studies addressing cultural differences as central to the experience. Developing cultural competence emerged as both a benefit and a challenge. Students' motivation and effort were critical for cultural adjustment, insight, and effective functioning in new contexts. Living abroad enhanced personal growth and understanding of multicultural care, often requiring unlearning of prior misconceptions. In relation to **global health**, international placements aimed to increase students' knowledge of healthcare systems, health challenges, and nursing practices in other countries. Reported benefits included knowledge transfer between countries, recognition of effective care models, and heightened awareness of global health issues. **Barriers to international experiences** were evident, as arranging and implementing placements proved complex, with students frequently reporting stress related to living in foreign and culturally unfamiliar environments. Communication difficulties were further compounded by cultural and linguistic differences, while financial constraints were consistently identified as a major barrier.

Mikkonen et al. (2016) underscored the **importance of positive intercultural mentoring** in international clinical learning, emphasizing that the presence of a supportive intercultural mentor was central to enhancing students' experiences. Mentors acted as intercultural mediators, facilitating students' adaptation, reducing stress, and fostering reciprocal learning. Reflection and dialogue were identified as vital processes, enabling students to process their clinical experiences while exploring intercultural differences. Mentors further observed that intercultural sensitivity nurtured greater empathy, with students beginning to articulate what it means to be "different" and how these insights could shape future nurse–patient relationships. In the context of **Encountering Lack of Knowledge, Skills and Time in Mentorship**, the need for dedicated, well-prepared, and time-available mentors proved crucial for supporting international students during demanding internships. In practice, however, mentors often faced time constraints, limited teaching skills, and challenges in communicating in a foreign language, which made their role stressful and exhausting. Intercultural differences further complicated mentor–student relationships, with mentors expressing dissatisfaction with inadequate institutional support and insufficient information about students' cultural backgrounds. **The Student's Own Role in Learning** was identified as a crucial factor shaping learning outcomes in the clinical environment. Students who were motivated, proactive, responsible, and receptive to feedback were more successful in adapting, overcoming language barriers, and maximizing their learning opportunities. In contrast, mentors found it difficult to support students who were less engaged, unmotivated, or inconsistent in clinical attendance, underscoring the importance of self-direction and commitment in international placements. **Students' language competence** was identified as a decisive factor in international clinical placements. Strong verbal and written skills enabled students to communicate effectively with patients and staff, complete documentation, and build positive mentor relationships. In contrast, inadequate proficiency created barriers, isolation, and in some cases failure in clinical practice. While language difficulties posed significant challenges, students also developed non-verbal communication strategies over time to aid their integration. **Integration of international and domestic students in the clinical environment** was regarded as crucial for fostering reciprocal learning and preventing discrimination. However, mentors reported instances of social isolation, rejection, and even bullying of international students due to language barriers and cultural differences. Facilitating shared experiences was considered an effective way to broaden global perspectives, build social networks, and reduce isolation, underscoring the mentor's pivotal role in supporting inclusion.

Following the approach of Elo and Kyngäs (2008), we conducted a content analysis to synthesize the selected studies, analyzing five systematic review articles. These are presented in Table 2 below, where categories, subcategories, and codes are defined." The main category identified was "International clinical placements as catalysts for cultural competence, personal growth, and professional development, mediated by barriers and facilitators". Within this, five subcategories emerged: (1) Cultural Learning and Competence; (2) Personal Growth and Identity; (3) Professional Development; (4) Barriers and Challenges; and (5) Facilitators of Success.

Cultural learning and competence was associated with cultural awareness, global perspectives, sensitivity, and the ability to adapt to diverse contexts (Browne et al., 2015; Johnston et al., 2022; Kulbok et al., 2012), though also linked to challenges such as culture shock and communication barriers (Kulbok et al., 2012; Johnston et al., 2022). Personal growth and identity referred to the development of confidence, resilience, reflection, and motivation, often described as transformative or life-changing experiences (Browne et al., 2015; Brown et al., 2016; Johnston et al., 2022). Professional development encompassed clinical knowledge, reflective practice, teamwork, leadership, and the shaping of professional identity through exposure to different healthcare systems (Johnston et al., 2022; Kulbok et al., 2012). Barriers and challenges were consistently reported, particularly financial constraints, language difficulties, limited institutional support, and stress associated with living abroad (Brown et al., 2016; Kulbok et al., 2012; Mikkonen et al., 2016). Conversely, facilitators of success included supportive mentoring, intercultural mediation, adequate preparation, financial aid, and integration with local students (Mikkonen et al., 2016; Browne et al., 2015; Brown et al., 2016).

Overall, the findings underscore that while international clinical placements present notable challenges, they also offer profound opportunities for fostering cultural competence, personal transformation, and professional growth when supported by appropriate structures and mentorship (Browne et al., 2015; Brown et al., 2016; Johnston et al., 2022; Kulbok et al., 2012; Mikkonen et al., 2016).

Table 2. Content analysis of research findings

<table>
<tr><th>Category</th><th>Subcategory</th><th>Codes</th></tr>
<tr><td rowspan="5">International clinical placements as catalysts for cultural competence, personal growth, and professional development, mediated by barriers and facilitators.</td><td>Cultural Learning and Competence</td><td>Cultural awareness, global perspectives, cultural sensitivity, adaptation, reduced bias, unlearning misconceptions, Campinha-Bacote's model, Bennett's continuum, culture shock, ethical dilemmas.</td></tr>
<tr><td>Personal Growth and Identity</td><td>Confidence, maturity, resilience, reflection, spirituality, worldview shifts, relationship-building, self-reflection, motivation for self-challenge, helping others, professional identity.</td></tr>
<tr><td>Professional Development</td><td>Clinical knowledge, reflective practice, teamwork, leadership, enhanced nursing/midwifery skills, professional identity, exposure to effective models, global professional outlook.</td></tr>
<tr><td>Barriers and Challenges</td><td>Limited financial support, high costs, lack of bursaries, language barriers, reliance on interpreters, isolation, family separation, stress of living abroad, inadequate institutional support, administrative burden, limited knowledge transfer to local contexts.</td></tr>
<tr><td>Facilitators of Success</td><td>Supportive mentors, intercultural mediation, reflection and dialogue, empathy, reciprocal learning, role models, adequate preparation, grants/financial aid, institutional champions, supportive academic environments, shared experiences with local students, integration strategies.</td></tr>
</table>

DISCUSSION

Our findings suggest that international clinical placements act as a powerful catalyst for the cultural competence, personal growth and professional development of nursing and midwifery students. However, these benefits are also limited by various barriers and other factors that either enhance or limit the overall impact of such experiences. Importantly, the evidence highlights the importance of mobility for both students and academics, and sustainable internationalization requires reciprocal collaboration at multiple levels.

Participation in international placements fostered cultural awareness, global perspectives, and cultural sensitivity. Students reported reduced bias, greater openness to difference, and the unlearning of misconceptions (Louis, White, & Brown, 2025; Shali, Bakhshi, & Hasanpour, 2024; Grinberg & Nissim, 2025; Streitwieser, Lomer & van der Wende, 2020). Culture shock and ethical dilemmas were also frequently encountered, serving both as challenges and opportunities for growth. These findings support previous research indicating that cultural immersion can be transformative but also emotionally and ethically demanding (Johnston, McKenna, Malik, & Reisenhofer, 2023; Streitwieser, Lomer, & van der Wende, 2020). This synthesis of mobility in nursing education highlights important benefits for nursing students and academic staff. Students gain cultural and linguistic capability, resilience, and the capacity to translate theory into practice. Multiple studies report gains in cultural competence and global awareness; for example, students completing placements in Cambodia described that the experience deepened their understanding of global health issues relevant to multicultural care in Australia and broadened their perspectives on working across cultures (Tuckett & Crompton, 2014). Similarly, immersive observation during short-term placements enabled students to compare health systems and translate insights into culturally responsive practice. During a two-week placement in Tanzania, students discerned shared humanistic foundations—"the basic elements of love and care are the same"—despite differing clinical routines (Michael et al., 2012; Ferranto, 2015; Jacob, Seif & Munyaw, 2023). International placements contributed substantially to students' confidence, maturity, and resilience. Reflective processes and encounters with unfamiliar spiritual and cultural contexts often shifted students' worldviews, prompting deeper self-reflection and the development of empathy. Such experiences motivated students to challenge themselves and reinforced their professional identity. These findings echo earlier studies that link international mobility with enhanced self-awareness and identity formation in healthcare professionals (Button et al., 2005; Jansen et al., 2021; Racine, 2023; Ulvund, Dadi, & Sundal, 2023).

Beyond personal and cultural gains, students developed advanced clinical knowledge, teamwork, leadership skills, and reflective practice. Exposure to diverse healthcare systems broadened their professional outlook and provided models of effective care delivery that could be adapted to their home contexts. Professional identity was reinforced not only through technical competence but also through adaptability, empathy, and critical reflection. This supports findings by Maltby and

Abrams (2009), who argue that international experiences can enrich both technical and relational aspects of professional practice.

Despite these benefits, students faced significant barriers. Financial constraints—including high costs and limited bursaries—were the most frequently cited limitations. Language barriers, reliance on interpreters, feelings of isolation, and separation from family also presented major challenges. Administrative burdens and inadequate institutional support compounded these difficulties. Furthermore, participants highlighted the limited transferability of some experiences to local contexts, which has been observed in prior studies examining international knowledge exchange (Buckner et al., 2014).

Where supportive structures were in place, students achieved more positive outcomes. Mentorship, intercultural mediation, opportunities for structured reflection, and dialogue proved critical for overcoming cultural shock and linguistic challenges. Institutional champions, adequate preparation, and financial support further facilitated success. Shared experiences with local students and reciprocal learning reinforced integration and empathy, echoing earlier evidence that peer collaboration enhances intercultural competence (Papadopoulos, 2006). Ergonomic aspects of mobility are intrinsically linked to learning outcomes and safety. Students and higher education teachers are confronted with unfamiliar equipment, spatial constraints, and documentation systems, which increase both physical load (e.g., strain related to patient handling) and cognitive load (new procedures, language, IT). Structured preparatory training, mentoring support, and standardized protocols are essential for safe work practices and patient safety (ASPHP, 2023). Students and staff, however, face parallel challenges. While students struggle with financial, linguistic, and informational barriers, staff often confront time constraints, limited institutional recognition, and insufficient funding. When staff mobility is undervalued, opportunities for international collaboration diminish, limiting the sustainability of student programs. Equal recognition of staff participation—through workload allocation, funding, and career incentives—is therefore essential (de Wit, 2019).

Academic staff also accrue important advantages from participation in mobility and collaborative teaching abroad, including refinement of pedagogical practice, heightened cultural awareness, and the expansion of international professional networks (de Wit, 2019; Nogueiro et al., 2022; Kafarski & Kazak, 2022). Staff contribute significantly by modelling intercultural sensitivity and embedding global health perspectives into curricula, thereby helping students translate theory into practice, broaden their professional outlook, and reinforce the outcomes of cultural learning, personal growth, and professional development identified in this review. Faculty-to-faculty exchanges and joint placements can further reinforce sustainability of programs and ensure reciprocity with host institutions (Knight, 2015). Sustainable internationalization requires reciprocity, meaning that benefits must extend not only to visiting students but also to host institutions and academic staff. Reciprocity ensures equity and long-term value by generating mutual benefits and supporting the capacity of both sending and host institutions. Faculty engagement plays a crucial role in this process, as the active involvement of academic staff in building and maintaining partnerships fosters continuity, meaningful knowledge exchange, and culturally sensitive program design.

A dual focus on student and staff mobility enhances global academic networks and deepens international collaboration, moving beyond the traditional emphasis on student exchanges alone. Increasingly, sustainable internationalization is also linked to broader sustainability goals, as universities integrate environmental, social, and educational sustainability into their international activities (Leask, 2015; Lourenço & Paiva, 2024). At the policy level, mobility contributes to universal health coverage and the Sustainable Development Goals by supporting knowledge exchange and workforce adaptability (McCarthy et al., 2020; Indicators, OECD, 2023). To maximize these benefits, institutions must embed global perspectives in curricula, provide adequate support structures, and ensure that programs prevent “brain drain” from low-resource settings.

This discussion confirms that international clinical placements hold considerable potential in shaping culturally competent, personally resilient, and professionally confident healthcare professionals. Yet this potential is not automatic; it requires systematic institutional support, targeted preparation, and reciprocal partnerships that recognize the contributions of both students and staff. By embedding intercultural perspectives into curricula, strengthening faculty and student exchanges, and fostering long-term, equitable collaboration with host institutions, international mobility can contribute not only to professional growth but also to sustainable, globally relevant nursing education.

CONCLUSION

Faculty and student mobility in nursing presents substantial opportunities for educational enrichment, fostering intercultural exchange, and the advancement of global health outcomes. However, realizing the full potential of these initiatives requires deliberate efforts to overcome structural and systemic barriers (including financial limitations, curricular rigidity, and disparities in access), promote equity in access, and strengthen the quality and sustainability of mobility programs. Furthermore, to harness the transformative potential of mobility experiences, it is essential to ensure meaningful engagement through adequate cultural preparation, guided reflection, and structured debriefing. The following sections will provide an in-depth examination of these complex dimensions, incorporating real-world case studies and policy strategies designed to promote effective, equitable, and sustainable international mobility within nursing education.

REFERENCES

Adhikari, R., & Smith, P. (2023). Global nursing workforce challenges: Time for a paradigm shift. *Nurse Education in Practice*, *69*, 103627. DOI: 10.1016/j.nepr.2023.103627 PMID: 37018998

AMSTAR. (2025, July). AMSTAR checklist. [from: https://amstar.ca/Amstar_Checklist.php]. *Access*, *28*, •••.

ASPHP. (2023). Safe Patient Handling and Mobility (SPHM) Education in Health Care Student Curriculum: A White Paper. [Internet]. The Association of Safe Patient Handling Professionals Access 1. october 2025,from www.ASPHP.org

Bjørnnes, A. K., Torbjørnsen, A., Thordardottir, B. S. A., Lund, A., Hovland, O. J., & Skarpaas, L. S. (2025). Exploring intentions: Factors influencing international study decisions in healthcare bachelor's degree programs. *BMC Medical Education*, *25*(1), 555. DOI: 10.1186/s12909-025-07136-4 PMID: 40247245

Brown, M., Boateng, E. A., & Evans, C. (2016). Should I stay or should I go? A systematic review of factors that influence healthcare students' decisions around study abroad programmes. *Nurse Education Today*, *39*, 63–71. DOI: 10.1016/j.nedt.2015.12.024 PMID: 27006034

Browne, C. A., Fetherston, C. M., & Medigovich, K. (2015). International clinical placements for Australian undergraduate nursing students: A systematic thematic synthesis of the literature. *Nurse Education Today*, *35*(10), 1028–1036. DOI: 10.1016/j.nedt.2015.05.012 PMID: 26059923

Buckner, E. B., Anderson, D. J., Garzon, N., Hafsteinsdóttir, T. B., Lai, C. K. Y., & Roshan, R. (2014). Perspectives on global nursing leadership: International experiences from the field. *International Nursing Review*, *61*(4), 463–471. DOI: 10.1111/inr.12139 PMID: 25411072

Button, L., Green, B., Tengnah, C., Johansson, I., & Baker, C. (2005). The impact of international placements on nurses' personal and professional lives: Literature review. *Journal of Advanced Nursing*, *50*(3), 315–324. DOI: 10.1111/j.1365-2648.2005.03395.x PMID: 15811111

Carayon, P., Kleinschmidt, P., Hose, B.-Z., & Salwei, M. (2020). Human factors and ergonomics in health care and patient safety from the perspective of medical residents. In *Textbook of Patient Safety and Clinical Risk Management* [Internet]. Springer. Published online: December 15, 2020. Access 1. october 2025, from https://www.ncbi.nlm.nih.gov/books/NBK585616/

Cunningham, S. (2020). Challenges of outward facing mobility opportunities for nursing students: Pre and periCOVID19. *European Journal of Open & Distance Learning*, *1*(1), 89–94. DOI: 10.17932/EJOH.2020.022/ejoh_v01i1008

De Wit, H. (2019). Internationalization in higher education, a critical review. *SFU Educational Review*, *12*(3), 9–17. DOI: 10.21810/sfuer.v12i3.1036

Dobrowolska, B., McGonagle, I., Jackson, C., Kane, R., Cabrera, E., Cooney-Miner, D., Di Cara, V., Pajnkihar, M., Prlić, N., Sigurdardottir, A. K., Kekuš, D., Wells, J., & Palese, A. (2015). Clinical practice models in nursing education: Implication for students' mobility. *International Nursing Review*, *62*(1), 36–46. DOI: 10.1111/inr.12162 PMID: 25559068

Elo, S., & Kyngäs, H. (2008). The qualitative content analysis process. *Journal of Advanced Nursing*, *62*(1), 107–115. DOI: 10.1111/j.1365-2648.2007.04569.x PMID: 18352969

European Education and Culture Executive Agency. (2023, November 28). *Erasmus+ programme guide 2024 (Version 1)*. Erasmus+. Access 21. july 2025, from: https://erasmus-plus.ec.europa.eu/sites/default/files/2023-11/2024-Erasmus%2BProgramme-Guide_EN.pdf

European University Association. (2024). *Trends 2024 – European higher education institutions in times of transition* [PDF]. EUA. Access 21. july 2025, from: https://www.eua.eu/images/publications/Publication_PDFs/Trends_2024.pdf

European University Foundation. (2022). *Making mobility the norm: Mobility report* (Project No. 20191DE01KA203005031) [PDF]. Evropska univerzitetna fundacija. https://uni-foundation.eu/uploads/2022_NORM_Mobility%20Report.pdf

Ferranto, M. L. G. (2015). A qualitative study of baccalaureate nursing students following an eight-day international cultural experience in Tanzania: Cultural humility as an outcome. *Procedia: Social and Behavioral Sciences*, *174*, 91–102. DOI: 10.1016/j.sbspro.2015.01.631

Galan-Lominchar, M., Roque, I. M.-S., Cazallas, C. C., Mcalpin, R., Fernández-Ayuso, D., & Ribeiro, A. S. F.GalanLominchar. (2024). Nursing students' internationalization: Virtual exchange and clinical simulation impact cultural intelligence. *Nursing Outlook*, *72*(2), 102137. DOI: 10.1016/j.outlook.2024.102137 PMID: 38340388

Ghimire, A., & Neupane, M. S. (2025). Navigating global mobility: A comparative study of nursing education in Nepal and Australia. *International Journal of Nursing Education Scholarship*, *22*(1), 20240108. Advance online publication. DOI: 10.1515/ijnes-2024-0108 PMID: 40643086

Green, W., & Whitsed, C. (Eds.). (2015). *Critical perspectives on internationalising the curriculum in disciplines: Reflective narrative accounts from business, education and health* (Vol. 28). Sense/Springer., DOI: 10.1007/978-94-6300-085-7

Grinberg, K., & Nissim, S. (2025). Cultural competence among nursing students: Exploring differences across academic stages. *BMC Nursing*, *24*(1), 640. DOI: 10.1186/s12912-025-03246-y PMID: 40468297

Indicators, OECD. (2023). Education at a Glance 2022. *link]. Acesso em março de.*

Jacob, A., Seif, S., & Munyaw, Y. (2023). Perceptions and experiences of diploma nursing students on clinical learning. A descriptive qualitative study in Tanzania. *BMC Nursing*, *22*(1), 225. DOI: 10.1186/s12912-023-01362-1 PMID: 37391811

Jansen, M. B., Lund, D. W., Baume, K., Lillyman, S., Rooney, K., & Nielsen, D. S. (2021). International clinical placement–Experiences of nursing students' cultural, personal and professional development; a qualitative study. *Nurse Education in Practice*, *51*, 102987. DOI: 10.1016/j.nepr.2021.102987 PMID: 33610023

Johnston, J., McKenna, L., Malik, G., & Reisenhofer, S. (2022). Reported outcomes of nursing or midwifery students participating in international educational programs in their pre-registration education: A narrative systematic review. *Nurse Education Today*, *111*, 105320. DOI: 10.1016/j.nedt.2022.105320 PMID: 35276538

Johnston, J., McKenna, L., Malik, G., & Reisenhofer, S. (2023). Recognizing and adapting to cultural differences: Influence of international educational programs on future nursing and midwifery practice. *Journal of Transcultural Nursing*, *34*(6), 423–430. DOI: 10.1177/10436596231198276 PMID: 37740536

Kafarski, K., & Kazak, J. K. (2022). Erasmus staff mobility in the building of a European network: The case of a Central European university. *Sustainability (Basel)*, *14*(9), 4949. DOI: 10.3390/su14094949

Knight, J. (2012). Concepts, rationales, and interpretive frameworks in the internationalization of higher education. In Deardorff, D. K., de Wit, H., Heyl, J. D., & Adams, T. (Eds.), *The SAGE Handbook of International Higher Education* (pp. 27–42). SAGE Publications., DOI: 10.4135/9781452218397.n2

Kulbok, P. A., Mitchell, E. M., Glick, D. F., & Greiner, D. (2012). International experiences in nursing education: A review of the literature. *International Journal of Nursing Education Scholarship*, *9*(1), 1–21. DOI: 10.1515/1548-923X.2365 PMID: 22628353

Leask, B. (2015). *Internationalizing the curriculum*. Routledge. DOI: 10.4324/9781315716954

Louis, K. S., White, A., & Brown, A. (2025). Nursing Students' Enhanced Cultural Competence After Study Abroad: A Mixed-Methods Study. *The Journal of Nursing Education, 64*(3), 185–191. DOI: 10.3928/01484834-20250108-01 PMID: 40048603

Lourenço, A., & Paiva, M. O. (2024). Globalization of higher education: The internationalization from a multifactorial perspective. In *Building resiliency in higher education: Globalization, digital skills, and student wellness* (pp. 285–305). IGI Global Scientific Publishing. DOI: 10.4018/979-8-3693-5483-4.ch016

Mackavey, C. L., Henderson, C., & Stout, T. (2024). Stepping outside national borders: International active learning educational collaboration events. *International Nursing Review, 71*(1), 5–12. DOI: 10.1111/inr.12927 PMID: 38156728

Maltby, H. J., & Abrams, S. (2009). Seeing with new eyes: The meaning of an immersion experience in Bangladesh for undergraduate senior nursing students. *International Journal of Nursing Education Scholarship, 6*(1). Advance online publication. DOI: 10.2202/1548-923X.1858 PMID: 19883373

McCarthy, C., Boniol, M., Daniels, K., Cometto, G., Diallo, K., Lawani, A. D., & Campbell, J. (2020). State of the World's Nursing 2020: Investing in education, jobs, and leadership. *Geneva: World Health Organization*. Access 21. july 2025, from: https://web.archive.org/web/20200407162231/https://www.who.int/publications-detail/nursing-report-2020

Michael, R., Della, P., Banner, C., Duckworth, S., & Nilson, T. (2012). The role of the photo novella in examining cultural competency in perioperative settings. *ACORN: The Journal of Perioperative Nursing in Australia, 25*(1), 20-24, 26.

Mikkonen, K., Elo, S., Tuomikoski, A. M., & Kääriäinen, M. (2016). Mentor experiences of international healthcare students' learning in a clinical environment: A systematic review. *Nurse Education Today, 40*, 87–94. DOI: 10.1016/j.nedt.2016.02.013 PMID: 27125155

Morley, L., Alexiadou, N., Garaz, S., González-Monteagudo, J., & Taba, M. (2018). Internationalisation and migrant academics: The hidden narratives of mobility. *Higher Education, 76*(3), 537–554. DOI: 10.1007/s10734-017-0224-z

Nogueiro, T., Saraiva, M., Jorge, F., & Chaleta, E. (2022). The Erasmus+ Programme and Sustainable Development Goals—Contribution of mobility actions in higher education. *Sustainability (Basel), 14*(3), 1628. DOI: 10.3390/su14031628

OECD. (2020). *Education at a glance 2020: OECD indicators*. OECD Publishing., DOI: 10.1787/69096873-

Papadopoulos, I. (Ed.). (2006). *Transcultural health and social care: development of culturally competent practitioners*. Elsevier Health Sciences.

Pathway, F. (2025, July). Fulbright program empowers global nursing education: Strategic insights on international collaboration, curriculum innovation, and talentshortage solutions. *Forward Pathway*. [from: https://www.forwardpathway.us/fulbright-program-empowers-global-nursing-education-strategic-insights-on-international-collaboration-curriculum-innovation-and-talent-shortage-solutions]. *Access*, *21*, •••.

Perez-Encinas, A., De Filippo, D., De La Torre, E. M., & Alonso, D. (2023). *Research competence framework: Competence frameworks in international student mobility* (Erasmus Careers Project No. 101049436). Erasmus Careers Consortium. Access 21. july 2025, from: https://project.erasmuscareers.org/documents/ResearchCompetenceFramework.pdf

Racine, L. (2023). International clinical experiences may increase cultural competency and support nurses' personal and professional development. *Evidence-Based Nursing*, *26*(4), 153–153. DOI: 10.1136/ebnurs-2022-103690 PMID: 37160348

Ryan, J. (2011). Teaching and learning for international students: Towards a transcultural approach. *Teachers and Teaching*, *17*(6), 631–648. DOI: 10.1080/13540602.2011.625138

Sailsman, S. (2021). EnglishAsASecondLanguage (ESL) nursing students' academic integration: A review of literature. *Nursing Education Perspectives*, *42*(3), 152–156. DOI: 10.1097/01.NEP.0000000000000731 PMID: 33861530

Shali, M., Bakhshi, F., & Hasanpour, M. (2024). Culture of patient care among international nursing students: A focused ethnographic study. *BMC Nursing*, *23*(1), 163. DOI: 10.1186/s12912-024-01807-1 PMID: 38448913

Sharplin, G., Clarke, J., & Eckert, M. (2025). *Assessing the global sustainability of the nursing workforce: A survey of national nurses' association presidents within the International Council of Nurses* (Report prepared for the International Council of Nurses by the Rosemary Bryant AO Research Centre). University of South Australia. Access 21. july 2025, from: https://www.icn.ch/sites/default/files/2025-04/ICN_NNA-Presidents-Survey-Report_EN_FINAL.pdf

Shea, B. J., Reeves, B. C., Wells, G., Thuku, M., Hamel, C., Moran, J., Moher, D., Tugwell, P., Welch, V., Kristjansson, E., & Henry, D. A. (2017). AMSTAR 2: A critical appraisal tool for systematic reviews that include randomised or non-randomised studies of healthcare interventions, or both. *BMJ (Clinical Research Ed.)*, *358*, j4008. DOI: 10.1136/bmj.j4008 PMID: 28935701

Streitwieser, B., Lomer, S., & van der Wende, M. (2020). Universities as global actors: The challenge of internationalization, sustainability, and global responsibility. *Higher Education Policy*, *33*(3), 393–409. DOI: 10.3390/su6053043

Tuckett, A., & Crompton, P. (2014). Qualitative understanding of an international learning experience: What A ustralian undergraduate nurses and midwives said about a Cambodia placement? *International Journal of Nursing Practice*, *20*(2), 135–141. DOI: 10.1111/ijn.12142 PMID: 24713009

Ulvund, I., Dadi, G. B., & Sundal, H. (2023). Nurses benefit from international clinical placement as nurse students: A qualitative study. *Nurse Education Today*, *121*, 105663. DOI: 10.1016/j.nedt.2022.105663 PMID: 36481523

University of Primorska, Faculty of Health Sciences. (2022). *BENEFITS: Better and more effective nursing education for improving transcultural nursing skills* (Project 20191TR01KA203076879). Erasmus+ KA2 Cooperation Projects. Access July 21, 2025 from: https://www.upr.si/en/up--environment/projects-of-the-university-of-primorska/erasmus-ka2-cooperation-projects/benefits-better-and-more-effective-nursing-education-for-improving-transcultural-nursing-skills

World Health Organization. (2016). *Nurse educator core competencies*. WHO. Access 27. july 2025, from: https://iris.who.int/bitstream/handle/10665/258713/9789241549622-eng.pdf?sequence=1

World Health Organization. (2020, April 6). *The state of the world's nursing 2020: Investing in education, jobs and leadership* [PDF]. WHO. Access 27. july 2025, from: https://www.who.int/publications/i/item/9789240003279

Chapter 4
Faculty and Student Mobility in Nursing:
Opportunities, Barriers, and Impacts

R. Velmurugan
https://orcid.org/0000-0002-7925-9757
Karpagam Academy of Higher Education, Coimbatore, India

R. Bhuvaneswari
https://orcid.org/0009-0003-9396-6129
Dr. Mahalingam College of Engineering and Technology, Pollachi, India

Maksud A. Madraswale
https://orcid.org/0000-0001-9565-0775
Presidency University, Bangalore, India

S. Senthilkumar
https://orcid.org/0000-0003-1968-6877
Skyline University, Nigeria

ABSTRACT

The globalization of healthcare underscores the importance of faculty and student mobility in nursing education, defined as movement across institutional and cultural boundaries to enhance learning, practice, and research. Such mobility fosters knowledge exchange, skill development, and cultural competence, vital for a globalized healthcare environment. Students gain adaptability and cross-cultural awareness, while faculty benefit from exposure to diverse pedagogies and research methods. Despite challenges such as financial, institutional, and cultural barriers, mobility strengthens professional growth, curriculum innovation, and global partnerships. It

DOI: 10.4018/979-8-3373-5931-1.ch004

enhances clinical competence, research collaboration, and global health outcomes. With supportive policies, funding, and technology-enabled exchanges, mobility can develop a culturally competent, innovative, and globally engaged nursing workforce.

INTRODUCTION

International collaborations, facilitated pedagogical conversations, and diversification of research agendas through incorporation of different perspectives are some of the ways through which professional development in nursing education is promoted (Garner et al., 2008; Kunaviktikul & Turale, 2020). These exchanges are critical to the construction of robust curricula informed by the global contexts and the growth of the nursing scholarship beyond the national boundaries (Kunaviktikul & Turale, 2020). The growth of the global interaction of the faculty also helps to perfect the teaching strategies and share the best practices in clinical teaching and research (Cavalcante et al., 2018). Regardless of the difficulties of different national legislations and qualification standards, faculty mobility can result in the standardisation of nursing training as well as improve the quality of nurse training on a larger scale, as well as promote the transfer of evidence-based knowledge into clinical practice (Kraaij et al., 2022). The internationalisation of nursing education has received serious momentum since the late twentieth century, as it was the case in Canadian universities which have experienced a strong growth in such operations during the past decades (Ogilvie et al., 2007). These programmes often manage to incorporate organized programmes like the Fulbright Scholarship where faculty members are allowed to teach and conduct research in foreign countries, thereby promoting professional growth and cross-cultural educational collaborations (Salman, 2018). International collaborations in nursing are essential to the development of cultural competence and are vital in normalising the international education programmes of nurses, yet contextual factors and cultural awareness moderate their success (Morley & Cunningham, 2021). An exploration into cultural diversity and taking into consideration scoping time is thus necessary in the formation of effective global alliances (Morley & Cunningham, 2021). Through this, such collaborations will eventually provide an equalized and globalized quality of nursing education, the gaps in nursing education among nations can be closed, and adaptably respond to the changing healthcare needs (Kraaij et al., 2022; Morley & Cunningham, 2021). Academic institutions are becoming more aware of the benefits of international partnerships in the faculty and the student, and study-abroad programs have begun to be incorporated into nursing programs to facilitate global awareness and clinical flexibility (Pedersen et al., 2023). Such active integration helps eliminate educational gaps between countries and preconditions the development of a globally competent nurse staff, increasing their sensitivity to various healthcare demands (Muraraneza et al., 2023). International collaboration between academic institutions and international development agencies in the development of international nursing curricula is another critical move towards establishing global collegiality among the nursing faculty and professionals (Sochan, 2008). Such partnerships are going beyond curriculum formulation to include common research projects and experience in clinical practice thus enhancing an appreciation of the global health issues and possible solutions to these problems. These initiatives are especially essential in those parts of the world where the nursing and midwifery education is shifting towards competency-based curriculum where well-skilled faculty is required to adopt new teaching methods and can utilize emerging technologies (Muraraneza et al., 2023). These types of partnerships do not only enable collaboration of the scholarly experiences but also create a space that supports the co-creation of the knowledge, which would result in the curricula that are globally applicable but also locally flexible (Morley & Cunningham, 2021). Faculty mobility combined with student mobility is a holistic model that can equip a nursing workforce that is capable of traversing the intricacies of the international healthcare environments (Morley & Cunningham, 2021). These efforts, therefore, play a major role in the evolution of a strong and culturally sensitive nursing profession, which is able to face various health challenges across the world. The holistic approach is not only transforming the quality of nursing education but also has direct results in the patient care through the creation of an internationally conscious and highly competent nursing staff. Curriculum internationalisation in nursing is thus essential in dealing with the health disparities in the world and equipping nurses to work in various cultures and clinical settings. Additionally, these international initiatives emphasize the role of training students to be more responsible in the attainment of fair care and universal health cover and often incorporate global clinical experiences into their curricula (Dohrn et al., 2018). These experiences are essential in shaping global health competencies, which are being considered critical in the modern nursing practice and in dealing with complex health matters (Wilson et al., 2012). In particular, a global learning community that investigates the issue of patient safety has shown favorable student results that boost competencies due to the online sessions and real-life experience of nursing students across the nations (Sanford et al., 2021).

OPPORTUNITIES IN FACULTY AND STUDENT MOBILITY

Those opportunities include the academic, professional, cultural, and personal aspects, which can make the nursing workforce more comprehensive and globally conscious (Guedes et al., 2018). The academic possibilities involve exposure to various pedagogical practices, curriculum models and research paradigms that disrupt the traditional methods and instill critical thinking abilities (Rukholm et al., 2009). A more profound insight into the global health problems can also be gained through this exposure at the time when they are usually disregarded in more localized educational settings (Morley & Cunningham, 2021). International nursing education experiences of this nature are also critical towards the development of adaptability and cultural sensitivity (which are fundamental qualities in nurses who work in a growing multicultural healthcare setting) (Myhre, 2011) (Geale et al., 2015). Moreover, global cooperation, including the one observed in Collaborative Online International Learning courses, enhances the learning experience of students by allowing virtual interactions and opening up new vistas of international health (Jenssen et al., 2023). The same collaborative online environments also offer the students an opportunity to interact with peer students in other cultures, intercultural communication and problem-solving skills, without necessarily having to travel physically (Appel et al., 2023). Besides, global health competencies, such as cultural, cross-cultural skills development is also a significant outcome of the students involved in the global experiences, equipping them with the skills necessary to meet the health needs of the world (Ventura et al., 2014). Professional networking opens opportunities of working with international colleagues, which can result in future research, clinical practice, and policy formulation. It may lead to improved professional opportunities, specialization, and management positions in global healthcare institutions, resolving acute problems with the shortage of the workforce (Ho et al., 2023) (Im and Broome, 2018). Besides, through these networks, innovative practices and technological developments can be shared, which further elevates the quality of nursing care to a higher level all over the world. In addition to professional benefits, cultural experiences enable the students and faculty to experience new cultural backgrounds, thus become culturally competent and mindful of other cultures to deliver patient-centred care in various environments (Leung et al., 2020). The experiences will make a person appreciate more the cultural nuance of health beliefs and practices, and this aspect is critical to cross-cultural communication and comprehensive patient care. The exposure also creates self awareness, empathy and cultural humility which are part of delivering compassionate and individualised care (Appel et al., 2023). The mentioned experiences, particularly those abroad, have been reported to speed up personal development, testing the resiliency and flexibility of students in high-stakes learning contexts (Morley & Cunningham, 2021). As an example, Collaborative Online International Learning has been demonstrated to be an effective tool to promote global competence across the international borders through virtual cultural interaction and foster cross-cultural awareness among nursing students (Jenssen et al., 2023) (Appel et al., 2023). Even without actual travel, these virtual international experiences can become very effective in developing cultural competency and awareness (Wu et al., 2021) (Jenssen et al., 2023). This strategy has been successful in assisting students in improving their professional practice and management of patients, which means that there is a high commitment and perceived benefit of such activities (Appel et al., 2023). These overseas clinical placements also enable undergraduate nursing students to be exposed to diverse healthcare practices, and culture and hence, compound their knowledge on global health (Browne et al., 2015). Such immersion leads to the formation of intercultural sensitivity, which is a very necessary quality in nurses who will inevitably have to deal with diverse populations of patients and foreign coworkers to work in an increasingly interconnected world (Appel et al., 2023) (Leathers et al., 2018). This can go further than clinical competence, developing a better self-awareness and knowledge of cultural identity, one has not been aware of before (Morley & Cunningham, 2021). This self-reflection and reflective thinking are essential in establishing transcultural nursing learning experiences which are not spontaneous, but instead nurtured by a committed pedagogical practice (Leyva-Moral et al., 2023). Thus, the employment of the modern methods of learning, including online classes, simulations, and role-plays, can contribute to developing culturally competent care and the traits that directly correlate with transcultural nursing, including such a notion as cultural humility (Leyva-Moral et al., 2023). Coupled with immersive global experiences and reflection, this cultural humility empowers nurses with a more profound insight into the needs and viewpoints of varied patients since it is no longer a matter of cultural competence (Fernandez, 2020). Faculty mobility, specifically, enables teachers to incorporate the various teaching techniques and programs into their institutions of origin and, therefore, enhance the learning experiences of every student and bring educational programs in line with international standards (Morley & Cunningham, 2021). The integration is essential in dealing with the absence of a systematic integration of cultural competence in nursing education in several parts (Leyva-Moral et al., 2023). Moreover, faculty exchange may result in the creation of new research projects, which would allow developing a global approach to researching healthcare challenges and making a contribution to the evidence-based practice on a global scale.

BARRIERS TO FACULTY AND STUDENT MOBILITY

Although the advantages are clear, mobility in nursing between the faculty and students is facing considerable obstacles that hinder its application and success. These barriers include financial and administrative issues to professional licensure and accreditation concerns in different jurisdictions (Kraaij et al., 2022). Cultural differences and language barriers also pose a problem to the integration and effectiveness of mobile faculty and students in new environments (Kraaij et al., 2022). Additionally, the lack of international standards of nursing education and regulatory frameworks complicates the process of qualification and clinical competency recognition, hence compromising smooth mobility (Kraaij et al., 2022). As an example, despite the fact that international student placements began to be taken seriously in the 1990s, a comprehensive implementation in all nursing schools and countries is yet to be achieved, and some countries, like the United Kingdom, on the one hand, show significantly low mobility rates among nursing students compared to other fields (Turale et al., 2020; Morley & Cunningham, 2021). Financial strains, such as tuition fees, travelling expenses, living costs, etc., are often used as the great deterrent to students and staff who want to experience international experiences, since funding opportunities and scholarship programmes to support nursing mobility are rather scarce (Ramos-Ramos et al., 2024). That is especially the case with the students who belong to low- and middle-income countries since the economic consequences of international education may be an obstacle, worsening rather than mitigating global health inequities (Ho et al., 2023). The bureaucratic hurdles, including visa requests, institutional approvals, credit movement, etc., only contribute to the hardships, often causing widespread delays and administrative overheads on both sides of the divide (Borrelli et al., 2021). Also, the regulatory barriers associated with professional licensure and acknowledgment of scholarly credentials across international boundaries are significant challenges that require harmonisation of standards to support easier transfer of nursing professionals (Morley & Cunningham, 2021). Such systemic factors are further complicated by pragmatically oriented factors like finding a proper home and experiencing the unknown healthcare systems that can further discourage potential participants (Borrelli et al., 2021). The issue of culture also takes a timely dimension because students who are foreign-born frequently face the challenges of teaching practices that differ radically in their countries of origin, as didactic teaching methods and rote learning may be at the forefront (Merry et al., 2021). This mismatch may trigger both academic and social problems often worsened by a sense of loneliness, social isolation, and discrimination (Merry et al., 2021). The issue of ensuring a uniform quality in foreign placements is further magnified by the difference in the nursing roles and scope of practice in various countries and creates confusion among the students (Morley & Cunningham, 2021). It is essential to build effective relations between home and host institutions, therefore, to reduce these obstacles and make sure that quality assurance measures, the correspondence of curricula and support systems are put in place to make the transcultural learning experience truly enriching (Morley & Cunningham, 2021).

IMPACTS OF FACULTY AND STUDENT MOBILITY

Faculty and student mobility have far-reaching effects that touch on not only personal growth but also affect the entire healthcare structure in the world and the nursing community at large. It will involve improving the ability of the healthcare workforce, encouraging linguistic and cultural diversity within nursing professionals, and encouraging the sharing of new ideas that enhance nursing practice (Merry et al., 2021). Through such interactions, a global understanding of the issue of healthcare and solutions is achieved and thus nurses are able to deal with complex health disparities as well as implement evidence based interventions that are responsive to different populations. In addition, virtual international collaborative learning programs have been demonstrated to significantly improve international and global competencies of nursing students and thus equip them with a globally networked healthcare environment (Jung et al., 2021). These programs help form the global outlook in academic and practice learning and understand that successful transcultural teaching depends on the effectiveness of partnerships (Morley & Cunningham, 2021). Nevertheless, to accomplish this goal, sufficient support systems and guidelines regarding the distribution of academic credit and assessment processes are required, so that the various learning experiences one faces when becoming mobile apply to the identified competencies (Morley & Cunningham, 2021).

Moreover, the effective mobility programmes require effective regulatory, administrative, and quality assurance systems that are locally and internationally applicable (Morley & Cunningham, 2021). Another significant hindrance to the provision of staff in the healthcare sector is the brain drain phenomenon, i.e., the migration of high-skilled professionals in their home countries, which is especially concerning with respect to the developing countries (Valdez et al., 2024). This highlights the need to have balanced policies that do not harm the current workforce shortages in the vulnerable areas. The only solution to these complexities is to take a multipronged approach that incorporates harmonised regulatory frameworks and mutual recognition agreements aimed at ensuring the smooth integration of mobile nurses into the various healthcare systems (Kraaij et al., 2022). In addition to regulatory efforts, the implication to individual learners is enormous, with international experiences fostering the development of cultural competence and a more in-depth comprehension of health disparities that are vital in practice in a more diverse patient base (Morley & Cunningham, 2021). These experiences also spur critical thinking about challenging health topics in resource-constrained environments, which eventually builds partnerships between sending and receiving institutions (Morley & Cunningham, 2021). This will increase the cultural competence awareness among nurses, who will be ready to work with an increasingly diverse patient base and help make healthcare more inclusive (Morley & Cunningham, 2021; Leyva-Moral et al.,

2023). This international contact also becomes a driving force towards attracting potential students, and it expands the international reach of nursing education further (Pedersen et al., 2023). Moreover, the programmes will help the participants see and apply diverse methods of healthcare delivery, hence, facilitating the process of global nursing practices and policies refinement.

Individual Level Impacts

However, these collaborations demand a careful maneuvering of regulatory, administrative, and quality-assurance processes that may be implemented on the local and international levels (Morley & Cunningham, 2021). There are further difficulties with standardisation of the curricular content, control processes, and assessment schemes, which are complicated by the differences in the competence of the staff in different institutions (Morley & Cunningham, 2021). Although the introduction of cultural diversity into nursing programmes can be recognized as a valuable resource, as the enhancement of learning opportunities, the practical use of internationalisation policies is often faced with challenges based on the incompatibility of professional standards and the lack of pedagogical competence among junior faculty members (Laugaland et al., 2021). Additionally, the increased enrolment of international nursing students globally accelerates the necessity to have strong support systems that can help students face the unique problems, including challenges of gender identity, sexual orientation, and being a foreign-born scholar (Merry et al., 2021). These issues highlight why there should be holistic support systems that integrate academic, psychological, and social resources to enable these heterogeneous groups of students achieve successful adaptation and retention (Morley & Cunningham, 2021; Keogh & Russel -Roberts, 2008).

Institutions are increasingly integrating the principles of equity, diversity, and inclusion into their compulsory requirements, forcing them to consider how they can properly equip foreign-born students with their skills and expertise to take the first job after their graduation, be that in the host country or their home country (Merry et al., 2021). This entails intellectual-property issues and fair-contract-based structures of faculty who are engaged in international terms, hence, enlightening institutional policy and academic freedom (Introduction, n.d.). Nevertheless, this kind of integration is often incompatible with system-wide barriers and implicit biases, which have been embedded in recruitment and retention procedures and may continue to promote inequities despite the targeted institutional priorities (Introduction, n.d.). To resolve these systemic problems, it is necessary to provide a collective response to eliminate past biases, redesign old policies and build an inclusive academic environment where faculty and students regardless of their backgrounds will thrive and make significant contributions to the nursing field (Introduction, n.d.). These attempts involve designing gender-sensitive interventions at both structural and curricular levels to draw and maintain a diverse student population and take into account the distinct set of issues that international and migrant students can face, and which may be gendered (Merry et al., 2021). Such interventions should take into consideration the complex interaction of gender roles, cultural norms, and perceived discrimination that often affects international and migrant nursing students in particular, in the context of an occupation traditionally defined as feminine and low-status (Merry et al., 2021). These efforts must also incorporate particular issues affecting foreign-born male nurses and those who may be discriminated against due to religious clothing, including the hijab, to create an authentic inclusive learning and professional experience (Merry et al., 2021). In order to explore these subtle gender-related issues and coping strategies of various international and migrant nursing students, further empirical research is necessary (Merry et al., 2021). The development of inclusive and supportive learning experiences that recognize and respond to these gendered experiences and adjust resources and support systems to meet the needs of foreign-born students in diverse ways should be prioritized by academic institutions (Merry et al., 2021).

Institutional Level Impacts

On an institutional level, strong international relationships can be created through the mobility programmes, which result in the establishment of transcultural curricula and mutual research projects that advance the quality and scope of nursing education worldwide (Morley & Cunningham, 2021; Pedersen et al., 2023). Such partnerships also have the potential to encourage exchange of best practices in pedagogy and clinical training that eventually has benefit to the participating institutions and the respective student bodies (Morley & Cunningham, 2021). Moreover, these exchanges enable universities to create innovative regulatory, administrative, and quality assurance frameworks that are locally and internationally both appropriate (Morley & Cunningham, 2021). The alignment of the strategy guarantees that the educational content, monitoring and evaluation plans are aligned with international standards, but they are relevant to local healthcare demands (Morley & Cunningham, 2021). In addition, these international interactions improve the status and reputation of universities with the indication of the willingness to internationalise and become academically high, thus drawing a more varied and talented group of students and staff (Abdul-Rahaman et al., 2022). Also, an active institutional motivation, expressed through mission statements, action plans, and sources of commitment, is essential to develop an inclusive and equitable educational setting that fosters diversity and a feeling of belongingness in international and migrant students (Merry et al., 2021). The latter may necessitate structural change of the support services to include not only academic and psychological counselling but also the socio-cultural and economic peculiarities of this demographic (Merry et al., 2021). These support systems will play a central role in reducing the effects of cultural shock, language barriers, and financial stressors, which are quoted as major barriers to academic achievement and personal well-being among the international student populations (Merry et al., 2021). It is important to note that foreign-born nursing students are highly stressed because of their foreign nationality, which is why it is necessary to develop all-encompassing interventions such as mentorship programmes and community-building forums that promote resilience and persistence in their academic activities (Merry et al., 2021; Ischer et al., 2013). Such proactive institutional strategy does not only enhance student performance but also makes the institution a pioneer in international health education, thus appealing to wider range of international talents (Merry et al., 2021). Such a wider range of talents will diversify the learning environment and foster intercultural awareness as well as equip every student to thrive in a more globalised world (Brito et al., 2025).

Societal Level Impacts

The effects are experienced at a societal level, whereby these partnerships would provide a globally competent nursing workforce that is better placed to handle universal health problems such as pandemics, climate change, and care delivery disparities (Ho et al., 2023). Mobility initiatives eventually can lead to better patient outcomes and health equity in the global healthcare setting by developing a workforce that is more culturally sensitive and aware of various healthcare systems. These efforts also enhance international collaboration in health by making people have a common comprehension of health issues and have an international collaboration to work on them. Additionally, incorporating the concepts of diversity, equity, and inclusion in these programs is a key to developing actually a representative and responsive nurse workforce capable of supporting an ever-more diverse patient demographic (Merry et al., 2021). Such an increase in cultural competence, which is achieved due to the exposure to diverse healthcare settings, is directly reflected in a positive change in patient care, especially among marginalized and underrepresented groups (Morley & Cunningham, 2021). This is especially relevant because the problems of international and migrant students are being identified as challenging to solve, as their life experiences include a complicated combination of gender, cultural background, and academic adaptation (Merry et al., 2021). Thus, effective programs should include support systems that would support these complex issues, such as customized academic materials and culturally competent mental health services (Merry et al., 2021). These holistic practices are essential towards enabling mutual cultural awareness and appreciation of diversity amongst all the players, and the foundation of more robust international health collaboration (Morley & Cunningham, 2021). These international partnerships should be sustained with the help of strategic funding and properly designed projects to grow the global nursing education foundation and have a visible contribution to global health and educational challenges (Morley & Cunningham, 2021). One of the most critical points of these collaborative efforts is relating students to the world and diversifying their insights regarding best practices and contributing to enhancing patient outcomes together (Jenssen et al., 2023). This nursing school globalization is essential to help future nurses meet the cultural competency and worldview required to help handle complex health issues efficiently (Kunaviktikul and Turale, 2020). It also makes sure that the nursing research and practice are kept informed by multicultural experiences and results in more inclusive and effective solutions to healthcare worldwide (Kulicki, 2006; Morley and Cunningham, 2021). The possible ways of such internationalization are multiple innovative solutions, such as the collaborative online international learning programs, that provide convenient channels of intercultural interchange and the formation of globalized visions in nursing education (Appel et al., 2023). Moreover, such a commitment to internationalization promotes capacity building in the global health through the acquisition of skills and knowledge by nurses, particularly low-income countries, and partnerships that are vital in the realization of global health goals (Kunaviktikul & Turale, 2020).

STRATEGIES TO OPTIMIZE MOBILITY BENEFITS

In order to make the most of faculty and student mobility, strategic interventions are needed to deal with the challenges inherent in the process and take advantage of the opportunities that internationalization presents (Morley & Cunningham, 2021; Brito et al., 2025). These involve coming up with globalized curricula, the identification of qualifications between borders and ensuring strong support networks to international faculty and students hence increasing the internationalization activities of the institutions of higher learning (Dias et al., 2020). Also, it is essential to promote inter-institutional agreements and build transparent credentialing procedures to ease the process of academic and professional recognition, thus leading to the easier transition of individuals affected by cross-border educational and clinical experiences (Morley & Cunningham, 2021). Moreover, the adoption of digital pedagogy, including the use of e -learning devices and blended learning are protective and adaptable substitutes of conventional mobility, especially to individuals who do not have an opportunity to move abroad (Urstad et al., 2021). These new strategies are able to expand the scope of involvement in international education, enabling more nursing student and staff to attain exposure to international health views without the logistical and monetary strains of the physical move (Msomphora, 2024). These online platforms have the potential to deliver experience of virtual exchange where the students can work on international projects and interact with various healthcare case studies and thus, widen their international health competencies without the need to move physically. As an example, the Collaborative International Online Learning programs can offer students of nursing significant interaction with international learners and support self-awareness, empathetic, and cultural humility (Appel et al., 2023).

Besides, university members may use such online resources to participate in collaborative academic and research projects with colleagues abroad and, as such, foster the exchange of knowledge and create a global community of practice (Montegrico et al., 2022; Ilieva and Ilieva, 2024). The virtual modalities have a particular role in overcoming the digital divide, as they enable institutions in resource-poor environments to gain access to the expertise and educational opportunities worldwide, which will further advance in creating a more equalized internationalization (Ilieva and Tsiligiris, 2024). These strategies reiterate that it is important to tap into the power of technology to increase access to the global nursing education to create a more inclusive and connected learning experience (Dovrat, 2023). In such a way, the process of internationalization of nursing curricula becomes more achievable, and a greater number of students and faculty are able to interact with different pedagogical solutions and clinical practices (Ho et al., 2023; Morley & Cunningham, 2021). The strategic use of these digital tools also facilitates the acquisition of critical aspects of digital literacy in nursing professionals, a skill that is considered vital in addressing the changing world in healthcare provision (Ho et al., 2023).

FUTURE DIRECTIONS AND POLICY IMPLICATIONS

The future policy frameworks should focus on the mechanisms to finance, harmonise regulatory frameworks, and support structures that are sensitive to culture so that the maximum potential of international nursing mobility can be realised. This would involve the resolution of gaps in the labour laws and accreditation frameworks that currently form major hurdles to the smooth academic and career transfer to mobile nurses (Introduction, n.d.). Moreover, policymaking should aim to foster the formation of international relationships that anticipate cultural empathy and reciprocity, and get beyond one-sided knowledge dissemination to actually collaborative learning processes (Morley & Cunningham, 2021). Moreover, the facilitation of the intentional growth and sustainability of the targeted initiatives through the systematic organization of projects in the form of international champions in nursing is compulsory to achieve a noticeable effect on the global health and educational priorities (Morley & Cunningham, 2021).

It is also necessary to introduce planetary health and digital literacy into nursing programs which will prepare nurses to operate in an environment that is rapidly changing and provide them with the required skills to promote health and prevent diseases in the twenty-first century because it makes them competent in both aspects (Ho et al., 2023). Besides, the curricula must go beyond the country-specific demands to embrace a more holistic global education programme to ensure that nurses are equipped to practise effectively in the country and across the borders (Ho et al., 2023). Virtual exchange programmes, like Collaborative Online International learning, can effectively help achieve the purchase of global health perspectives and intercultural competence without necessarily traveling physically, thereby alleviating the effects of accessibility and cost barriers (Jenssen et al., 2023; Appel et al., 2023). These virtual programmes can be easily used to incorporate a macro-level approach in the curriculum, which should be used to supplement the micro-level international placements in the case that the latter is feasible (Morley & Cunningham, 2021). Combined with a desire to decolonise the curriculum, as well as to encourage moral deliberations in international placements, these efforts offer a rare chance to correct historical power imbalances and to develop, indeed, equitable global health relationships (Beck, 2023; Morley & Cunningham, 2021).

This holistic solution will ensure that nursing education is responsive to the global health issues and that the workforce that is produced is able to work around varied healthcare environments and also provide sustainable health outcomes around the world. A flexible governance by all parties is the key to an agile and adaptive nursing curriculum that enhances nurse competency and congruity between educational goals and the needs of nursing on the global scale (Efendi et al., 2021). Moreover, these programmes can be extended and maintained on a larger scale through the cultivation of international champions in nursing through carefully planned, funded projects and have significant impact on the global demands of health and education (Morley & Cunningham, 2021). Lastly, a holistic global outlook that introduces transcultural concepts into the curriculum and hands-on experiences is still a fundamental requirement that can equip nursing students with the complexity of global healthcare better (Morley & Cunningham, 2021; Ho et al., 2023).

CONCLUSION

Finally, globalization of healthcare is offering opportunities and challenges to nursing education; strategic plans such as faculty and student mobility are the most important to prepare a globally competent and culturally sensitive nursing workforce (Morley & Cunningham, 2021). This mobility contributes to the educational results and career advancement, as well as making a great contribution to healthcare service provision and equity in health among the population of various categories (Mohammadi et al., 2020). It will be necessary to continue to focus on these initiatives in order to prepare future generations of nurses with the skills and insights needed to operate in an increasingly global health environment, which is becoming an increasingly interconnected and complex environment. An integrated strategy will make nursing education responsive to the changing health requirements in the world, especially in areas like digital literacy, and planetary health (Ho et al., 2023). Furthermore, the competencies that need to be tackled, particularly following such events as the COVID-19 pandemic, will be crucial to equip a responsive nursing workforce that can react to global health crises in the future and workforce mobilization (Ho et al., 2023).

Nevertheless, certain issues are persistent, such as insufficient time of face-to-face communication during the pandemic and that nurses in other countries need to be supported by the government over an extended period (Efendi et al., 2021). All these international connections would be necessary to lead learning efforts and speed up the process of a deeper understanding of cultural sensitivity and cultural diversity, and strengthen the macro-level approach to health delivery (Morley & Cunningham, 2021). Thus, in the future, studies ought to examine the long-term effects of virtual mobility on acquiring skills and developing a professional career and explore novel ways to achieve sustainable international clinical placements that would take into account the views of local stakeholders and foster reciprocal learning (Beck, 2023). Moreover, it is essential to assess the long-term effectiveness of practice audit tools designed in the global partnerships to secure the long-term quality of student nurse placements, despite the impact of such phenomena as a pandemic that requires adaptation methods (Morley & Cunningham, 2021).

Also, a primary literature review showed that there was a severe absence of transcultural concepts that govern international placement exchanges, indicating a gap that needs to be filled to increase effectiveness of global nursing education (Morley & Cunningham, 2021). This gap highlights the need to come up with sound, internationally sensitive regulatory and quality-assurance systems that cut across many dimensions, including curriculum design to faculty proficiency, and thus guarantee the uniformity of global placements (Morley & Cunningham, 2021). These mechanisms play an important role in standardization of course materials, tracking student progress, and assessing results in a variety of international partnerships (Morley & Cunningham, 2021). Extensive models of this nature play a crucial role in enhancing cultural sensitivity and diversity respect amongst the students, and eventually training them to respond to health disparities in resource-deficient environments (Morley & Cunningham, 2021). Good collaborations between learning institutions and the host organizations are the basis of enhancing transcultural learning and offering quality consistency in global learning programmes in nursing (Morley & Cunningham, 2021). In fact, such collaborations are also important in encouraging sustainable health-system change, especially in resource-constrained areas, through improved training and service delivery (Edwards et al., 2021). Grants, including those offered by programs like Erasmus+ and Turing scheme, are essential in helping to maintain these international networks and alleviate the resource disparity between the collaborating organizations (Morley & Cunningham, 2021). These financing systems represent an ongoing pattern of student outward mobility, which helps to create a community of practice that is not limited to institutions or countries (Morley & Cunningham, 2021). Effective management hierarchies in such partnerships, with distinct workstreams are also key in enhancing partner ownership, autonomy, and voice, and they empower the collaborative setting (Morley & Cunningham, 2021). These frameworks with drawing on prior international experience improvements assist performance and cultural sensitivity besides facilitating international capabilities and managing inequalities (Morley & Cunningham, 2021). As an example, regulatory organizations, like the UK Nursing and Midwifery Council, require strict education audit and oversight of international placements, required to comply with the quality standards and achieve better outcomes in students (Beck, 2023; Morley & Cunningham, 2021).

REFERENCES

Abdul-Rahaman, N., Arkorful, V. E., & Okereke, T. (2022). Academic integration in higher education: A review of effective institutional strategies and personal factors [Review of *Academic integration in higher education: A review of effective institutional strategies and personal factors*]. *Frontiers in Education, 7*. Frontiers Media. DOI: 10.3389/feduc.2022.856967

Appel, H. B., Martínez-Fernández, M. C., & Fernández-Martínez, E. (2023). Implementation of COIL in mental health education: Outcomes of a collaboration between Spain and the United States nursing students. *Journal of Virtual Exchange, 65*, 65–82. Advance online publication. DOI: 10.21827/jve.6.39836

Beck, K. (2023). Local people's perceptions of international clinical placements in low- and middle-income countries: A literature review [Review of *Local people's perceptions of international clinical placements in low- and middle-income countries: A literature review*]. *International Journal of Nursing Studies Advances, 5*, 100165. Elsevier BV. DOI: 10.1016/j.ijnsa.2023.100165

Borrelli, S., Walker, L., Coolin, K., Fumagalli, S., Kärema, A., Konstantinidis, S., Mets-Oja, S., Nespoli, A., Smit, A.-M., van Oost, M., & Spiby, H. (2021). Midwifery students' perspectives of physical and virtual mobility activities including preferences for e-learning: A cross-sectional survey. *Nurse Education Today, 109*, 105214. DOI: 10.1016/j.nedt.2021.105214 PMID: 34799193

Brito, E., Neves, M. P. C. C. D., Gomes, N., & Lopes, N. (2025). Inclusion and Internationalization: Perception of Higher Education Students. *Interchange, 56*(3-4), 259–283. Advance online publication. DOI: 10.1007/s10780-025-09544-3

Browne, C., Fetherston, C., & Medigovich, K. (2015). International clinical placements for Australian undergraduate nursing students: A systematic thematic synthesis of the literature [Review of *International clinical placements for Australian undergraduate nursing students: A systematic thematic synthesis of the literature*]. *Nurse Education Today, 35*(10), 1028. Elsevier BV. DOI: 10.1016/j.nedt.2015.05.012

Cavalcante, I. M. da S., Guedes, G. F., & Püschel, V. A. de A. (2018). Nursing international student mobility in the University of São Paulo. *Revista Brasileira de Enfermagem, 71*(suppl 4), 1619–1625. DOI: 10.1590/0034-7167-2017-0754 PMID: 30088632

Dias, G. P., Barbosa, B., Santos, C. A., Pinheiro, M. M., Simões, D., & Filipe, S. (2020). Between promises and pitfalls: The impact of mobility on the internationalization of higher education. *Journal of Further and Higher Education, 45*(1), 79–94. DOI: 10.1080/0309877X.2020.1735321

Dohrn, J., Desjardins, K., Honig, J., Hahn-Schroeder, H., Ferng, Y., & Larson, E. (2018). Transforming nursing curricula for a global community. *Journal of Professional Nursing, 34*(6), 449–453. DOI: 10.1016/j.profnurs.2018.02.001 PMID: 30527692

Dovrat, L. (2023). *Virtual exchanges in Israel: Faculty experiences of implementing a transformative pedagogy. 3*(2). DOI: 10.21428/8c225f6e.4530bc4d

Edwards, R., Patrician, P. A., Bakitas, M., & Markaki, A. (2021). Palliative care integration: a critical review of nurse migration effect in Jamaica [Review of *Palliative care integration: a critical review of nurse migration effect in Jamaica*]. *BMC Palliative Care, 20*(1). BioMed Central. DOI: 10.1186/s12904-021-00863-7

Efendi, F., Haryanto, J., Indarwati, R., Kuswanto, H., Ulfiana, E., Has, E. M. M., & Chong, M. C. (2021). Going Global: Insights of Indonesian Policymakers on International Migration of Nurses. *Journal of Multidisciplinary Healthcare, 3285*, 3285–3293. Advance online publication. DOI: 10.2147/JMDH.S327962 PMID: 34858031

Fernandez, K. R. (2020). Developing Cultural Humility During Short-Term Study Abroad Immersion. *International Journal of Studies in Nursing, 5*(3), 48. DOI: 10.20849/ijsn.v5i3.764

Garner, B., Metcalfe, S. E., & Hallyburton, A. (2008). International collaboration: A concept model to engage nursing leaders and promote global nursing education partnerships. *Nurse Education in Practice, 9*(2), 102–108. DOI: 10.1016/j.nepr.2008.10.011 PMID: 19059008

Geale, S., Beament, T., Gibson, N., Fowler, A., Baker, M., & Smith, G. (2015). International Practicum: Not just another overseas jaunt—Supporting learning objectives and the development of graduate attributes. *Journal of Nursing Education and Practice, 5*(11). Advance online publication. DOI: 10.5430/jnep.v5n11p96

Guedes, G. F., Cavalcante, I. M. da S., & Püschel, V. A. de A. (2018). *International academic mobility: the experience of undergraduate nursing students. 52*. https://doi.org/DOI: 10.1590/s1980-220x2017039403358

Ho, K. H. M., Cheng, H. Y., McKenna, L., & Cheung, D. S. K. (2023). Nursing and midwifery in a changing world: Addressing planetary health and digital literacy through a global curriculum. *Nursing Open, 11*(1), e2075. Advance online publication. DOI: 10.1002/nop2.2075 PMID: 38268246

Ilieva, J., & Tsiligiris, V. (2024). Globally Engaged and Locally Relevant—Revisiting Higher Education. In *BRILL eBooks* (p. 379). Brill., DOI: 10.1163/9789004713901_101

Im, E., & Broome, M. E. (2018). Introduction: Women's Leadership in Asian Culture. *Asian/Pacific Island Nursing Journal, 3*(2), 39–41. DOI: 10.31372/20180302.1093 PMID: 31037252

Jenssen, U., Bochenek, J., King, T. S., Steindal, S. A., Hestvold, I. V., & Morrison-Beedy, D. (2023). Impact of COIL: Learning From Student Nurses in Norway Who Collaborated With U.S. Students. *Journal of Transcultural Nursing, 35*(1), 74–82. DOI: 10.1177/10436596231209043 PMID: 37933746

Jung, D., Gagné, J. C. D., Choi, E., & Lee, K. (2021). An Online International Collaborative Learning Program During the COVID-19 Pandemic for Nursing Students: Mixed Methods Study. *JMIR Medical Education, 8*(1), e34171. Advance online publication. DOI: 10.2196/34171 PMID: 34982035

Keogh, J. J., & Russel-Roberts, E. (2008). Exchange programmes and student mobility: Meeting student's expectations or an expensive holiday? *Nurse Education Today, 29*(1), 108–116. DOI: 10.1016/j.nedt.2008.07.006 PMID: 18782646

Kraaij, J. van, Veenstra, M., Stalpers, D., Schoonhoven, L., Vermeulen, H., & Oostveen, C. van. (2022). Uniformity along the way: A scoping review on characteristics of nurse education programs worldwide [Review of *Uniformity along the way: A scoping review on characteristics of nurse education programs worldwide*]. *Nurse Education Today, 120*, 105646. Elsevier BV. DOI: 10.1016/j.nedt.2022.105646

Kunaviktikul, W., & Turale, S. (2020). Internationalizing nursing curricula in a rapidly globalizing world. *Nurse Education in Practice, 43*, 102704. DOI: 10.1016/j.nepr.2020.102704 PMID: 31991380

Laugaland, K. A., Billett, S., Akerjordet, K., Frøiland, C. T., Grealish, L., & Aase, I. (2021). Enhancing student nurses' clinical education in aged care homes: A qualitative study of challenges perceived by faculty staff. *BMC Nursing, 20*(1), 111. Advance online publication. DOI: 10.1186/s12912-021-00632-0 PMID: 34174881

Leathers, J., Davidson, H., & Desai, N. (2018). Interprofessional education between medical students and nurse practitioner students in a Global Health course. *BMC Medical Education, 18*(1), 200. Advance online publication. DOI: 10.1186/s12909-018-1307-y PMID: 30119625

Leung, D., Chan, E. A., Wong, A. K. C., Reisenhofer, S., Stenberg, M., Sze, C. P., Lai, K., Cruz, E., & Carlson, E. (2020). Advancing pedagogy of undergraduate nursing students' cultural awareness through internationalization webinars: A qualitative study. *Nurse Education Today, 93*, 104514. DOI: 10.1016/j.nedt.2020.104514 PMID: 32659533

Leyva-Moral, J. M., Tosun, B., Gómez-Ibáñez, R., Navarrete, L., Yava, A., Aguayo-González, M., Dirgar, E., Checa-Jiménez, C., & Bernabeu-Tamayo, M. D. (2023). From a learning opportunity to a conscious multidimensional change: A metasynthesis of transcultural learning experiences among nursing students. *BMC Nursing, 22*(1), 356. Advance online publication. DOI: 10.1186/s12912-023-01521-4 PMID: 37798717

Merry, L., Vissandjée, B., & Verville-Provencher, K. (2021). Challenges, coping responses and supportive interventions for international and migrant students in academic nursing programs in major host countries: a scoping review with a gender lens [Review of *Challenges, coping responses and supportive interventions for international and migrant students in academic nursing programs in major host countries: a scoping review with a gender lens*]. *BMC Nursing, 20*(1). BioMed Central. DOI: 10.1186/s12912-021-00678-0

Mohammadi, N., Dorri, S., & Abedi, A. (2020). Nursing education in the path of globalization: Promotion or challenge? [Review of *Nursing education in the path of globalization: Promotion or challenge?*]. *Journal of Education and Health Promotion, 9*(1), 269. Medknow. DOI: 10.4103/jehp.jehp_775_19

Montegrico, J., Cornelius, J. B., Downing, C., Fradelos, E. C., Machuca-Contreras, F., Oducado, R. M., & Resna, R. W. (2022). International nurse education research collaboration during the COVID-19 pandemic: Researchers' perspectives. *Nurse Education Today, 120*, 105606. DOI: 10.1016/j.nedt.2022.105606 PMID: 36343419

Morley, D. A., & Cunningham, S. (2021). Global partnerships in nursing – A qualitative study in lessons for success. *Nurse Education in Practice, 54*, 103069. DOI: 10.1016/j.nepr.2021.103069 PMID: 34058464

Msomphora, M. R. (2024). Bridging borders: Global insights and challenges in internationalising higher education using a decade-long case study. *International Journal of Educational Research Open, 8*, 100402. DOI: 10.1016/j.ijedro.2024.100402

Muraraneza, C., Mukamana, D., Katende, G., Bazirete, O., & Wolvaardt, L. (2023). Global partnerships in transformation of nursing and midwifery education in Africa: A systematic scoping review protocol. *Research Square (Research Square)*. DOI: 10.21203/rs.3.rs-3145480/v1

Myhre, K. (2011). Exchange students crossing language boundaries in clinical nursing practice. *International Nursing Review, 58*(4), 428–433. DOI: 10.1111/j.1466-7657.2011.00904.x PMID: 22092320

Ogilvie, L., Paul, P., & Burgess-Pinto, E. (2007). International Dimensions of Higher Education in Nursing in Canada: Tapping the Wisdom of the 20th Century While Embracing Possibilities for the 21st Century [Review of *International Dimensions of Higher Education in Nursing in Canada: Tapping the Wisdom of the 20th Century While Embracing Possibilities for the 21st Century*]. *International Journal of Nursing Education Scholarship, 4*(1). De Gruyter. DOI: 10.2202/1548-923X.1306

Pedersen, M. L., Gildberg, F. A., Baker, J., & Tingleff, E. B. (2023). A Review of Ethnic Disparities in Restrictive Mental Health Practices [Review of *A Review of Ethnic Disparities in Restrictive Mental Health Practices*]. *Research Portal Denmark.* Technical University of Denmark. https://local.forskningsportal.dk/local/dki-cgi/ws/cris-link?src=sdu&id=sdu-a108e4b6-bd44-4687-a043-cf0ae357167e&ti=A%20Review%20of%20Ethnic%20Disparities%20in%20Restrictive%20Mental%20Health%20Practices

Ramos-Ramos, A., Rodríguez-Suárez, C.-A., Díaz-González, C. de la M., Soriano, J. V., Berenguer-Pérez, M., & la Torre, H. G. (2024). Academic and Employment Preferences of Nursing Students at the University of Las Palmas of Gran Canaria: A Cross-Sectional Study. *Nursing Reports, 14*(4), 3328–3345. DOI: 10.3390/nursrep14040241 PMID: 39585132

Rukholm, E., Stamler, L. L., Talbot, L. R., Bednash, G., Raines, F., Potempa, K., Nugent, P., Clark, D. J. M., Bernhauser, S., & Parfitt, B. (2009). Scaling up the global nursing health workforce: Contributions of an international organization [Review of *Scaling up the global nursing health workforce: Contributions of an international organization*]. *Collegian Journal of the Royal College of Nursing Australia, 16*(1), 41. Elsevier BV. DOI: 10.1016/j.colegn.2009.01.001

Salman, K. (2018). The Fulbright Journey: Reflections on a Challenging and Rewarding Experience in Saudi Arabia by a Nursing Professor. *Journal of Professional Nursing, 35*(4), 335–340. DOI: 10.1016/j.profnurs.2018.10.004 PMID: 31345516

Sanford, J., Argenbright, C., Sherwood, G., Jordan, P., Herrera, M., Bengtsson, M., Moriyama, M., Lui, L., & McDonald, M. (2021). Student outcomes of an international learning collaborative to develop patient safety and quality competencies in nursing. *Journal of Research in Nursing : JRN, 26*(1-2), 81–94. DOI: 10.1177/1744987120970606 PMID: 35251228

Sochan, A. (2008). Relationship building through the development of international nursing curricula: a literature review [Review of *Relationship building through the development of international nursing curricula: a literature review*]. *International Nursing Review, 55*(2), 192. Wiley. DOI: 10.1111/j.1466-7657.2007.00595.x

Turale, S., Kunaviktikul, W., & Mesukko, J. (2020). Giving undergraduate nursing students international experiences: Issues and strategies. *Nursing and Health Sciences, 22*(3), 830. DOI: 10.1111/nhs.12722

Urstad, K. H., Navarro-Illana, E., Oftedal, B., Whittingham, K., Alamar, S., Windle, R., Løkken, A., Taylor, M. G., Larsen, M. H., Narayasanamy, M., Sancho-Pelluz, J., Navarro-Illana, P., & Wharrad, H. (2021). Usability and value of a digital learning resource in nursing education across European countries: A cross-sectional exploration. *BMC Nursing, 20*(1), 161. Advance online publication. DOI: 10.1186/s12912-021-00681-5 PMID: 34488724

Valdez, G. F. D., Genuino, R.-B. M. J., Babate, F. J., Bernardo, M., Biluan, F.-C. A. P., & Santos, M. (2024). A Global Survey of Filipino Nurses' Motivations, Challenges, and Aspirations. *Research Square (Research Square)*. DOI: 10.21203/rs.3.rs-5218786/v1

Ventura, C. A. A., Mendes, I. A. C., Wilson, L., de Godoy, S., Tamí-Maury, I., Zárate-Grajales, R. A., & Salas-Segura, S. (2014). Global health competencies according to nursing faculty from Brazilian higher education institutions. *Revista Latino-Americana de Enfermagem, 22*(2), 179–186. DOI: 10.1590/0104-1169.2996.2400 PMID: 26107823

Wilson, L., Harper, D. C., Tamí-Maury, I., Zarate, R., Salas, S. P. E., Farley, J. E., Warren, N., Mendes, I. A. C., & Ventura, C. A. A. (2012). Global Health Competencies for Nurses in the Americas. *Journal of Professional Nursing, 28*(4), 213–222. DOI: 10.1016/j.profnurs.2011.11.021 PMID: 22818191

Wu, A., Maddula, V., Singh, J., Sagoo, M. G., Chien, C. L., Wingate, R., Kielstein, H., Traxler, H., Brassett, C., Waschke, J., Vielmuth, F., Sakurai, T., Zeroual, M., Olsen, J., El-Batti, S., Viranta, S., Kitahara, S., Keay, K. A., Kunzel, C., & Noël, G. (2021). Alternatives to Student Outbound Mobility—Improving Students' Cultural Competency Skills Online to Improve Global Health Without Travel. *Medical Science Educator*, *31*(4), 1441–1451. DOI: 10.1007/s40670-021-01332-9 PMID: 34123512

Chapter 5
Interdisciplinary Team in Geriatric Hip Fracture Care:
A Clinical Rehabilitation Model

Anna Pantouvaki
https://orcid.org/0000-0002-6657-9049
Hellenic Mediterranean University, Greece

Michail Zografakis Sfakianakis
https://orcid.org/0000-0002-5376-9580
Hellenic Mediterranean University, Greece

ABSTRACT

Falls in people over the age of 65 is the most important factor of geriatric injuries leading to serious conditions, to increased death rates and serious socio-economic consequences. Hip fractures due to fall is an increased phenomenon, which quite regularly leads to secondary falls within six months after surgery, with all consequences that follows. Therefore, it is quite crucial to enhance the best treatment procedure for managing hip fracture after a fall, eliminating the incidence of further falls and improving the quality of patient's life. The multicomponent nature of geriatric hip fracture care demands a paradigm of a healthcare pathway from traditional single medical approaches to comprehensive multidisciplinary models. It is proved by various researchers that this phenomenon is being managed better by a multidisciplinary team, therefore it is quite crucial to design hip fracture rehabilitation plan and fall prevention strategies, based on cross border healthcare partnerships. This would ensure to implement strong and common healthcare policies in elderly care. Successful implementation strategies addressing these barriers typically include interprofessional education and team-building, communication protocols, and

DOI: 10.4018/979-8-3373-5931-1.ch005

data-driven quality improvement with transparent outcome reporting. The role of advanced practice nurses and specialized care coordinators has emerged as crucial in recent studies. These professionals play a binding role in multidisciplinary teams together, ensuring that assessment findings translate into actionable care plans, facilitating communication across specialties and care transitions, and providing continuity for patients' healthcare plan in complex healthcare systems. The evidence increasingly suggests that dedicated orthogeriatric coordinators in multidisciplinary teams are not optional enhancements but rather essential substitute for high-quality hip fracture care.

INTRODUCTION

The global demographic increase in elderly populations presents a significant challenge for healthcare systems worldwide, particularly in managing hip fractures in geriatric patients. International organizations, including the World Health Organization and various national health services, are increasingly called upon to analyze and address this phenomenon, ensuring healthy aging and contributing to improved quality of life for individuals over 65 years of age, their families, and society at large.

This chapter examines how nursing partnerships can advance evidence-based rehabilitation practices for geriatric hip fracture care through international collaboration, knowledge exchange, and multidisciplinary approaches (Lasater et al., 2016). Contemporary research and clinical evidence demonstrate how nurses can help in leading innovative care models that integrate precision healthcare principles, cultural competency, and interdisciplinary collaboration to improve functional outcomes and prevent secondary complications (Lasater et al., 2016). The chapter presents a framework for collaboration between healthcare providers that addresses the complex needs of elderly patients with hip fractures and international collaboration could advance evidence-based care for elderly populations and promote global health equity and professional development.

The complexity of hip fracture rehabilitation extends beyond immediate surgical intervention and requires expertise in geriatric assessment, fall prevention, nutritional management, psychological support, and long-term care planning. This multidimensional nature of care presents both challenges and opportunities for nursing professionals to lead innovative, collaborative approaches that leverage international expertise and evidence-based practices. These challenges could be addressed through nursing partnerships which improve shared knowledge, standardized protocols, and collaborative research initiatives. By examining successful models of international collaboration in hip fracture care, this chapter demonstrates how nursing professionals can reshape practice standards, improve patient outcomes, and contribute to global health equity through strategic partnerships beyond geographical boundaries (Groos et al., 2025).

The nursing profession's central role in coordinating care, advocating for patients, and implementing evidence-based interventions positions nurses as ideal leaders in developing and implementing cross-border collaborative frameworks for geriatric hip fracture care. This chapter explores partnerships can transform practice through knowledge exchange, joint research initiatives, and the development of culturally responsive care models that address the unique needs of diverse elderly populations (Groos et al., 2025, Swift et al., 2016).

The multidimensional aspect of geriatric hip fracture care demands a paradigm shift from traditional single specialty approaches to comprehensive multidisciplinary models. Recent evidence has increasingly demonstrated that the biological, psychological, and social complexity of elderly hip fracture patients cannot be adequately addressed by orthopaedic surgeon alone. The multifaceted nature of these patients characterized by frailty, polypharmacy, cognitive impairment, nutritional deficits, and multiple comorbidities necessitates expertise from diverse healthcare professionals working in coordinated fashion from the moment of hospital admission through long-term follow-up.

A systematic review examining the performance indicators in hip fracture care, found that early comprehensive geriatric assessment was associated with improved outcomes in 86% of patient-reported measures and 70.78% of reported clinical outcomes derived from hospital records. This substantial body of evidence demonstrates that early geriatric assessment within 72 hours of admission reduces significantly preoperative waiting time, medical and surgical complications, length of hospital stay and mortality at various postoperative times. These findings highlight that comprehensive geriatric assessment is not merely an adjunct to surgical care, but rather a fundamental component of evidence-based hip fracture management.

The Hip-POS (Hip-Padua Osteosarcopenia) fracture liaison service model, introduce contemporary integrated approaches. This model systematically incorporates assessment of muscle status alongside bone health, recognizing that the concept of sarcopenia with the coexistence of osteoporosis is critical for accurately estimating fracture risk and optimizing recovery. In the first five months of implementation, the Hip-POS program demonstrated dramatic improvements in treatment rates, with patients receiving anti-fracture therapy increasing from approximately 40% to 80%, and vitamin D and calcium supplementation rising from 29.6% to 81%. Such systematic approaches address the well-documented secondary fracture prevention gap, that leaves the majority of hip fracture patients untreated for underlying bone fragility, thereby exposing them to imminent risk of subsequent fractures due to absence of following-up monitoring (Arcidiakono et al., 2025).

GLOBAL EPIDEMIOLOGY OF HIP FRACTURES

According to the International Osteoporosis Society, by 2034 the increase in the population over 75 years of age in Greece will reach 23.7% in men and 21% in women, with an increased likelihood of fragility fracture (IOF 2021). By 2050, population growth in Greece for those over 60 years of age will reach 40.40%. Data from the Hellenic Statistical Authority for 2014 indicate that 53.5% of people between 65 and 74 years of age and 74.6% of people over 75 years of age report limitations in their functional capacity. As a result of the increasing percentage of the aging population and the coexistence of frailty syndrome, chronic diseases, and physical inactivity, which lead to loss of autonomy, independence, and reduced functional activity, falls in old age become increasingly common. Falls represent a major public health problem due to their high incidence in the elderly and their serious consequences, including fractures, loss of autonomy, reduced independence, increased need for care, and mortality (WHO falls, 2020).

Hip fractures are the most common and frequent injury, associated with falls, over the age of 65 years old and is naturally associated with the aging process. This represents a major public health problem, as hip fractures are associated with significant loss of mobility, increased mortality rates, and a substantial burden on national health systems. Hip fractures from falls occur in 95% of cases, while 25% of older people who experience such a fracture die within the first year. It is estimated that 1,600,000 hip fractures occur worldwide each year, with 300,000 resulting in hospitalization, and this number is expected to increase as the aging population grows progressively. According to the International Osteoporosis Organization, while in 2010 there were an estimated 158,000,000 fragility fractures, by 2040 this number is estimated to double due to demographic increases in the population (Gerdhem, 2013). It is expected that by 2050 there will be an increase in hip fractures of 310% in men and 240% in women (IOF 2021). The phenomenon of hip fractures is directly related to age, especially after 65 years, and is more common in women than in men. Women appear to be 2-3 times more prone to hip fractures than men (Gibson et al., 2014; Kanis et al., 2012). Interestingly, the incidence of hip fractures varies depending on country and geographical region, with the highest rates occurring in Western countries. This is likely due to lifestyle factors, aging populations, and different healthcare system conditions. However, hip fracture rates are also increasing in developing countries as living conditions continue to improve (Tsuda, 2017; Kanis et al., 2012).

As the average age of the population continues to increase worldwide, the incidence of hip fractures is expected to continue rising. This makes the implementation of early rehabilitation and fall prevention strategies even more critical. Public health efforts are focused on improving bone health through screening, information, and education, as well as promoting healthier lifestyles, with the aim of reducing the likelihood of hip fractures in the geriatric population. Collaboration among healthcare providers ensures that individuals receive holistic care, addressing their medical, physical, and environmental needs. Rehabilitation strategies as well as prevention care improve patients' outcomes and the quality of health care services (Baumann et al., 2022).

PREDISPOSING FACTORS FOR FALLS IN THE ELDERLY

Understanding the predisposing factors that contribute to falls is essential for addressing this phenomenon and the injuries that result. The epidemiology of hip fractures in older adults is associated with multifactorial reasons, including normal aging, lifestyle factors, and underlying health problems. Endogenous factors concern the medical history and clinical picture of the patient and can be related either to the natural progression of aging and its effects on the human body and behaviour, or to pathological health problems. Age-related changes include decreased muscle mass and strength affecting balance and mobility, delayed nervous system responses such as decreased reflexes and impaired proprioception and neuromuscular coordination, and reduced joint flexibility and elasticity with limited range of motion that makes maintaining balance difficult (Pizzonia et al., 2021).The presence of chronic diseases combined with the aging process makes recovery from fall-related injuries more difficult. Conditions that increase fall risk include osteoporosis, neurological disorders such as Parkinson's disease, stroke, and dementia. Biomarkers also play an important role in fall risk assessment, as they can contribute to predicting fall risk, understanding underlying causes, and guiding appropriate interventions (Veronese & Maggi, 2018).

Research suggests that certain biomarkers can serve as indicators of physiological changes or conditions that increase fall risk. For example, low vitamin D levels are associated with muscle weakness, balance disorders, and increased fall risk. Inflammatory markers, such as C-reactive protein (CRP), indicate chronic inflammation that can negatively impact muscle and bone health, increasing fall likelihood. Hormonal biomarkers, such as estrogen and testosterone, play crucial roles, as hormonal imbalance, especially in older adults, can lead to loss of muscle and bone mass. Biomarkers related to muscle condition, such as creatinine and myostatin, are important indicators of reduced muscle strength and function, which are critical for maintaining balance and preventing falls (Calvani et al., 2015).

Nutritional status also influences fall risk. Conditions such as diabetes mellitus are associated with factors that increase fall risk, including poor blood circulation, muscle weakness, and dizziness. Vision disorders such as cataracts, glaucoma, and optic nerve degeneration reduce visual acuity and spatial perception, increasing fall risk (Arkley et al., 2019; Uriz-Otano & Malafarina, 2015). Cognitive deficits such as dementia affect perception, attention, and orientation, increasing fall risk. Polypharmacy (taking multiple medications) can cause dizziness, confusion, and hypotension, provoking falls. Balance and gait problems, unsteady gait, poor posture, and foot deformities affect joint mobility and individual stability, thus increasing fall risk (Uriz-Otano & Malafarina, 2015).

Exogenous factors that could predispose individuals to falls include unsafe home environments. The phenomenon of falls is often due to factors such as insufficient lighting, slippery, wet, or polished floors, fixed obstacles such as loose carpets or heavy furniture in walkways, and lack of supports such as grab bars in bathrooms and on stairs. Inappropriate footwear affects balance, and environmental obstacles outside the home, including uneven terrain, potholes, and bad weather conditions (ice, rain, snow), affect stability. The multifactorial nature of falls implicates the involvement of different healthcare providers to assess, diagnose, prevent, and manage fall risk factors (Damián et al., 2013; Francis-Coad et al., 2018).

SECONDARY FALLS AFTER A HIP FRACTURE SURGERY

After a hip fracture, older adults are at higher risk of further falls. Research data shows that 20-50% of patients who have suffered a hip fracture experience at least one additional fall within the first year of the initial injury. The risk is highest in the first months after the fracture, as patients are in the recovery process, presenting with muscle weakness, reduced mobility, balance disorders, and fear of falling. Secondary falls after hip fracture pose serious risks to the health and independence of older adults. Their consequences can be severe, causing new injuries and additional complications in rehabilitation. Secondary falls lead to prolonged overall hospitalization and increased recovery time, resulting in dependence on caregivers and higher hospitalization and rehabilitation costs. Recurrent falls are burdensome for both patients and their family environments. Secondary falls also significantly increase the likelihood of negative functional outcomes, including death (Davis et al., 2020).

STRATEGIES FOR PREVENTING FALLS

Falls in older adults are among the most important causes of limited mobility and increased mortality due to the presence of many predisposing factors. However, many of these factors can be eliminated or reduced through implementation of appropriate prevention strategies. By choosing the right techniques and interventions, healthcare providers can influence important internal factors such as muscle strength, visual impairment, cognitive dysfunction, and medication management. Simultaneously, it is equally important to address external factors by creating safe outdoor environments, adapting home spaces, and ensuring appropriate clothing and footwear to reduce fall risk (Francis-Coad et al., 2018; Zinger et al., 2023).

Special exercise programs, ergonomic and environmental adaptations, and education are key axes of intervention to prevent falls and promote quality of life. By implementing these strategies, it is possible to reduce the risk of new falls, improve elderly individuals' quality of life, and maintain their independence. Basic principles of fall prevention strategy include bone health management, fall prevention programs, physical activity, and lifestyle adjustments. Implementing these measures can significantly reduce the risk of falls and fractures, improving quality of life for older adults (Andreasen et al., 2025, Bilik et al., 2017). A multifaceted aspect of rehabilitation approach is required, incorporating falls risk assessment, physical therapy sessions, medication screening and review, environmental modifications and patient education (Muusse et al., 2023).

CLINICAL PRACTICE IN HIP FRACTURE REHABILITATION

Standard Clinical Practice

The provision of healthcare to patients with hip fracture surgery depends on many factors and includes various stages of rehabilitation to regain functional activity. A classic rehabilitation model in daily clinical practice is subdivided into stages depending on the patient's age, clinical picture, and treating physician's instructions (de Sire et al., 2021). Nurses, as primary or clinical caregivers, are in the optimal position not only to identify fall risks but to provide ongoing monitoring and support to patients that enhances fall prevention (Swift et al., 2016).

Surgical factors, including the type of surgery after hip fracture, significantly affect the risk of complications (Zhou et al. 2023). Delaying surgery after hip fracture increases the risk of complications such as infections, embolisms, and increased mortality. Intraoperative complications may occur during surgery, including significant blood loss requiring transfusion and leading to hemodynamic instability, or difficulties managing anesthesia, especially in patients with cardiovascular or respiratory problems (Venegas-Sanabria et al. 2018).

Postoperative complications are common and can include pneumonia, urinary tract infections, or wound infections (Venegas-Sanabria et al., 2018). Respiratory complications such as pneumonia, pulmonary embolism, and respiratory failure are more common in patients with reduced mobility or pre-existing respiratory diseases. Cardiovascular complications can include myocardial infarction, arrhythmias, or heart failure (Assouline et al., 2021). Patients who remain immobilized after surgery and whose early mobilization is delayed are at higher risk of developing deep vein thrombosis (DVT) and pulmonary embolism (PE), with high mortality rates. Postoperative delirium is common in the elderly and can cause prolonged hospitalization, reduced mobility, additional complications, and increased mortality (Venegas-Sanabria et al., 2018).

Kidney damage can result from inadequate fluid management, pre-existing kidney disease, or drug toxicity, further increasing infection and mortality risk. Inadequate nutrition before and after surgery can delay wound healing, increase infection risk, and weaken the immune system. Malnourished patients have increased risk of pressure ulcers, poor wound healing, and other infections (Marcantonio et al., 2000).

Social factors also play significant roles. Individuals who live alone or lack social support face difficulties in recovery and have increased risk of complications and mortality. Individuals of low socioeconomic status may experience delayed treatment seeking, inadequate postoperative care, and higher risk of complications and mortality (Borgström et al., 2020; Malafarina et al., 2017).

Postoperative Care and Hospital Environment

Postoperative care and rehabilitation after hip fracture are crucial for successful patient recovery. Prolonged hospitalization is often an indication of complications such as infections, delayed recovery time, and comorbidities. Long hospitalization is associated with increased mortality risk (Liem et al., 2013). Multidisciplinary collaboration, proper management of complications, and enhancement of mobility should be key priorities in caring for elderly patients after hip fracture.

Key elements of an effective rehabilitation program include regaining mobility so patients can walk and move independently, strengthening muscle and regaining balance for stability and reducing new fall risk, helping patients perform daily activities with less dependence on caregivers, managing postoperative pain and inflammation to promote faster wound healing and facilitate mobilization, and preventing secondary complications such as deep vein thrombosis, pressure ulcers, and muscle atrophy. A well-organized and individualized rehabilitation program can reduce morbidity and mortality while increasing patient functional capacity (Fernandez et al., 2015; O'Connor & Switzer, 2022; Pfeufer et al., 2020).

Prevention of Secondary Falls

Prevention of secondary falls after hip fracture requires a multifactorial approach including early mobilization, medication management, adjustments to family environment, patient education, psychological support, and long-term physical activity. Early intervention and a holistic multidisciplinary approach are essential to reduce secondary fall risk, improve functional outcomes, and promote quality of life for older adults recovering from hip fracture (Conley et al., 2020; Sherrington & Tiedemann, 2015; Zinger et al., 2023).

One of the most scientifically documented exercise programs for fall prevention is the Otago Exercise Program (OEP), which is particularly effective in older adults, including those recovering from recent hip fracture. This program aims to improve patient muscle strength, balance, and walking ability and appears particularly helpful in helping individuals regain self-confidence, maintain independence, and prevent future falls (Albornos-Muñoz et al., 2024; Martins et al., 2018).

Multidisciplinary Rehabilitation Models: International Perspectives

The emergence of orthogeriatric care models represents a paradigm shift in hip fracture management that emphasizes collaborative, interdisciplinary approaches to care. These models, successfully implemented in various international settings, demonstrate the effectiveness of coordinated care that integrates orthopaedic expertise with geriatric assessment and management principles (Van Heghe, 2022).

From a nursing perspective, orthogeriatric models create opportunities for advanced practice nurses to assume leadership roles in coordinating complex care plans, conducting comprehensive geriatric assessments, and managing the multifaceted needs of elderly patients with hip fractures. International partnerships allow nurses to learn from successful orthogeriatric implementations, adapt models to local contexts, and contribute to the evidence base supporting these approaches. Nurses play an essential role in the ongoing function of the interdisciplinary team as they facilitate the communication and coordination between healthcare professionals, ensuring patients' healthcare benefits (Muusse et al., 2023).

The development and implementation of evidence-based rehabilitation protocols for hip fracture patients requires systematic approaches to literature review, protocol development, implementation science, and outcome evaluation. International nursing partnerships provide opportunities to pool resources, expertise, and patient populations to conduct high-quality research that informs clinical practice guidelines. The Otago Exercise Program represents one example of an evidence-based intervention that has been successfully adapted and implemented across different countries and healthcare systems (Martins, 2018).

Nursing leadership in implementing and evaluating such programs through international partnerships can contribute to the global evidence base while ensuring cultural adaptation and local relevance. Cross-border nursing research collaborations can address critical knowledge gaps in hip fracture rehabilitation, such as optimal timing for intervention initiation, effectiveness of home-based versus facility-based programs, and identification of patient populations most likely to benefit from specific interventions. By leveraging international partnerships, nurses can conduct large-scale studies with diverse populations that provide more robust evidence for clinical decision-making (Groos et al., 2025).

Clinical Approaches

A comprehensive multifactorial rehabilitation program is crucial to ensure optimal patient functional capacity and independence. A well-designed rehabilitation program is vital in preventing secondary falls, which are considered among the most important consequences after hip fracture surgery. These programs focus on improving strength, balance, coordination, and mobility while also addressing psychological factors, offering reinforcement, social support, and education in fall prevention strategies (Pfeufer et al., 2020; Yee et al., 2022). By following holistic multidisciplinary rehabilitation programs, the risk of future falls can be significantly reduced and functional outcomes improved. Based on this philosophy, such rehabilitation programs can be effective in preventing future falls if they include a combination of methodical approaches such as pharmaceutical management, rehabilitation strategies, ergonomic adaptations, and patient education.

Fall prevention programs should offer psychological support to reduce fear of falling. A rehabilitation program should include psychological support and specialized strategies for assessing and addressing this fear, as patients often avoid moving or walking, leading to muscle weakness and balance problems. Programs such as cognitive training or other psychological support can help patients cope with their fear and regain confidence in their ability to move safely. Encouraging patients to take small steps, slowly engage in physical activity, and progressively increase walking time and distance can help reduce fear of falling and improve functional activities (Yee et al., 2022).

Informing and educating patients and their caregivers about secondary fall risk and the importance of rehabilitation is also a feature of fall prevention programs. This information should include fall prevention techniques, information on how to avoid falls, specific transfer and mobility techniques, how to get up after a fall, and correct use of assistive devices (Diong et al., 2016). Educating patients about the importance of compliance regarding instructions, prescribed exercises and the continuous attendance at physical therapy sessions to maintain mobility and strength, enhances prevention results. Information about the role of nutrition in patient recovery and administration of supplements such as vitamin D and calcium for bone health are essential. Management of comorbidities and other conditions such as osteoporosis, diabetes, or hypertension is crucial to improve quality of life (Selaković et al., 2024).

The involvement of family members or caregivers in the rehabilitation process ensures that patients will have adequate support and assistance during mobilization, exercise, and daily activities. Frequent medical follow-up and recording of patient assessments are important. Regular appointments with healthcare professionals, including physiotherapists, physicians, and other specialists, help ensure patient participation and compliance in the rehabilitation process and identify risk factors for falls, allowing early intervention when necessary (Freiberger et al., 2012).

For patients with a history of hip fractures and evidence of bone health problems, implementing fall prevention procedures is essential, which may include medication and nutritional supplements. In many communities and countries, group-based fall prevention programs are often offered. Participation in exercise programs such as Step or Tai Chi groups, which have been shown effective in reducing fall rates by improving balance and self-confidence, should be encouraged (Lee & Lee, 2022).

Future Clinical Perspectives And Technology Integration

As the elderly population increases, the rate of secondary falls is expected to increase dramatically. The need for further research and interventions is crucial to assess which strategies are most effective in reducing secondary fall likelihood, especially in high-risk populations such as those with cognitive deficits or increased frailty. Technology can play an important role through various means, such as wearable sensors to detect mobility patterns and smart home devices to prevent falls. The integration of technology in hip fracture rehabilitation offers opportunities for international nursing partnerships to develop and evaluate innovative approaches to healthcare services. Telemedicine, mobile health applications, and virtual reality rehabilitation offer solutions to overcome geographical barriers, resource constraints, and access limitations that affect recovery of elderly patients with hip fractures (Swift et al., 2016).

Nursing expertise in patient education, behaviour modification, and technology adoption makes nurses ideal multidisciplinary team members in developing and implementing technology-enhanced rehabilitation programs. Cross-border nursing partnerships can develop innovative approaches to hip fracture rehabilitation that maintain quality of care and significantly improve outcomes for older individuals who have sustained hip fractures, reducing the likelihood of new falls and complications based on cross-border collaboration (Lasater et al., 2016).

Fall prevention strategies through International collaboration

International nursing partnerships can facilitate the development and implementation of comprehensive fall prevention programs that address multiple risk factors through coordinated, evidence-based interventions. The multifactorial nature of fall risk, encompassing physiological, psychological, environmental, and social factors, requires comprehensive assessment and intervention approaches that benefit from international knowledge exchange. Nurses' expertise in health promotion, patient education, and community-based interventions positions them as leaders in developing culturally appropriate fall prevention strategies that can be adapted across different healthcare systems and populations. Cross-border partnerships enable multidisciplinary teams to share successful fall prevention models, conduct comparative effectiveness research, and develop standardized assessment tools that facilitate risk evaluation across different clinical settings. The development of international databases and outcome registries can support evidence-based decision-making and quality improvement initiatives that benefit elderly populations globally (Baek et al., 2023).

Secondary Fall Prevention and Rehabilitation

Secondary fall prevention, focused on preventing subsequent falls among individuals who have already experienced a fall or hip fracture, represents a critical area where nursing expertise can significantly impact outcomes. The high rate of secondary falls, with 20-50% of hip fracture patients experiencing additional falls within the first year, demonstrates the urgent need for effective prevention strategies (Zinger et al., 2023). International nursing partnerships can facilitate the development and evaluation of comprehensive secondary prevention programs that integrate rehabilitation exercises, environmental modifications, medication management, and psychological support. Sharing successful models, such as multidisciplinary fall prevention clinics and community-based exercise programs, can accelerate the adoption of evidence-based practices across different healthcare systems (Sherrington & Tiedemann, 2015; WHO Falls, 2020).

The nursing role in secondary fall prevention is essential in individual patient care, family education and caregiver training, and community engagement initiatives to create supportive environments for elderly individuals at risk for falls. Cross-border partnerships enable nurses to understand cultural differences, share educational resources, and collaborate on research initiatives that examine the effectiveness of different prevention strategies across diverse populations (Lasater et al., 2016).

Nursing Contribution in Hip Fracture Care

Nursing-sensitive outcomes in hip fracture care encompass a broad range of indicators that reflect the quality and effectiveness of nursing interventions throughout the care continuum. These outcomes include functional recovery measures, fall prevention effectiveness, medication compliance, nutritional status improvement, psychological well-being indicators, and patient satisfaction scores. The complexity of measuring and improving nursing contribution across different healthcare systems presents opportunities for international nursing partnerships to develop standardized assessment tools, share best practices, and conduct comparative effectiveness research. Nurses' unique position in healthcare systems, providing continuous patient care and coordinating multidisciplinary interventions, makes them ideally suited to lead initiatives that improve nursing-sensitive outcomes through international collaboration. By sharing expertise in areas such as pain management, mobility assessment, fall risk evaluation, and family education, nursing partnerships can enhance the quality of care provided to elderly patients with hip fractures worldwide (Groos et al., 2025; Lasater et al., 2016).

A CLINICAL MULTIDISCIPLINARY MODEL: EVIDENCE FROM PRACTICE

Study Design and Implementation

A prospective, randomized, controlled trial was conducted in a general hospital in Crete island, to investigate the effect of a specialized rehabilitation program, including a modified Otago exercise program and educational lectures on nutritional behaviour and ergonomic management, on improving functional capacity and reducing secondary falls in elderly people after hip fracture surgery (Albornos-Muñoz et al., 2024; Martins et al., 2018).The study investigated the effectiveness of the intervention program, in reducing muscle atrophy, reducing fear of falls, and improving the biomarker values too. A total of 100 patients aged 65 and older who had sustained hip fractures due to falls and subsequently underwent surgical treatment were assessed eight weeks after surgery. A multidisciplinary team comprising an orthopaedic surgeon, an internal medicine specialist, a physiotherapist, and a nurse conducted evaluations to determine each patient's suitability for a rehabilitation program (Table 1).

Table 1. Interdisciplinary team

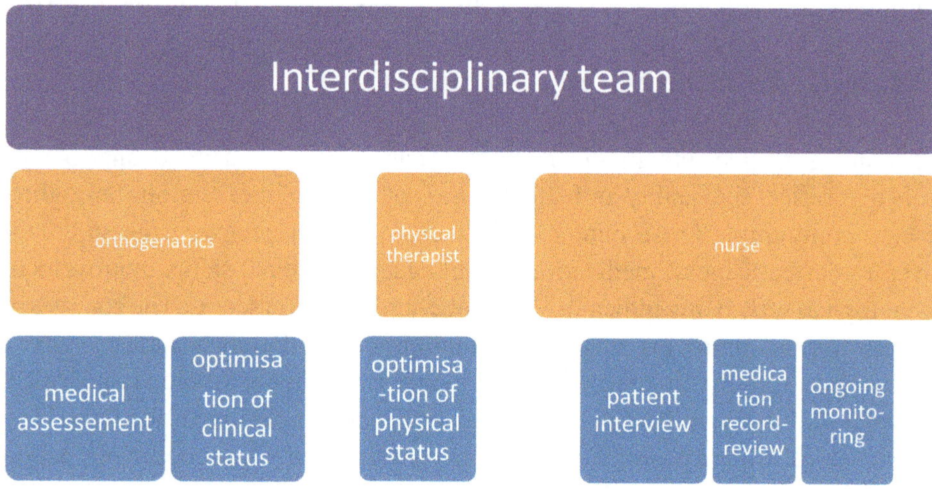

Based on these assessments, 36 individuals identified as being at high risk for recurrent falls, muscle weakness, and fear of falling were selected to participate in the study. All participants underwent blood testing at two and six months post-surgery to evaluate specific biomarkers. Nutritional supplements, including vitamin B12, vitamin D, and magnesium, were administered when deemed necessary (Dadgari et al., 2016; Lee et al. 2018).

Participants were randomly assigned to either the control or intervention group in a 1:1 ratio using computer-generated randomization software. Both groups were assessed using standardized questionnaires (EQ-5D-5L, SARC-F, MSRA-7, LEFS, and FES-1) along with objective measures such as the Sit-to-Stand Test, Timed Up and Go, grip strength via Jamar dynamometer, and the 4-meter walking test. Evaluations were conducted at two, six, and nine months after surgery, with a follow-up telephone interview at 12 months (Backes et al., 2015; Billis et al., 2011; Bohannon & Wang 2019; Mehta et al., 2016; Pantouvaki et al., 2023; Perez et al., 2020; Stasi et al., 2013; Tsekoura 2020; Yfantopoulos et al., 2001; Wald et al, 2020).

The intervention group followed a structured rehabilitation program beginning two months post-surgery, including a modified version of the Otago Exercise Program consisting of 12 sessions lasting 45 to 60 minutes each, aimed at enhancing balance and muscle strength. Additionally, participants attended educational sessions on nutrition, proper body mechanics, and exercise program (Ftouh et al., 2011; Hayward-Livingston et al. 2024).

Results

The number of subjects submitted in the referred study was 32 patients, 26 women and 6 men with an average of 76,8 ± 6,4 years old. After completion of the study all measurements were statistically analyzed (Mauchly test) and the most important data will be reported in next. So in summary, analyzing the measurements of LEFS score, it is found that there is a significant increase in intervention group between 2 and 6 months (F=8,715, p=0,006). The analysis of the SARC-F questionnaire showed significant improvement in muscle mass at 6 months in the intervention group (mean score decreased from 5.44 at 2 months to 1.31 at 6 months, compared to control group decrease from 6.44 to 4.50). MSRA-7 was used additionally to assess pre=screening of sarcopenia. During Mauchly test, the analysis showed a decrease of MSRA-7 score in intervention group while there was an increase of MSRA-7 score in control group (F = 9,800, p = 0,004) between 2 and 6 months time.

The FES-1 questionnaire, indicative of patient independence and secondary fall prevention, showed significant improvement in fear of falling at 6 months in the intervention group (mean score decreased from 45.25 at 2 months to 24.06 at 6 months and maintained at 21.94 at 9 months), whereas no reported improvement occurred in the control group (mean scores remained elevated at 42.69 at 6 months and 34.69 at 9 months).

Quality of life assessment, using the EQ-5D-5L questionnaire, revealed significant effects of the intervention program at 6, 9, and 12 months compared to the control group. The intervention group showed substantial improvement (mean score increased from 53.13 at 2 months to 75.63 at 6 months, 80.00 at 9 months, and 80.63 at 12 months), while the control group showed more modest improvement (from 48.38 to 57.81 at 6 months, 61.25 at 9 months, and 61.38 at 12 months). A multicomponent intervention program which includes a modified exercise program and educational lectures on nutrition and ergonomic issues has a positive effect in functional outcomes and prevention of secondary falls after a hip fracture surgery. And this is the result of collaboration of an interprofessional healthcare team.

DISCUSSION

The management of patients with hip fracture after a fall represents a common and serious problem in the elderly that concerns national health systems, with high epidemiological evidence that is constantly reinforced due to the increasing geriatric population. As the age limit increases, the presence of factors related to aging and causing falls in the population increases, including osteoporosis, frailty, sarcopenia, malnutrition, dyskinesia, and lack of independence (Hayward-Livingston et al. 2024,

Yee et al. 2022). Various systematic reviews have been conducted in recent years, which have provided evidence for the superiority of orthogeriatric care models. Van Heghe et al. (2022) in a comprehensive systematic review and meta-analysis, including 37 studies with 37,294 hip fracture patients, demonstrated that orthogeriatric care significantly reduced length of stay, in-hospital mortality, one-year mortality and delirium incidence. The authors noted moderate-quality evidence supporting these findings, with the integrated care model showing particularly strong effects on reducing in-hospital mortality by 35%.

The consistency of benefits across diverse healthcare systems and populations is particularly noteworthy. Studies from high-income countries including Norway, Germany, Italy, the Netherlands, and the United Kingdom, as well as emerging evidence from middle-income settings in China and Latin America, demonstrate that the principles of comprehensive geriatric assessment and multidisciplinary coordination translate across different healthcare contexts. This generalizability suggests that the core components of orthogeriatric care, early geriatric assessment, systematic management of comorbidities and geriatric syndromes, coordinated surgical and medical care, early mobilization, and comprehensive discharge planning, are representing universally best practices rather than single specific interventions (Feng et al 2024).

The economic evidence for multidisciplinary care has also strengthened considerably. While the upfront costs of establishing orthogeriatric services may appear substantial, multiple cost-effectiveness analyses from the past five years demonstrate favorable cost-utility ratios. Ginsberg et al. (2013), in an analysis updated and validated by subsequent studies, showed that comprehensive orthogeriatric care uses 23% fewer resources per patient compared to standard care while increasing disability-adjusted life years by 0.226 per patient. These data are derived through multiple mechanisms such as reduced length of stay, fewer complications requiring intensive interventions, decreased readmission rates, reduced need for institutional placement, and prevention of secondary fractures through systematic bone health management.

The results of the present study highlight the multidimensional nature of rehabilitation for surgically treated hip fractures from falls, as the physiological deterioration that individuals may experience due to aging emerges, in combination with predisposing factors for falls such as sarcopenia, fragility, cachexia, malnutrition, depression, or comorbidities. Frequent and regular monitoring of patients with this clinical profile, supervised exercise with specific instructions, and proper information and education of patients on issues related to treatment lead to encouraging results for recovery of patients' functional capacity in a shorter period of time.

Classic postoperative rehabilitation care begins on the first postoperative day with the aim of restoring mobility, avoiding postoperative complications, and improving patient gait and functional independence. The degree of improvement depends on various factors concerning both the patient and the rehabilitation program followed. Early mobilization is considered essential, as it enhances patient self-confidence and psychology, reduces mortality rate, and increases mobility (Selaković et al. 2024).

Modern models of healthcare for geriatric patients with hip fracture involve multidisciplinary teams of many specialties or organized departments that constitute models called "Orthogeriatric units" of rehabilitation (Mitchell et al. 2019, Pioli et al. 2018). The role of these teams is the coordinated rehabilitation of patients, which initially includes recording and assessment of the patient's medical file and predisposing factors for possible secondary falls. The implementation of progressive and individualized exercise postoperatively is the basic prerequisite for improving the mobility, strength and function of the affected hip. The type of exercises, duration and intensity are the elements that show heterogeneity in the various research studies, regarding the proposed rehabilitation programs, while the importance of continued exercise immediately after hospitalization has not been investigated (Pfeufer et al. 2020).

Recording predisposing factors for falls related to the patient's medical picture, such as vision disorders, nutritional deficiencies (vitamin, calcium, vitamin D), or the presence of osteoporosis are resolved by the respective specialties, while problems related to lack of strength, balance, gait disorders, proprioception, and coordination are resolved by the rehabilitation team. Management of patients with hip fracture using an orthogeriatric model has positive effects on reducing time to surgery and hospitalization, as well as reducing mortality rate during hospital stay. The potential medical and postoperative complications of patients are significantly reduced due to systematic and interdisciplinary monitoring. Implementation of a standard orthogeriatric model is associated with reduced management costs for patients with hip fracture due to reduced length of hospital stay and postoperative complications observed (Van Heghe et al. 2022). The role of nurses in coordination of communication and collaboration of this team could be vital.

Nutritional assessment and intervention represent critical components of hip fracture rehabilitation where precision healthcare approaches can significantly improve outcomes. The relationship between nutritional status, muscle mass preservation, and functional recovery creates opportunities for personalized nutritional interventions based on individual metabolic profiles, genetic factors, and lifestyle preferences (Fernandez, Griffin and Costa 2015). Nursing expertise in nutritional assessment, patient education, and behavior modification positions nurses as leaders in implementing precision nutrition approaches that consider individual needs, preferences, and constraints. Cross-border partnerships enable the sharing of innovative approaches, collaborative research initiatives, and development of implementation frameworks that support sustainable nutritional care improvements.

International nursing partnerships can facilitate the development and validation of nutritional assessment tools, intervention protocols, and outcome measures that support evidence-based nutritional care for elderly patients with hip fractures. Sharing successful nutritional intervention models, considering cultural dietary preferences and resource availability, can improve the quality and effectiveness of nutritional care across different healthcare systems (Muusse et al. 2023, Swift 2016).

Medication management represents a critical area where precision healthcare approaches can reduce adverse events, improve therapeutic effectiveness, and enhance patient outcomes among elderly individuals with hip fractures. The complexity of polypharmacy in elderly populations, combined with age-related changes in drug metabolism and increased risk for adverse drug events, creates opportunities for personalized medication management approaches (Middleton et al. 2017).

Despite the significant evidence base research, serious implementation gaps exist globally. A report from the Global Fragility Fracture Network indicated that while over 70% of hospitals in Belgium and Ireland have implemented a type of orthogeriatric care, uptake remains below 55% in many high-income countries and is virtually absent in most low and middle-income settings. This implementation gap represents a critical opportunity for health systems improvement, particularly given the optimal increase in hip fractures alone between 2018 and 2050 (CDC, Falls, 2019).

Recent innovations in orthogeriatric care delivery offer promising solutions to implementation barriers. Telemedicine and remote monitoring technologies, accelerated by the COVID-19 pandemic, have demonstrated feasibility for providing specialist geriatric input to remote or resource-limited settings. The Hip-POS model's incorporation of bioelectrical impedance analysis for sarcopenia assessment represents an example of integrating objective, reproducible measurement tools into routine clinical workflows. Such innovations may help standardize care quality across different settings and facilitate comparative effectiveness research (Arcidacono et al 2025).

The role of advanced practice nurses and specialized care coordinators has emerged as particularly crucial in recent studies because of their binding role in multidisciplinary teams together, ensuring and providing continuity for patients navigating complex healthcare systems. Nursing partnerships can facilitate sharing of medication management protocols, adverse event monitoring systems, and patient education strategies that improve medication safety and effectiveness. Development of standardized assessment tools for medication-related risk factors, combined with culturally appropriate patient education materials, can enhance the quality of pharmaceutical care across different healthcare systems. Nursing expertise in medication administration, patient monitoring, and adverse event recognition positions nurses as leaders in implementing precision approaches to medication management that consider individual patient factors, cultural preferences, and healthcare system constraints. Cross-border partnerships enable collaborative research initiatives that examine medication effectiveness, safety profiles, and optimization strategies across diverse populations (Groos et al. 2023).

Based on the evidence based literature, there are some suggestions to be made as essential components of a high-quality geriatric hip fracture care in healthcare services that would be considered in implementing policy strategies.

An early systematic geriatric assessment is suggested in hip fracture patients aged 65 and above within 24 hours of admission. This assessment should include screening validated tools for the fall risk evaluation like the Berg Balance Scale or equivalent measures, for the nutritional status using the Mini Risk Sarcopenia Assessement and Sarc-F questionnaires, for the medication review with emphasis to polypharmacy, for the assessment of pre-fracture functional status and social support, and bone health evaluation including calcium, vitamin D, and causes of osteoporosis (Eamer et al. 2018, Ellis et al. 2017).

A coordinated surgical and medical collaboration is suggested also, as an essential part of a multidisciplinary team, to prepare patients for surgery and to minimize delays, targeting surgical intervention within 48 hours for medically stable candidates. Implement shared decision-making protocols between orthopaedic surgeons, anesthesiologists, and geriatricians regarding surgical timing, anaesthetic approach, and perioperative management. Utilize multimodal pain management strategies incorporating the appropriate anaesthesia method, guided by individual patient factors and risk assessment, and avoidance of NSAIDs in frail elderly patients at risk for various medical complications (Groos et al. 2023).

Some more considerations for clinical status of the patients are suggested to be considered also for holistic approach and better functional outcomes. So, delirium prevention strategies as environmental orientation, minimization of unnecessary catheterization and physical restraints, appropriate pain management without oversedation and early mobilization according to guidelines are quite essential and managed in parallel. The implementation of venous thromboembolism prophylaxis, with consideration of both pharmacological and mechanical measures tailored to individual bleeding risk and prevention pressure ulcers through regular repositioning, appropriate support surfaces, early mobilization, and optimization of nutritional status are some of the points too (NICE 2023).

An integrated rehabilitation program should be initiated with physiotherapy sessions when medically feasible postoperatively, with weight-bearing exercises appropriate to the surgical fixation method. A progressive mobilization protocol with clear functional goals, incorporating balance training, strengthening exercises for lower extremities, and gait training with appropriate assistive devices should be introduced. Engaging also occupational therapists for activities of daily living retraining, home safety assessment and modifications, adaptive equipment recommendations, and caregiver education regarding safe transfer techniques and fall prevention strategies is quite essential (McDonough et al. 2021).

A comprehensive discharge planning on admission day, with early identification of post-acute care needs and available resources is quite vital for reassessing patients. Following -up appointments should be arranged periodically after the orthopaedic surgery, while primary care and specialized services are needed, including fracture liaison services for osteoporosis management. Instructions should be given regarding medications, precautions, warning signs requiring medical attention, and rehabilitation expectations (NICE 2023).

A research in identifying barriers and facilitators to orthogeriatric care implementation in different healthcare systems and cultural contexts should be interpreted globally. More research investigating the relationship between acute care quality, including orthogeriatric involvement, and long-term cognitive outcomes, particularly prevention of delirium-associated cognitive decline must be delivered. Studies examining secondary fracture prevention effectiveness and the optimal integration of fracture liaison services with acute orthogeriatric care. Development and validation of implementation toolkits and quality improvement frameworks adaptable to varied settings should be settled. Studies examining the role of policy interventions, financial incentives, and regulatory requirements in promoting adoption of evidence-based hip fracture care models should be introduced with nurses to bind the roles. Longitudinal studies examining functional trajectories, quality of life, and survival beyond one year after hip fracture are necessary (Dreinhofer et al. 2018, Pinto et al. 2022).

A systematic improvement in hip fracture care quality requires supportive policy frameworks and resource allocation based on several fundamental rules. Quality standards and monitoring must be developed with national or regional hip fracture registries to collect standardized data on processes and outcomes, enabling quality improvement. It is recognized that time and expertise is required for comprehensive care coordination, discharge planning, and post-acute follow-up. It should also be developed specialized training for hip fracture liaison nurses and care coordinators, physical and occupational therapists with geriatric orthopaedic expertise, and clinical pharmacists with geriatric specialization. The interprofessional education in medical, nursing, and allied health curricula should be introduced to grow collaborative practice skills from early training stages. Implement strategies to reduce geographic disparities and ensure culturally appropriate care through language services, culturally tailored educational materials, and diverse workforce representation should be introduced as well in healthcare services (Feng et al. 2024).

CONCLUSION

Hip fractures represent the most common injury after a fall in the elderly requiring hospitalization and surgical rehabilitation. The majority of these fractures are fragility fractures with high risk of secondary falls that further complicate patient rehabilitation and increase chances of motor deficiency or mortality. This represents a major socioeconomic issue that concerns both the scientific community and national health systems worldwide, as it causes decline in functional capacity with attendant high morbidity and mortality. The presented study, based on the latest scientific data and new international recommendations regarding management of patients after hip fracture, investigated the effectiveness of a multicomponent rehabilitation model that aims to restore functional capacity and independence while managing most of the predisposing factors for falls mentioned in research and scientific literature.

From the recording and analysis of examined variables, the effect of a multifactorial rehabilitation program that includes a specialized exercise program and educational lectures on topics related to nutrition and ergonomic adjustments was positive in terms of recovery of functional activity and prevention of secondary falls. The intervention was particularly effective at 6 months after surgical repair, a period described by researchers as critical for occurrence of new falls. The results of this study, carried out in a clinical environment with collaboration of an interdisciplinary team, are encouraging for proper management of patients over 65 years of age with hip fractures that have undergone surgery and reinforce international proposals for holistic management standards for these patients.

Further research is necessary on larger numbers of patients with common standards of assessment, treatment, and management in different clinical settings and geographical distributions to draw safe conclusions and provide appropriate guidelines for correct and comprehensive rehabilitation of patients at national and global levels. Recent research data has identified several common barriers to orthogeriatric care strategy because of different professional approaches and concerns between orthopaedic surgery and geriatric medicine, inadequate reimbursement for multidisciplinary team activities, workforce shortages in geriatric medicine and specialized rehabilitation professionals and resistance to changing established practice patterns. However, the rehabilitation program implemented could constitute a proposal for operation of interdisciplinary teams in healthcare units and institutions, based on principles of high-quality management policy for provision of health services.

This chapter demonstrates that international nursing partnerships could offer substantial opportunities to advance evidence-based rehabilitation practices for geriatric hip fracture care. By collaborative research, knowledge exchange, and shared clinical protocols, nurses can lead transformative initiatives that improve patient outcomes across different healthcare systems. The integration of precision healthcare principles, cultural competency, and interdisciplinary approaches positions nursing professionals at the forefront of global efforts to address the challenges of hip fracture management in aging populations.

Future directions for cross-border nursing partnerships should focus on developing standardized assessment tools, conducting large-scale comparative effectiveness research, implementing technology-enhanced rehabilitation programs, and creating sustainable frameworks for knowledge exchange that promote global health equity and professional development. Through these collaborative efforts, the nursing profession can continue to reshape practice standards and contribute to improved quality of life for elderly patients with hip fractures worldwide.

REFERENCES

Albornos-Muñoz, L., Blanco-Blanco, J., Cidoncha-Moreno, M. Á., Abad-Corpa, E., Rivera-Álvarez, A., López-Pisa, R. M., Caperos, J. M., Baz, M. P. R., Moneo, A. B., González, L. P., Skelton, D. A., Todd, C., Townley, R., Hidalgo, P. L. P., Blasco, O. C., Agusti, M. C. S., Rich-Ruiz, M., Pisano, A. C. G., Xamena, J. M., & Moreno-Casbas, M. T. (2024). Efficacy of the Otago-Exercise-Programme to reduce falls in community-dwelling adults aged 65-80 when delivered as group or individual training: Non-inferiority-clinical-trial. *BMC Nursing*, *23*(1), 705. DOI: 10.1186/s12912-024-02310-3 PMID: 39354514

Andreasen, C., Dahl, C., Frihagen, F., Borgen, T. T., Basso, T., Gjertsen, J.-E., Figved, W., Wisløff, T., Hagen, G., Apalset, E. M., Stutzer, J. M., Lund, I., Hansen, A. K., Nissen, F. I., Joakimsen, R. M., Syversen, U., Eriksen, E. F., Nordsletten, L., Omsland, T. K., & Solberg, L. B. (2025). Fracture liaison service (FLS) is associated with lower subsequent fragility fracture risk and mortality: NoFRACT (the Norwegian capture the fracture initiative) [Preprint]. *Osteoporosis International*, *36*(3), 501–512. Advance online publication. DOI: 10.1007/s00198-024-07376-y PMID: 39808195

Arkley, J., Dixon, J., Wilson, F., Charlton, K., Ollivere, B. J., & Eardley, W. (2019). Assessment of Nutrition and Supplementation in Patients With Hip Fractures. *Geriatric Orthopaedic Surgery & Rehabilitation*, *10*, 2151459319879804. Advance online publication. DOI: 10.1177/2151459319879804 PMID: 31667002

Assouline, B.. (2021). Preoperative exercise training to prevent postoperative pulmonary complications in adults undergoing major surgery: A systematic review and meta-analysis with trial sequential analysis. In *Annals of the American Thoracic Society* (pp. 678–688). American Thoracic Society., DOI: 10.1513/AnnalsATS.202002-183OC

Backes, M., Dingemans, S. A., Schep, N. W. L., Bloemers, F. W., Van Dijkman, B., Garssen, F. P., Haverlag, R., Hoogendoorn, J. M., Joosse, P., Mirck, B., Postma, V., Ritchie, E., Roerdink, W. H., Sintenie, J. B., Soesman, N. M. R., Sosef, N. L., Twigt, B. A., Van Veen, R. N., Van der Veen, A. H., & Schepers, T. (2015). Wound infections following implant removal below the knee: The effect of antibiotic prophylaxis; the WIFI-trial, a multi-centre randomized controlled trial. *BMC Surgery*, *15*(1), 1–6. DOI: 10.1186/1471-2482-15-12 PMID: 25972101

Baek, H., Han, K., Cho, H., & Ju, J. (2023). Nursing teamwork is essential in promoting patient-centered care: A cross-sectional study. *BMC Nursing*, *22*(1), 433. Advance online publication. DOI: 10.1186/s12912-023-01592-3 PMID: 37978376

Baumann, I., Wieber, F., Volken, T., Rüesch, P., & Glässel, A. (2022). Interprofessional Collaboration in Fall Prevention: Insights from a Qualitative Study. *International Journal of Environmental Research and Public Health, 19*(17), 10477. Advance online publication. DOI: 10.3390/ijerph191710477 PMID: 36078195

Bilik, O., Damar, H. T., & Karayurt, O. (2017). Fall behaviors and risk factors among elderly patients with hip fractures. *Acta Paulista de Enfermagem, 30*(4), 420–427. DOI: 10.1590/1982-0194201700062

Billis, E., Strimpakos, N., Kapreli, E., Sakellari, V., Skelton, D. A., Dontas, I., Ioannou, F., Filon, G., & Gioftsos, G. (2011). Cross-cultural validation of the Falls Efficacy Scale International (FES-I) in Greek community-dwelling older adults. *Disability and Rehabilitation, 33*(19–20), 1776–1784. DOI: 10.3109/09638288.2010.546937 PMID: 21219254

Bohannon, R. W., & Wang, Y. C. (2019). Four-Meter Gait Speed: Normative Values and Reliability Determined for Adults Participating in the NIH Toolbox Study. *Archives of Physical Medicine and Rehabilitation, 100*(3), 509–513. DOI: 10.1016/j.apmr.2018.06.031 PMID: 30092204

Borgström, F., Karlsson, L., Ortsäter, G., Norton, N., Halbout, P., Cooper, C., Lorentzon, M., McCloskey, E. V., Harvey, N. C., Javaid, M. K., & Kanis, J. A. (2020). Fragility fractures in Europe: Burden, management and opportunities. *Archives of Osteoporosis, 15*(1), 59. Advance online publication. DOI: 10.1007/s11657-020-0706-y PMID: 32306163

Calvani, R. *et al.* (2015) "Biomarkers for physical frailty and sarcopenia: State of the science and future developments," *Journal of Cachexia, Sarcopenia and Muscle*. Wiley Blackwell, pp. 278–286. Available at: https://doi.org/.DOI: 10.1002/jcsm.12051

CDC. (2019). Available at URL: https://www.cdc.gov/falls/prevention/index.html

Conley, R. B., Adib, G., Adler, R. A., Åkesson, K. E., Alexander, I. M., Amenta, K. C., Blank, R. D., Brox, W. T., Carmody, E. E., Chapman-Novakofski, K., Clarke, B. L., Cody, K. M., Cooper, C., Crandall, C. J., Dirschl, D. R., Eagen, T. J., Elderkin, A. L., Fujita, M., Greenspan, S. L., & Kiel, D. P. (2020). Secondary Fracture Prevention: Consensus Clinical Recommendations from a Multistakeholder Coalition. *Journal of Bone and Mineral Research : the Official Journal of the American Society for Bone and Mineral Research, 35*(1), 36–52. DOI: 10.1002/jbmr.3877 PMID: 31538675

Dadgari, A., Hamid, T. A., Hakim, M. N., Chaman, R., Mousavi, S. A., Hin, L. P., & Dadvar, L. (2016). Randomized control trials on Otago Exercise Program (OEP) to reduce falls among elderly community dwellers in Shahroud, Iran. *Iranian Red Crescent Medical Journal, 18*(5). Advance online publication. DOI: 10.5812/ircmj.26340 PMID: 27478629

Damián, J., Pastor-Barriuso, R., Valderrama-Gama, E., & de Pedro-Cuesta, J. (2013). Factors associated with falls among older adults living in institutions. *BMC Geriatrics, 13*(1), 6. DOI: 10.1186/1471-2318-13-6 PMID: 23320746

Davis, J. C., Khan, K. M., Hsu, C. L., Chan, P., Cook, W. L., Dian, L., & Liu-Ambrose, T. (2020). Action Seniors! Cost-Effectiveness Analysis of a Secondary Falls Prevention Strategy Among Community-Dwelling Older Fallers. *Journal of the American Geriatrics Society, 68*(9), 1988–1997. DOI: 10.1111/jgs.16476 PMID: 32472567

de Sire, A., Invernizzi, M., Baricich, A., Lippi, L., Ammendolia, A., Grassi, F. A., & Leigheb, M. (2021). Optimization of transdisciplinary management of elderly with femur proximal extremity fracture: A patient-tailored plan from orthopaedics to rehabilitation. *World Journal of Orthopedics, 12*(7), 456–466. DOI: 10.5312/wjo.v12.i7.456 PMID: 34354934

Diong, J., Allen, N. and Sherrington, C. (2016) "Structured exercise improves mobility after hip fracture: A meta-analysis with meta-regression," *British Journal of Sports Medicine*. BMJ Publishing Group, pp. 346–355. Available at: https://doi.org/.DOI: 10.1136/bjsports-2014-094465

Dreinhofer, K. E., Mitchell, P. J., Bégué, T., Cooper, C., Costa, M. L., Falaschi, P., Hertz, K., Marsh, D., Maggi, S., Nana, A., Palm, H., Speerin, R., & Magaziner, J. (2018). A global call to action to improve the care of people with fragility fractures. *Injury, 49*(8), 1393–1397. DOI: 10.1016/j.injury.2018.06.032 PMID: 29983172

Eamer, G., Taheri, A., Chen, S. S., Daviduck, Q., Chambers, T., Shi, X., & Khadaroo, R. G. (2018). Comprehensive geriatric assessment for older people admitted to a surgical service. *Cochrane Database of Systematic Reviews*, 1.

Ellis G, *et al.* (2017). Comprehensive geriatric assessment for older adults admitted to hospital. *Cochrane Database Syst Rev*. Sep 12;9:CD006211.

Feng, J. N., Zhang, C., Li, B., Zhan, S., Wang, S., & Song, C. (2024). Global burden of hip fracture: The Global Burden of Disease Study. *Osteoporosis International, 35*(1), 41–52. DOI: 10.1007/s00198-023-06907-3 PMID: 37704919

Fernandez, M. A., Griffin, X. L., & Costa, M. L. (2015). Management of hip fracture. *British Medical Bulletin, 115*(1), 165–172. DOI: 10.1093/bmb/ldv036 PMID: 26311503

Francis-Coad, J., Etherton-Beer, C., Burton, E., Naseri, C., & Hill, A. M. (2018). Effectiveness of complex falls prevention interventions in residential aged care settings: A systematic review. *JBI Evidence Synthesis, 16*(4), 973–1002. PMID: 29634516

Freiberger, E., Häberle, L., Spirduso, W. W., & Rixt Zijlstra, G. A. (2012). Long-term effects of three multicomponent exercise interventions on physical performance and fall-related psychological outcomes in community-dwelling older adults: A randomized controlled trial. *Journal of the American Geriatrics Society, 60*(3), 437–446. DOI: 10.1111/j.1532-5415.2011.03859.x PMID: 22324753

Ftouh, S., Morga, A., & Swift, C. (2011). Management of hip fracture in adults: Summary of NICE guidance. *BMJ (Clinical Research Ed.), 342*(jun21 3), d3304. Advance online publication. DOI: 10.1136/bmj.d3304 PMID: 21693526

Gerdhem, P. (2013). Osteoporosis and fragility fractures. *Best Practice & Research. Clinical Rheumatology, 27*(6), 743–755. DOI: 10.1016/j.berh.2014.01.002 PMID: 24836333

Gibson, A. A., Hay, A. W., & Ray, D. C. (2014). Patients with hip fracture admitted to critical care: Epidemiology, interventions and outcome. *Injury, 45*(7), 1066–1070. DOI: 10.1016/j.injury.2014.02.037 PMID: 24680801

Groos, S. S., Tan, S. M., Linn, A. J., Kuiper, J. I., van Schoor, N. M., van Weert, J. C. M., & van der Velde, N. (2025). Multidisciplinary care pathways for falls prevention in older adults: Visualizing the needs of primary care-based health care professionals. *European Geriatric Medicine, 16*(1), 229–236. DOI: 10.1007/s41999-024-01142-3 PMID: 39789364

Hayward-Livingston, A., Ozdag, Y., Kolessar, D., Weinberg, J., Pamul, A., Koury, K., & Balsamo, A. (2024). A 10-Year Experience of an Integrated Geriatric Hip Fracture Treatment Protocol: Outcomes at a Minimum 2-Year Follow-Up. *Geriatric Orthopaedic Surgery & Rehabilitation, 15*, 21514593241273155. Advance online publication. DOI: 10.1177/21514593241273155 PMID: 39130164

IOF. (2021). Available at URL: https://www.osteoporosis.foundation/health-professionals/fragility-fractures/falls-prevention.

Kanis, J. A., Odén, A., McCloskey, E. V., Johansson, H., Wahl, D. A., & Cooper, C. (2012). A systematic review of hip fracture incidence and probability of fracture worldwide. *Osteoporosis International, 23*(9), 2239–2256. DOI: 10.1007/s00198-012-1964-3 PMID: 22419370

Lasater, K., Cotrell, V., McKenzie, G., Simonson, W., Morgove, M. W., Long, E. E., & Eckstrom, E. (2016). Collaborative falls prevention: Interprofessional team formation, implementation, and evaluation. *Journal of Continuing Education in Nursing, 47*(12), 545–550. DOI: 10.3928/00220124-20161115-07 PMID: 27893917

Lee, H., & Lee, S. H. (2022). Effectiveness of Multicomponent Home-Based Rehabilitation in Elderly Patients after Hip Fracture Surgery: A Randomized Controlled Trial. *Journal of Personalized Medicine, 12*(4), 649. Advance online publication. DOI: 10.3390/jpm12040649 PMID: 35455765

Liem, I. S., Kammerlander, C., Suhm, N., Blauth, M., Roth, T., Gosch, M., Hoang-Kim, A., Mendelson, D., Zuckerman, J., Leung, F., Burton, J., Moran, C., Parker, M., Giusti, A., Pioli, G., Goldhahn, J., & Kates, S. L. (2013). Identifying a standard set of outcome parameters for the evaluation of orthogeriatric co-management for hip fractures. *Injury, 44*(11), 1403–1412. DOI: 10.1016/j.injury.2013.06.018 PMID: 23880377

Malafarina, V., Uriz-Otano, F., Malafarina, C., Martinez, J. A., & Zulet, M. A. (2017). Effectiveness of nutritional supplementation on sarcopenia and recovery in hip fracture patients. A multi-centre randomized trial. *Maturitas, 101*, 42–50. DOI: 10.1016/j.maturitas.2017.04.010 PMID: 28539168

Marcantonio, E. R., Flacker, J. M., Michaels, M., & Resnick, N. M. (2000). Delirium is independently associated with poor functional recovery after hip fracture. *Journal of the American Geriatrics Society, 48*(6), 618–624. DOI: 10.1111/j.1532-5415.2000.tb04718.x PMID: 10855596

Martins, A. C.. (2018). Does modified Otago Exercise Program improves balance in older people? A systematic review. In *Preventive Medicine Reports* (pp. 231–239). Elsevier Inc., DOI: 10.1016/j.pmedr.2018.06.015

McDonough, C. M., Harris-Hayes, M., Kristensen, M. T., Overgaard, J. A., Herring, T. B., Kenny, A. M., & Mangione, K. K. (2021). Physical therapy management of older adults with hip fracture. *The Journal of Orthopaedic and Sports Physical Therapy, 51*(2), CPG1–CPG81. DOI: 10.2519/jospt.2021.0301 PMID: 33522384

Mehta, S. P., Fulton, A., Quach, C., Thistle, M., Toledo, C., & Evans, N. A. (2016). Measurement properties of the Lower Extremity Functional Scale: A systematic review. *The Journal of Orthopaedic and Sports Physical Therapy*, *46*(3), 200–216. DOI: 10.2519/jospt.2016.6165 PMID: 26813750

Middleton, M., Wan, B., & da Assunçao, R. (2017). Improving hip fracture outcomes with integrated orthogeriatric care: A comparison between two accepted orthogeriatric models. *Age and Ageing*, *46*(3), 465–470. DOI: 10.1093/ageing/afw232 PMID: 27974304

Mitchell, P. J.. (2019). Quality Improvement Initiatives in Fragility Fracture Care and Prevention. In *Current Osteoporosis Reports* (pp. 510–520). Springer., DOI: 10.1007/s11914-019-00544-8

Muusse, J. S. C., Zuidema, R., van Scherpenseel, M. C., & te Velde, S. J. (2023). Influencing factors of interprofessional collaboration in multifactorial fall prevention interventions: A qualitative systematic review. *BMC Primary Care*, *24*(1), 116. Advance online publication. DOI: 10.1186/s12875-023-02066-w PMID: 37193995

NICE. (2023) Hip fracture management. Available at URL: https://www.nice.org.uk/guidance/cg124

O'Connor, M. I., & Switzer, J. A. (2022). AAOS clinical practice guideline summary: Management of hip fractures in older adults. *The Journal of the American Academy of Orthopaedic Surgeons*, *30*(20), e1291–e1296. DOI: 10.5435/JAAOS-D-22-00125 PMID: 36200817

Pantouvaki, A., Kastanis, G., Patelarou, E., Alpantaki, K., Kleisiaris, C., & Zografakis-Sfakianakis, M. (2023). Greek Translation, Cultural Adaptation and Validation of the Mini Sarcopenia Risk Assessment Questionnaire, to Evaluate Sarcopenia in Greek Elderly at a Hospital Setting. *Nursing Reports*, *13*(1), 404–411. DOI: 10.3390/nursrep13010037 PMID: 36976689

Pfeufer, D., Kammerlander, C., Stadler, C., Roth, T., Blauth, M., Neuerburg, C., Böcker, W., Zeckey, C., Lechleitner, M., & Gosch, M. (2020). Multidisciplinary inpatient rehabilitation improves the long-term functional status of geriatric hip-fracture patients. *European Journal of Medical Research*, *25*(1), 31. Advance online publication. DOI: 10.1186/s40001-020-00433-2 PMID: 32778164

Pinto, D., Alshahrani, M., Chapurlat, R., Chevalley, T., Dennison, E., Camargos, B. M., Papaioannou, A., Silverman, S., Kaux, J.-F., Lane, N. E., Morales Torres, J., Paccou, J., Rizzoli, R., Bruyere, O., Blank, R., Buehring, B., Cooper, C., Ferrari, S., Kanis, J. A., & Tüzün, Ş. (2022). The global approach to rehabilitation following an osteoporotic fragility fracture: A review of the rehabilitation working group of the International Osteoporosis Foundation (IOF) committee of scientific advisors. *Osteoporosis International*, *33*(3), 527–540. DOI: 10.1007/s00198-021-06240-7 PMID: 35048200

Pioli, G., Bendini, C., Pignedoli, P., Giusti, A., & Marsh, D. (2018). Orthogeriatric co-management – managing frailty as well as fragility. *Injury*, *49*(8), 1398–1402. DOI: 10.1016/j.injury.2018.04.014 PMID: 29921533

Pizzonia, M., Giannotti, C., Carmisciano, L., Signori, A., Rosa, G., Santolini, F., Caffa, I., Montecucco, F., Nencioni, A., & Monacelli, F. (2021). Frailty assessment, hip fracture and long-term clinical outcomes in older adults. *European Journal of Clinical Investigation*, *51*(4), e13445. Advance online publication. DOI: 10.1111/eci.13445 PMID: 33131066

Selaković, I., Mandić-Rajčević, S., Milovanović, A., Tomanović-Vujadinović, S., Dimitrijević, S., Aleksić, M., & Dubljanin-Raspopović, E. (2024). Pre-Fracture Functional Status and Early Functional Recovery are Significant Predictors of Instrumental Activities of Daily Living After Hip Fracture: A Prospective Cohort Study. *Geriatric Orthopaedic Surgery & Rehabilitation*, *15*, 21514593241255627. Advance online publication. DOI: 10.1177/21514593241255627 PMID: 38766275

Sherrington, C., & Tiedemann, A. (2015). Physiotherapy in the prevention of falls in older people. *Journal of Physiotherapy*, *61*(2), 54–60. DOI: 10.1016/j.jphys.2015.02.011 PMID: 25797882

Stasi, S., Papathanasiou, G., Korres, N., Marinakis, G., Chronopoulos, E., Baltopoulos, P. I., & Papaioannou, N. A. (2013). Validation of the Lower Extremity Functional Scale in community-dwelling elderly people (LEFS-Greek); Determination of functional status cut-off points using TUG test. *European Geriatric Medicine*, *4*(4), 237–241. DOI: 10.1016/j.eurger.2013.04.004

Swift, C., Ftouh, S., Langford, P., Chesser, T. S., & Johanssen, A. (2016). CMJv16n6-Swift(WITHOUT ITAL CORX). indd. [). www.nice.org.uk/]. *Clinical Medicine*, *16*(6), •••. PMID: 27927818

Tsekoura, M., ... (2020) "Cross-cultural adaptation and validation of the Greek Version of the SARC-F for evaluating sarcopenia in Greek older adults" Available at: http://www.ismni.org

Tsuda, T. (2017) "Epidemiology of fragility fractures and fall prevention in the elderly: a systematic review of the literature". Available at: https://journals.lww.com/c-orthopaedicpractice

Uriz-Otano, F., Uriz-Otano, J. I., & Malafarina, V. (2015). Factors Associated With Short-Term Functional Recovery in Elderly People With a Hip Fracture. Influence of Cognitive Impairment. *Journal of the American Medical Directors Association, 16*(3), 215–220. DOI: 10.1016/j.jamda.2014.09.009 PMID: 25441099

Van Egmond, M. A., van der Schaaf, M., Vredeveld, T., Vollenbroek-Hutten, M. M. R., van Berge Henegouwen, M. I., Klinkenbijl, J. H. G., & Engelbert, R. H. H. (2018). Effectiveness of physiotherapy with telerehabilitation in surgical patients: A systematic review and meta-analysis. *Physiotherapy*, *104*(3), 277–298. DOI: 10.1016/j.physio.2018.04.004 PMID: 30030037

Van Heghe, A.. (2022). Effects of Orthogeriatric Care Models on Outcomes of Hip Fracture Patients: A Systematic Review and Meta-Analysis. In *Calcified Tissue International* (pp. 162–184). Springer., DOI: 10.1007/s00223-021-00913-5

Venegas-Sanabria, L. C.. (2018). Factors associated with in-hospital complications in the elderly subjected to hip fracture surgery. *Revista Española de Geriatría y Gerontología*, *53*(3), 181–182. DOI: 10.1016/j.regg.2017.06.004 PMID: 28733077

Veronese, N., & Maggi, S. (2018). Epidemiology and social costs of hip fracture. *Injury*, *49*(8), 1458–1460. DOI: 10.1016/j.injury.2018.04.015 PMID: 29699731

Wald, P., Chocano-Bedoya, P. O., Meyer, U., Orav, E. J., Egli, A., Theiler, R., & Bischoff-Ferrari, H. A. (2020). Comparative Effectiveness of Functional Tests in Fall Prediction After Hip Fracture. *Journal of the American Medical Directors Association*, *21*(9), 1327–1330. DOI: 10.1016/j.jamda.2020.02.008 PMID: 32276783

WHO. Falls, (2020). Available at URL: https://www.who.int/news-room/fact-sheets/detail/falls

WHO. Healthy aging, (2020). Available at URL: https://www.who.int/news-room/questions-and-answers/item/healthy-ageing-and-functional-ability

Yee, D. K. H., Lau, T.-W., Fang, C., Ching, K., Cheung, J., & Leung, F. (2022). Orthogeriatric Multidisciplinary Co-Management Across Acute and Rehabilitation Care Improves Length of Stay, Functional Outcomes and Complications in Geriatric Hip Fracture Patients. *Geriatric Orthopaedic Surgery & Rehabilitation*, *13*, 21514593221085813. Advance online publication. DOI: 10.1177/21514593221085813 PMID: 35433103

Yfantopoulos, J. (2001, March-April). The Greek version of the EuroQol (EQ-5D) instrument. *Arch Hellen Med*, *18*(2), 180–191.

Zhou, Y.. (2023) “Different Surgical interventions for Unstable intertrochanteric fracture of the femur: Network meta-analysis.” Available at: https://doi.org/DOI: 10.21203/rs.3.rs-3258227/v1

Zinger, G., Sylvetsky, N., Levy, Y., Steinberg, K., Bregman, A., Yudkevich, G., & Peyser, A. (2023). Early benefits of a secondary fracture prevention programme. *Hip International*, *33*(2), 332–337. DOI: 10.1177/11207000211027476 PMID: 34180292

Chapter 6
Social Capital of the Patient and Its Influence on the Mental Well-Being and Quick Recovery

Julia Paulevna Bayer
https://orcid.org/0000-0002-1866-3633
Russian Academy of National Economy and Public Administration, Russia

ABSTRACT

In this chapter the author considers Social Capital Theory of Pierre Bourdieu, the Connected theory of Nicholas Christakis and James Fowler in order to help in finding out how social capital (that is - nurses, all social network of close relatives, friends, even followers in social media) matters in the process of passing through illness/surgery smoothly and recover faster. Also, the Theory of Social Capital as Functional Social Structure by James Coleman and a new approach to social capital of Robert Putnam are being considered by the author as constituent parts of contemporary approach to social capital.

INTRODUCTION

In this chapter let's discuss how social capital, state of being trusted and creative can help patients in a hospital to upgrade and recover faster and smoother.

Discussing opening up the creativity, we know many inspiring examples, when patients, being limited in their moves, make a great breakthrough in science, art, literature, etc and become famous each in their own field. Frida Kahlo, being limited with the spine trauma, started drawing incredibly beautiful art, releasing her psycho

DOI: 10.4018/979-8-3373-5931-1.ch006

traumas and fears. Dr. Joe Dispenza became famous because, being heavily injured in car accident, started testing the possibilities of the mind and thus creating the whole new theory in neuroscience and dedicating his life to this after successfully recovering through the self-created methods. The examples can go on and on. The reason we give these examples in our studies is to show that the perception of the illness matters. That the communication during challenging times matters.

If, through direct personal social interaction nurses drop these examples into the minds of their patients, they might be naturally triggered and inspired and will be eager to do the same and more. The social idea behind this is that we (scientists) should also help in shifting social norms and attitude towards the patients being in the hospital. Less pity and more support, more treating as social normal behaviour, when patients start creating, providing them with tools for it: books, colours for drawing, tools for writing, audio for listening music etc.

Let's consider why creativity of the patients is important. Being creative eliminates fear and anxiety that most of the patients have. Also, it lowers the level of depression that is also common for those, who are forced to break their usual life routine and are limited in the freedom of moving.

The face-to-face communication of the ones being in hospital is very limited. So that is why the nurses are the ones who implement the face-to-face communication every day, and have the power to influence the patients. Thus, nurses should get not only medical education, but also the basic social communicative skills. These communicative skills should include the understanding that they can influence the mental wellbeing of the patients and thus, shorten the time of the illness through providing with encouraging words and behaviour.

We consider nurses as important communicators that have the power to implement healing interactions. Which hard and soft skills should possess the regular nurse, which tools of communication she/he should use to encourage patients not only to heal physically but use the quiet time in the hospital to make a breakthrough, reconsider life and restart with more mindful approach. Communication with the nurses also implies social trust that patients should have established.

In this chapter we will consider *Social Capital Theory* of *Pierre Bourdieu*, the *Connected* theory of *Nicholas Christakis and James Fowler* to help us in finding out how not only nurses, but *all the social network of connections* matter in the process of passing through illness/surgery smoothly and recover faster, the *Theory of Social Capital as Functional Social Structure* by *James Coleman* and a *political approach of Robert Putnam*.

Social capital is a concept introduced by Pierre Bourdieu in 1980 that studies social connections that can serve as a resource for generating benefits. Social capital is considered as a collective asset formed through the establishment of friendly and honest relationships between individuals of the society and different social groups.

Pierre Bourdieu describes mutually beneficial relationships, thus, strengthening connections between group members occur through the constant increase of shared social capital. The more we share and establish these connections – the stronger the person feels and the more successful he/she is.

Pierre Bourdieu introduced the concept of *social capital* as part of his theory of different forms of capital that individuals employ to maintain and enhance their position in social space. In his famous essay "The Forms of Capital" (Bourdieu, 1986), Bourdieu defines social capital as "the aggregate of the actual or potential resources which are linked to possession of a durable network of more or less institutionalized relationships of mutual acquaintance or recognition". In other words, social capital comprises the resources accessible through social connections – it is the benefit one gains by virtue of membership in networks and groups. Bourdieu emphasized that these network-derived "profits" (resources and advantages) are the basis of the solidarity that binds group members together.

Importantly, he emphasizes that social networks do not arise naturally; they are actively constructed through investment strategies (of quality time together, regular efforts and so on) aimed at establishing, reproducing and maintaining beneficial relationships. In the original formulation, Bourdieu even noted that *"the profits which accrue from membership in a group are the basis of the solidarity which makes them possible"*, underlining the reciprocal relationship between network ties and the resources they yield.

Bourdieu's formulation of social capital is grounded in a broader concern with how different forms of capital perpetuate social inequality and power. Social capital, in his view, is an *individual attribute* (one's network-derived resources), not a collective good uniformly available to all members of a community. Indeed, we absolutely agree that every individual has his/her own life story, through which he/she meets different people with different talents, network of connections and thus power, so that they become constituent parts of personal social capital. By lucky coincidence we can meet a powerful person, who can speed up our social mobility to the level of saving us years and even decades of climbing the social ladder in usual conditional ways.

It is unevenly distributed because it depends on an individual's social ties, which in turn reflect that person's social position (status, class, etc.). Those in higher positions can typically accumulate more social capital, thereby furthering their advantage. Bourdieu saw the pursuit and use of social capital as largely instrumental – people invest in social relationships to secure benefits (such as information, influence, or support) that can ultimately be converted into other gains.

For example, through social capital one might gain access to economic capital (e.g. job opportunities, credit) or augment one's cultural capital (e.g. by connecting with those who have expertise, or prestigious, or power credentials). This convertibility means that, although social capital is not directly monetary, it can facilitate or get advantages in other currencies of power. Indeed, Bourdieu stated that all forms of capital are ultimately fungible and, under certain conditions, can be monetized, that is – transformed into economic capital.

Crucially, Bourdieu linked social capital to the *reproduction of inequality*. Social inequality is pre-determined by nature, as Russian-American sociologist stated in his famous work "Social mobility", published in 1927. As well as Sorokin stated, we can continue this line that everyone is being born with inequal social capital that is, having different connections, different opportunities and thus, different starting points from the birth date.

In this chapter we consider social capital as a support system for the patients being in a way isolated in hospitals.

In this chapter we will add more understanding to the social capital theory and suggest to consider social capital in several dimensions:

1. **First circle** - close circle of family and friends with intense, regular and deep quality communication
2. **Second circle** - wide circle of friends, acquaintances, followers, admirers that like the content, might not know you in person but follow you and get inspired from you.
3. **Third circle** - haters, who take their attention and energy through negative emotions they throw out in social media on others.

So, we assume that the patient, being in hospital in contemporary digital era, can keep interacting and lean on having support, good wishes and prayers from first and second circles. Obviously, the type of communication will be different: with first circle it will be intense and emotionally deep conversations, with the second circle – it will be massive support in responding on the situation in likes and comments. Third circle of haters will only counterbalance the situation. Actually, we can say that having a third circle, that is – haters, means that that the person moves to the level of celebrity in social hierarchy.

So, talking about moral, mental, emotional and psychological support, we can state that social capital of every patient will determine its presence, its intensity and number of contacts reaching out to a person. Social capital is, as Bourdieu states, is being partly given by the social position of the parents, but, and here we insist, it is being maintained and grown by the behavior and communicative strategies of the person him/herself.

So, we can determine the direct correlation of the social capital and the intensity of the support the patients receive during the isolated time in the hospital. And here we will turn to the "Connected" theory of Nicholas et al. (2009), the scientists that describe "the amazing power of social networks and how they shape our lives. Christakis, being a professor at Harvard University, underlines the three rules of life in the network. Let us dive into this theory and connect it with the unfolding discussion. So, the authors state that we choose "the structure of our networks in three important ways" (Christakis N., Fowler J., 2011).

So, that is, if we see this theory through the eyes of Bourdieu, the person him/herself determines the structure and quality of social capital he/she possesses, that is, as Christakis and Fowler state, *the rules* are the following.

Firstly, "we shape our network", that is - "we decide how many people we are connected to" that is, it's our personal choice the amount and quality of our social bonds, "we influence how densely interconnected our friends and family are", we determine the strength of the social bonds and also we control ourselves how central we are to the social network.

Secondly, is that "our network shapes us", that is, having an extra friend "may create all kinds of benefits for your health", this actually, strongly applied to our theme of mental wellbeing of the patients.

And *thirdly*, "our friends affect us" rule is that, if we put it short, we start copying the behavior of those people we communicate more often. In our case of the hospital, the roommates of the patients may have either positive or negative influence on each other.

Fourth rule is "friends' friends affect us". On the simple example of being infected with a germ or with a piece of gossip through communication. Also, we can say on the example of the attitude towards those being sick in the hospital – it can be perceived either as time to reconsider, recover, healing alone time or a reason to panic and affect with this attitude all the social circles and the patient and thus his/her mental health included.

Fifth rule states that "network has a life of its own". This case the author explains by very easily comprehended analogy: the taste of the cake transcends the simple sum of ingredients into something more complicated and advanced in taste and flavour.

So, to continue one of the feeling good factors is social capital of the patient.

Bourdieu's "master concepts" can be summarized as follows: *capital* refers to valued resources in different guises (economic capital as financial assets, *cultural capital* as educational credentials, knowledge, and cultural goods, *social capital* as network-derived resources, and *symbolic capital* as prestige or legitimate authority). A *field* is "a social space of objective relations between positions" – essentially, a structured context in which agents and their capital endowments interact and compete. And *habitus* refers to the internalized dispositions, habits, and ways of perceiving that individuals develop through their life experiences and social position (their "feel for the game" in a given field). Habitus and field are in a dialectical relationship: the field conditions what resources (capital) are effective, and habitus is the embodied history of one's position in fields, guiding how one uses capital.

Within this framework, social capital is one species of capital that individuals deploy in fields. Bourdieu emphasized that, actually, all forms of capital are interlinked and together reproduce the social structure. For example, a person's family background might endow them with substantial economic capital and cultural capital (e.g. elite education); these, in turn, enable that person to move in high-status social circles and accumulate social capital (connections to influential others). Conversely, having strong social capital (say, connections to employers or professors) can help an individual acquire cultural credentials or economic opportunities.

Bourdieu wrote that all forms of capital, being "organically related to positions in social space," tend to *reproduce themselves*: those who already possess capital can use it to secure more, and thus maintain or improve their position. Social capital in particular helps to *"embed the actor's position further"* in the social structure, as network ties yield ongoing benefits that reinforce one's status. This creates a feedback loop: "positions of actors are both the cause and the effect of all forms of past accumulations of capital, particularly social capital". In simpler terms, people who occupy advantaged positions can build extensive networks (high social capital), and those networks then provide further advantages that solidify the person's position.

Thus, social capital has a context-dependent and cumulative character in Bourdieu's theory. It is *"highly context-specific as a direct consequence of the relativity among the social, cultural, economic and symbolic fields"*. This is one reason Bourdieu was skeptical of treating social capital as an abstract quantity of a whole society – for him, it only has meaning relative to a particular field and social context, where the value of connections is defined by the field's structure.

It should be noted that Bourdieu's focus on the convertibility of capital also implies a hierarchy: he was often interpreted (and criticized) as privileging *economic capital* as the ultimately most "fundamental" form. Indeed, he argued that in the last instance, economic capital (accumulated labor or wealth) is the form into which other capitals can be ultimately converted. For example, cultural distinctions or social connections can often be monetized. Scholars have critiqued this view as reductionist for privileging economic capital as the ultimate source and eventual exchange form of all other capitals. Bourdieu was also critiqued for portraying social action as somewhat *"interest-bound"* or strategic (even when discussing cultural practices or social ties), which some saw as aligning too closely with rational-choice or utilitarian thinking (an ironic parallel with approaches he otherwise differed from). Nonetheless, the strength of Bourdieu's framework is its holistic integration of material and symbolic power: social capital, like cultural and economic capital, is one piece of a larger system explaining how inequality is produced and perpetuated.

He famously wrote that different forms of capital together "explain the structure and dynamics of differentiated societies". Social capital was, for Bourdieu, inseparable from this wider theory of practice – it cannot be divorced from concepts of habitus (which inclines individuals to cultivate certain networks) and field (which defines what networks are valuable and how capital can be used). This richness also makes Bourdieu's version of social capital relatively complex and nuanced. Later scholars have noted that Bourdieu's concept is deeply reliant on the context of a particular social space and resists simplifying or universalizing. This complexity may be why, for many years, researchers outside sociology tended to favor simpler notions of social capital, only more recently returning to Bourdieu's formulation as they grapple with issues of power and inequality in social networks.

Bourdieu's early work on social capital (first published in 1980) initially garnered limited attention in the English-speaking academy. However, by the late 1980s and 1990s, other theorists independently advanced their own formulations of social capital, often with quite different emphases. Notably, James S. Coleman and Robert D. Putnam became central figures in popularizing the concept, each orienting it toward different theoretical traditions. In turn, sociologists such as Alejandro Portes critically examined these formulations, clarifying the concept and cautioning against its misuse. It is useful to distinguish the major approaches: one review identifies *three* broad schools of thought on social capital, corresponding roughly to Bourdieu, Coleman, and Putnam.

The *first* approach (exemplified by Bourdieu) treats social capital same way as other forms of capital – economic, cultural, symbolic – as a resource that gives individuals competitive advantages and thus helps explain social stratification.

The *second* (exemplified by Coleman) merges sociological and economic viewpoints, focusing on how social ties function (through norms, trust, etc.) to produce benefits for individuals or groups, with an implicit assumption of rational actors utilizing these ties.

The *third* (exemplified by Putnam (1993) and communitarian thinkers) shifts the level of analysis to large collectives, defining social capital in terms of societal traits like trust, civic norms, and networks that improve the efficiency and cohesion of society as a whole. Below, we outline Coleman's and Putnam's contributions and how they diverge from – or build upon – Bourdieu's concept, followed by Portes' critical assessments and more recent theoretical developments.

James Coleman theory of Social Capital as Functional Social Structure

James Coleman, an American sociologist working within a rational-choice and functionalist paradigm, introduced social capital into modern sociological discourse with a distinct focus from Bourdieu's. In his influential 1988 article "Social Capital in the Creation of Human Capital," Coleman defined social capital by its function – "some aspect of social structure that facilitates certain actions of actors… within the structure". This definition sees social capital not as a personal asset per se, but as a feature of the social environment (relationships, networks, norms) that makes possible the achievement of goals that would be difficult in its absence. Coleman's approach is often described as "productivism" or instrumental: social capital is *productive* in the sense that it enables outcomes (much as physical or human capital do) that actors value. For example, a norm of mutual help or a network of obliging neighbors can help a person accomplish tasks or obtain resources that, alone, they could not – hence those social ties have "capital" value in enabling action.

Coleman explicitly sought to incorporate social capital into a theory bridging the micro-macro gap in sociology. He positioned his explanation in between two theoretical traditions: (1) a *functionalist* perspective (from Durkheim, Parsons, etc.) which emphasizes how social structures constrain and guide action, and (2) a *rational actor* perspective (from economics) which views individuals as goal-oriented and self-interested. In Coleman's view, social capital is a resource that inheres in the *structure of relations among actors* and can thus be used to explain both individual-level outcomes and collective-level phenomena.

He famously illustrated social capital through examples like the network of wholesale diamond traders who rely on trust to lend gems to each other – the trust and enforceable norms within that community constitute social capital that lowers transaction costs and facilitates their economic activity. Coleman identified several forms or sources of social capital, such as obligations and expectations (credit slips created by doing favors), norms and effective sanctions, and information channels (access to knowledge via contacts). These all describe how certain network structures (e.g. a tightly-knit community with strong norms of reciprocity) can yield tangible benefits to members. Notably, Coleman placed heavy importance on *"closure"* of social networks (i.e. a network where members are densely interconnected). He argued that closed networks foster strong norms and trust – for instance, if everyone in a community knows each other, a reputation for trustworthiness is enforced and obligations are more likely to be repaid. This emphasis on network closure and internal cohesion was later critiqued (as we shall see), but it was central to Coleman's understanding of how social structure produces value.

In comparison to Bourdieu, Coleman's formulation had a more *benign and collective* tone. While Bourdieu saw social capital as contributing to the exclusion of outsiders and the reproduction of elite advantage, Coleman treated social capital as, in many cases, a *public good*. He famously noted that parents who cultivate a strong community (say, by volunteering in a Parent-Teacher Association) generate social capital that benefits not just their own but all children in the school – because norms of educational support or trust among community members help everyone's kids. In Coleman's words, when individuals create social ties or uphold norms, "direct contributions by actors will benefit the whole". Strong families and communities build social capital through bonding ties, and "internal community social links" are seen as broadly beneficial. Unlike Bourdieu's zero-sum view, Coleman did not foreground the idea that one person's social capital could exclude another; instead, he was interested in how *social capital brings about integration and cooperation.* Indeed, Coleman saw social capital as a resource that *increases* social cohesion (he describes it as a *"bonding mechanism"* that adds to the integration of society). In his analysis, social capital often arises inadvertently as a byproduct of social organization (for example, a close-knit religious community may develop mutual aid practices that then constitute social capital).

In sum, Coleman's work was pivotal in moving social capital into mainstream sociological theory (especially in the United States) and highlighting its *functional role in facilitating action*, but it departed from Bourdieu by downplaying conflict and stratification. This set the stage for the next major interpretation by Putnam (2000), which took an even more collective, society-wide perspective.

Robert Putnam, a political scientist, further popularized social capital in the 1990s, giving it a communitarian and civic twist. Putnam's interest in the concept arose from questions about effective governance and democracy. In *"Making Democracy Work"* (1993) and later in the famous *"Bowling Alone"* article (1995) and book (2000), Putnam defines social capital in collective terms, as *"features of social organization, such as networks, norms, and trust, that facilitate action and cooperation for mutual benefit"*. This definition reflects Putnam's focus on *community-level properties* – unlike Bourdieu (individual resources) or Coleman (relations that benefit actors), Putnam speaks of social capital as an attribute of a community or nation, manifest in the prevalence of civic networks and a culture of trust and reciprocity. In Putnam's formulation, *social capital is essentially the glue of society*: communities high in social capital are those where people are civically engaged, trust one another, join together in associations, and cooperate for the common good.

A hallmark of Putnam's contribution was his empirical claim that social capital (so defined) has been in *decline* in modern societies, particularly in the United States late in the 20th century. He famously documented drops in indicators like voter turnout, membership in clubs and civic organizations, church attendance, and even informal socializing – encapsulated in the metaphor that Americans were "bowling alone" rather than in leagues. This decline in participation was linked, in Putnam's view, to eroding trust and civic engagement, which he saw as alarming for democracy.

Putnam's early study "Making Democracy Work" compared Italian regions and found that *regions with dense networks of civic associations and high interpersonal trust (i.e. high social capital) had much better governance and institutional perfor-*

mance. He extrapolated this idea to argue that social capital is a key determinant of effective democratic society: *"working together is easier in a community blessed with a substantial stock of social capital"*. If we extrapolate these statements of Putnam – we can assume that these two factors – high interpersonal trust and high social capital work the same way in smaller social institutes, that is – hospitals.

We should underline that *high social capital regions or societies purportedly enjoy not only better government but also faster economic growth and lower crime* – essentially a multitude of positive outcomes. This line of reasoning elevated social capital to a *diagnostic tool for societal health*, a measurable quantity that could explain why some societies prosper and others lag. For example, Putnam cited Francis Fukuyama's assertion that *social capital (especially generalized trust) is the sine qua non of stable liberal democracy and even a lubricant for modern economies*. Here we bump not only into the already known definition of *social capital*, but also into the definition of *trust*. Peter Sztompka (Sztompka, 2007) in his famous book "Trust as the Foundation of Society" underlines that, together with social connections *trust* has a special meaning because if we don't trust our social circles than we can't even get up from bed in the morning, we can't build family, friends, business connections and, talking about hospitals – we should trust surgeon to implement necessary procedures, nurses – to do the necessary care after and our relatives and friends that they will support us. Sztompka underlines that trust and refers to the earlier works of Luhmann – who said that it is not just belief, it "is being given in advance, like prepayment is being done counting on luck" (Luhmann, 1979).

In developing these ideas, Putnam built on Coleman's notion that social networks have value for society, but he explicitly moved to the *macro level*. He treated social capital as an *"aggregate trait"* – something a whole city, region or nation could possess in varying degrees, measurable via surveys of trust or counts of civic associations. Furthermore, Putnam introduced a now-famous distinction between *"bonding"* and *"bridging"* social capital (and later, scholars added "linking" social capital). *Bonding social capital* refers to ties within a homogeneous group – e.g. family, close friends, or an ethnic enclave – which bolster internal solidarity and support. *Bridging social capital* refers to ties that connect people across diverse social cleavages (such as class, race, religion, or other divides). *"The first type of capital expands networks while the second increases their cohesion"*.

Both types, according to Putnam, have benefits: bonding capital provides emotional and material support (a safety net within tight-knit groups), while bridging capital spreads information and fosters broader identities and reciprocity across society. However, they are not equally good for all outcomes – an excess of bonding without bridging can lead to factionalism or insularity, whereas bridging ties are often linked to generalized trust and a more inclusive society. Putnam argued that an ideal community would have a healthy balance of bonding and bridging social capital. For instance, strong bonds within a neighborhood are valuable, but if that neighborhood also has connections outward (bridging ties), it will be better integrated into the wider society. This bridging/bonding distinction was an important theoretical development that extended the social capital concept beyond what Bourdieu or Coleman had articulated, incorporating an understanding of *network structure diversity* into the conversation.

While Putnam's work sparked enormous interest across the social sciences and even policy circles, it too faced *substantial criticism*. Many scholars pointed out that Putnam's analyses often blur *cause and effect*. He sometimes treated social capital (measured by trust or association membership) as the cause of various good outcomes (good government, economic prosperity), but critics argued he failed to demonstrate the direction of causality. For example, does a high-trust society cause good government, or does effective, fair governance foster trust in institutions and among citizens? Putnam's famous finding that northern Italy had higher social capital (and better government) than the south could be interpreted in multiple ways – Portes (1998) and others noted that Putnam *"simply engages in an ex post facto analysis... reverberating the same tautological reasoning"*, effectively saying the north's success is due to its stock of social capital, which is inferred from the same success. This circularity (using outcomes to define the cause) makes it difficult to use social capital as a truly explanatory concept. Additionally, *measurement* issues plagued Putnam's approach: relying on proxy indicators like survey questions about trust or counting club memberships may not capture the full complexity of social capital, and such measures can be culturally biased or too coarse. Critics also charged that Putnam *romanticized the past* and glossed over factors like inequality, power, and context.

For instance, high levels of association membership in mid-20th-century America (Putnam's baseline for "good" social capital) coexisted with the exclusion of women and minorities from many civic opportunities – raising the question, *whose* social capital and whose cooperation are we measuring? Scholars like Foley and Edwards (1999) and Woolcock (2001) have emphasized that *context matters*: trust and networks mean different things in different environments, and national aggregates hide local variations.

Moreover, the "dark side" of social capital – something Bourdieu implicitly recognized – got little attention in Putnam's early work. Tight-knit communities can enforce negative norms (e.g. organized crime networks have high internal trust) or exclude others (e.g. high bonding capital in an ethnic group might coincide with suspicion toward outsiders). Putnam acknowledged some of these issues later and cautioned that social capital is not automatically benevolent.

Still, much of the critique centered on the *over-simplification* in the communitarian view: by treating social capital as an almost uniformly positive resource like a public virtue, one risks ignoring how it can also *reinforce inequality or work against outsiders*. Alejandro Portes succinctly noted that *"social capital, to be sure, is not all roses"* – it has downsides like any form of power (e.g. the capacity for exclusion, excess claims on group members, restrictions on individual freedoms, and downward leveling norms in tightly bonded groups). Putnam's framework was less equipped to theorize these negative consequences, whereas Bourdieu's was centered on them.

Despite these criticisms, Putnam's legacy was to firmly install social capital in the vocabulary of *public discourse* and a wide array of academic fields (from economics to public health to urban studies). His work led to an outpouring of empirical studies in the late 1990s and 2000s attempting to measure social capital at regional or national levels and link it to outcomes like economic growth, health indicators, crime rates, and so forth. This, as other scientists call it, *impressive wave of empirical research,* attests to the appeal of the concept.

However, as Portes (2000) and others warned, stretching the concept to ever larger aggregates and treating it as a causal variable in growth or governance can lead to conceptual dilution. If virtually any positive social trait (low corruption, high trust, many clubs) is dubbed "social capital," the term risks losing analytical precision. Portes argued that social capital is most useful when kept to its core meaning – the benefits of social ties – and used *"as shorthand for the positive consequences of sociability"* But *"excessive extensions of the concept may jeopardize its heuristic value"*. In essence, using "social capital" to explain national wealth or democratic stability might be going too far, since those phenomena have deep historical and structural roots (of which social networks and norms are only a part). This caution aligns with Bourdieu's insistence on context: social capital is embedded in concrete social structures, not an independent substance a society simply "has" or "lacks."

Alejandro Portes has been one of the key sociologists providing clarity and critique on social capital theory. In his influential 1998 article *"Social Capital: Its Origins and Applications in Modern Sociology,"* Portes reviews the definitions by Bourdieu, Coleman, and others, and commends Bourdieu's formulation as "arguably the most theoretically refined". Portes emphasizes that Bourdieu's analysis focused on how individuals deliberately construct and use networks for gain, linking the concept to power and instrumental action – aspects that later versions, especially Putnam's, downplayed. Portes contributed by *systematizing the concept*: he identified and illustrated several distinct *functions* of social capital (for example, as a source of social control, as support from family and kin, and as resources mediated by broader networks). These correspond to observable benefits like maintaining discipline and norms (social control), providing assistance to members (family support), and opening access to opportunities through connections (network-mediated benefits). Crucially, Portes (1998) also catalogued the *negative consequences* that often accompany these same processes. He outlined at least four downsides: (1)

exclusion of outsiders – a tightly bonded group can bar others from accessing the same resources; (2) *excess claims on group members* – those who have strong social capital within a group may face heavy obligations and constraints (e.g. pressure to share resources with less fortunate kin); (3) *restriction on individual freedoms* – strong group cohesion and norms can limit personal choice and innovation; and (4) *downward leveling norms* – in groups suffering adversity or marginalization, strong internal ties may enforce norms that impede members' success (for instance, peers discouraging someone from "getting above" their social station). By articulating these, Portes (1998) made it clear that *social capital is a double-edged sword*: the same network mechanisms that help some can harm others or have costs. This balanced perspective was a corrective to overly optimistic views.

Through the 2000s and 2010s, *social capital theory evolved and diversified* in its applications. Researchers have examined social capital in contexts ranging from schools (educational outcomes), workplaces (career advancement), public health (how community networks influence health behaviors and outcomes), to digital communities (online social capital). The core idea remains the value of social connections, but there is ongoing debate about how to properly *define and measure* social capital in these various domains. A review of the literature noted persistent *"conceptual ambiguity and misspecification"* – different studies often mean very different things by "social capital," and measures are not consistent.

For instance, one study might measure social capital by counting club memberships, another by trust surveys, another by network analysis of friendships, making it hard to compare results.

We can suggest to count social capital by directly asking respondents in the interview the number of close friends that they have and the number of followers in social media. This will give us a bigger picture about the level of tight social reliable connections as well as the level of influence a person has on others through the number of followers. This counts as well when we consider socializing art works being made in a hospital. So, for patients' *social capital* will mean both: having moral support during hard times as well as sharing their texts, videos, drawings and may be even music with the public they have available. Even through publishing their art (in whatever form on any public platform) their social capital can skyrocket, just because more and more people might get attracted to it. And together with social capital and creativity comes *trust* a base to create and as a foundation of any communication being implemented.

And now let's get back to the Connected theory. All the factors mentioned in this chapter – social capital, creativity and trust, should finally lead us to achieve happy states of mind. Though the authors state that "lasting happiness is difficult to achieve because people are on a "hedonic treadmill"" (Christakis & Fowler, 2009). And still out of this scientific study we get inspiring information that can be applied towards patients: happiness, they say, 50% is depending on our genes (this we, as sociologists, can't change), 10% being happy depend on the circumstances (this we already can change even in hospital environment) and 40% on what people choose to think and do. And obviously we can influence also the way of thinking by dropping the ideas of mental regulation, trust and creative self-expression into the minds of the patients, for example. Moreover, in their study, Christakis and Fowler found that a person is 45% more likely to be happy if a friend became happy in the previous six months, so we can state that happiness is contagious. Also we can assume that patterns of behavior that lead to happiness like being trusted and creative, are also easily spread even among patients that spend their time in one room in hospital.

CONCLUSIONS

In our chapter we studied how social circles – that is, social capital of every patient can contribute or hinder the recovery process. We also consider awakening of creativity as a part of a recovering process and social circles – as a potentially supportive environment for this.

In this chapter we unite the process of opening up the creativity with the amount of social surrounding and level of social trust and consider this to be supportive and beneficial environment to create and recover on the example of hospital.

The environment around the patient that either can either support or discourage the creativity, so we consider such definitions as social capital and social trust.

Pierre Bourdieu's theory of social capital remains a foundational reference point in sociology, emphasizing that social networks are not merely sociable niceties but forms of capital deeply enmeshed in power and inequality. We have seen how Bourdieu's original formulation – rooted in concepts of habitus, field, and conversion of capitals – framed social capital as a mechanism of *social reproduction* that advantages those already well-positioned. Later scholars like Coleman and Putnam reinterpreted social capital in more optimistic or collective lights: as a resource for productive ends or a vital ingredient of democratic society. Their contributions broadened the concept's appeal and application, but also invited critiques for oversimplifying or idealizing the social dimensions of cooperation. The dialogue between these perspectives, sharpened by analysts such as Portes (1998), has enriched our theoretical understanding: it forced recognition of social capital's *bright and dark sides*, its micro and macro manifestations, and the need for methodological rigor in its study.

In contemporary sociology, social capital is both widely applied and continually debated. It has been adapted to explain phenomena in diverse contexts – from how immigrant communities mobilize resources, to how "networking" on social media might yield advantages – yet scholars are careful to specify what aspect of social capital they mean (trust, networks, or resources) and to acknowledge the context-bound nature of its effects. In summary, Bourdieu's concept of social capital has evolved from a technical term in a theory of class stratification to a versatile (if sometimes nebulous) paradigm spanning multiple disciplines. Its core insight endures: *social relationships, and the resources flowing through them, are key to understanding both individual success, the fabric of social life* – all these factors become essential and crucial in the moments, when a person needs help in the hospital at least in moral support, and of course if we need the confirmation of whom to trust on the conducting surgery or to whom show the creative artwork that was done during the time being sick.

REFERENCES

Bourdieu, P. (1984). *Distinction: A Social Critique of the Judgment of Taste*. Harvard University Press.

Bourdieu, P. (1986). The Forms of Capital. In Richardson, J. G. (Ed.), *Handbook of Theory and Research for the Sociology of Education* (pp. 241–258). Greenwood Press.

Bourdieu, P., & Wacquant, L. (1992). *An Invitation to Reflexive Sociology*. University of Chicago Press.

Coleman, J. S. (1988). Social Capital in the Creation of Human Capital. *American Journal of Sociology*, *94*(Supplement), S95–S120. DOI: 10.1086/228943

Foley, M. W., & Edwards, B. (1999). Is it Time to Disinvest in Social Capital? *Journal of Public Policy*, *19*(2), 141–173. DOI: 10.1017/S0143814X99000215

Nicholas A.. Christakis, & Fowler, J. H. (2009). Connected: The Amazing Power of Social Networks and How They Shape Our Lives. HarperPress.

Portes, A. (1998). Social Capital: Its Origins and Applications in Modern Sociology. *Annual Review of Sociology*, *24*(1), 1–24. DOI: 10.1146/annurev.soc.24.1.1

Putnam, R. D. (1993). *Making Democracy Work: Civic Traditions in Modern Italy*. Princeton University Press.

Putnam, R. D. (2000). *Bowling Alone: The Collapse and Revival of American Community*. Simon & Schuster.

Woolcock, M. (2001). The Place of Social Capital in Understanding Social and Economic Outcomes. [Plus additional analyses by Woolcock & Narayan on "linking" social capital]. *Canadian Journal of Policy Research*, *2*(1), 11–17.

Chapter 7
Patient Safety in Health Professions Education: Educational Frameworks and Evaluation of Patient Safety in Nursing

Daniela Bartoníčková
https://orcid.org/0000-0003-0220-2944
Faculty of Health Sciences, Palacky University, Olomouc, Czech Republic

ABSTRACT

This chapter examines how patient safety is integrated into nursing education by synthesizing international competency frameworks and their corresponding measurement instruments. It reviews general frameworks—the National Patient Safety Education Framework (NPSEF), the World Health Organization's Patient Safety Curriculum Guide, the Canadian Safety Competencies Framework, and EUNetPaS—and nursing-specific models including Quality and Safety Education for Nurses (QSEN) and the Patient Safety Competency Frameworks (PSCF[a], PSCF[b]). The chapter maps core domains (teamwork, communication, human and system factors, risk management, and safety culture) to curricular design and clinical learning, and evaluates widely used tools (e.g., H-PEPSS, PaSNEQ, SAQ, HSOPS-NS, JCAT-NE) for their structure, validity, and applicability across various settings. The synthesis demonstrates how structured frameworks and validated instruments enable benchmarking, identify gaps, and advance a sustained culture of safety in nursing education and practice.

DOI: 10.4018/979-8-3373-5931-1.ch007

PATIENT SAFETY IN HEALTH PROFESSIONS EDUCATION

Calls to embed patient safety within the education of health professionals date back at least to the Institute of Medicine's landmark work at the turn of the century (Institute of Medicine [IOM] Committee on Quality of Health Care in America, 2000). *Health Professions Education: A Bridge to Quality* stated that graduates were not adequately prepared to deliver high-quality, safe care and articulated a competency-based instructional agenda: patient-centered care, team-based practice, evidence-based practice, quality improvement, and informatics (Institute of Medicine (U.S.) Committee on the Health Professions Education Summit, 2003). Since then, integrating patient safety content into undergraduate health curricula has become a global priority; nevertheless, the extent and regulatory oversight of such integration remain uneven across disciplines and jurisdictions, with nursing often lacking explicit curricular regulation compared to medicine (Kirwan et al., 2019).

Even before the IOM's 2003 call, the American Association of Colleges of Nursing (AACN) underscored that nurses should be equipped with competencies in patient safety and quality as part of the baccalaureate curriculum, identifying early domains such as critical thinking, health policy and systems, communication, disease management, ethics, and information technologies. These expectations were refined in *The Essentials of Baccalaureate Education for Professional Nursing Practice* (American Association of College of Nursing, 2006). Despite such momentum, early evaluations highlighted persistent curricular gaps. Attree, Cooke, and Wakefield (2008) observed that nursing programs frequently underemphasized patient safety and called for coordinated global action. Subsequent guidance proliferated to support the design of safety-oriented curricula (Kirwan et al., 2019).

The International Council of Nurses (ICN) subsequently issued a position statement emphasizing that patient safety is foundational to quality nursing care and should be addressed from initial qualification onwards. Priority domains include continuous quality improvement, environmental protection and risk management (including infection prevention and control), safe medication administration, equipment and workplace safety, clinical safety, safe care environments, and the development of integrated, evidence-based, and enabling infrastructures. ICN also delineated responsibilities for nurses and national nursing associations, including informing patients/families about risks; prompt reporting of adverse events; active participation in safety and quality evaluation; strengthening communication; fostering positive practice environments; supporting infection prevention programs; advocating standardized protocols; staffing and skill-mix adequacy; promoting education and research; establishing clear reporting policies and disclosure processes; creating national reporting systems to monitor, analyze, and learn from events; and reinforcing oversight through accreditation (International Council of Nurses [ICN], 2022).

In Europe, revision of Directive 2005/36/EC (amended by 2013/55/EU) set minimum training requirements for nurses. Article 31 (7) specifies core capabilities irrespective of training location, including independent nursing assessment and planning using current theoretical and clinical knowledge; organization and delivery of care; effective interprofessional collaboration; health promotion; immediate life-saving and adverse event response; counseling and support; quality assurance and evaluation; interprofessional communication; and analysis of care quality for professional development. The European Federation of Nurses Associations (EFN) operationalized these expectations through the EFN Competency Framework, defining competence as the intersection of knowledge, skills, attitudes, and values mobilized to address real situations, and mapping learning outcomes across subjects. Within quality and safety, proposed educational objectives include creating and maintaining safe care environments via quality assurance and risk management strategies; using appropriate tools to assess and identify actual/potential risks; and recording and communicating safety issues to relevant authorities (European Federation of Nurses Associations [EFNA], 2015).

Despite EU Council recommendations to include patient safety across undergraduate and postgraduate training, nursing education providers have not consistently operationalized this agenda. A 27-country RANCARE study reported that safety content is often unspecified in nursing curricula and tends to emphasize instrumental competencies (e.g., infection control, hand hygiene, medication and transfusion administration, fall prevention, occupational health and safety), while human factors and sociocultural aspects are underrepresented or hidden within courses (Boucaut & Cusack, 2016; Kirwan et al., 2019; Lee et al., 2020). Consequently, students may not sufficiently develop critical thinking and related capabilities in these areas. Internationally, despite logistical barriers, some countries—notably the United States, the United Kingdom, and Australia—have made substantive progress in curricular integration (Mansour et al., 2018). Crucially, authors argue that instruction encompassing human factors and sociocultural aspects must begin early in undergraduate nursing education (Mansour et al., 2018). Rather than adding yet another discrete course to congested programs, educators should embed patient safety competencies throughout curricula (Leotsakos et al., 2014). Integrative reviews further recommend a systems-oriented approach and deliberate cultivation of a safety culture in how students are taught and supervised (Bedgood & Mellott, 2021). Nevertheless, consistent with prior studies (e.g., Kirwan et al., 2019; Lee et al., 2020; Lukewich et al., 2015; Mansour et al., 2012), safety content in many bachelor-level programs remains implicit, and sociocultural aspects are insufficiently implemented. Tella et al. (2015) additionally underscore the importance of educating for safety culture within clinical placements.

Educational Frameworks & Evaluation of Patient Safety in Nursing

Among frameworks designed to support the integration of patient safety into nursing curricula, two have achieved particular prominence internationally—the WHO Patient Safety Curriculum Guide and Quality and Safety Education for Nurses (QSEN)—though the literature identifies six frameworks overall (Bartoníčková et al., 2023). For analytic clarity, these could be grouped into general frameworks (applicable across health professions, including nursing) and nursing-specific frameworks (developed explicitly for nursing). All frameworks define safety-relevant domains and associated competencies that nursing students should master before qualification.

General Educational Frameworks

Among the educational frameworks for implementing patient safety in the curricula of health professions programs—including nursing—are the Australian National Patient Safety Education Framework (NPSEF) (basis for the WHO Patient Safety Curriculum Guide), the Canadian Safety Competencies Framework (SCF), and the framework of the European Network for Patient Safety (EUNetPaS). The educational areas derived from these frameworks comprise a list of competencies for health professionals (Table 1) about patient safety. This sub-chapter elaborates on the individual general educational frameworks for health professions fields, including nursing.

Australian National Patient Safety Education Framework (NPSEF)

The Australian National Patient Safety Education Framework was created by the Australian Commission on Safety and Quality in Health Care, in cooperation with the national Ministry of Health, in 2005. The aim was to intensify efforts to improve the safety and quality of healthcare and reduce the occurrence of adverse events in the delivery of care. The NPSEF interprets the knowledge, skills, behaviors, attitudes, and performances required of health professionals to assume responsibility for providing safe care. It was developed based on an extensive literature review and designed to assist organizations in creating educational curricula and developing new programs or auditing existing ones, with the programs grounded in students' competencies in patient safety. Foundational principles were also established, including: safety is everyone's responsibility; patient orientation; the importance of the health care consumer perspective; an emphasis on quality of care; simplicity, flexibility, and accessibility; general applicability; standardized and comprehensible language; evidence-based practice; and relevance for institutional education (Australian Commission on Safety and Quality in Health Care [ACSQHC], 2005). Patient safety is defined as *"the prevention of harm caused by errors of commission and omission. The process by which an organization ensures safer care for patients. The process should include: risk assessment; identification, reporting, and analysis of incidents; the ability to learn from incidents, to follow up on them, and to implement solutions that minimize the risk of recurrence."* (Australian Commission on Safety and Quality in Health Care, 2005).

The primary objective of the NPSEF was to summarize the competencies that a health professional should possess in relation to providing safe care, regardless of the individual's position or role within the organization. The NPSEF, therefore, includes 22 competencies grouped into seven key learning areas (domains) as follows:

- Communicating Effectively
- Using Evidence and Information
- Identifying, Preventing, and Managing Adverse Events and Near Misses
- Working Safely
- Being Ethical
- Continuing Learning
- Specific Issues (Australian Commission on Safety and Quality in Health Care, 2005)

The framework's content matrix is divided into four educational levels from basic to organizational, with each level described by learning objectives and the required knowledge, skills, behaviors, and attitudes (Australian Commission on Safety and Quality in Health Care, 2005; Walton et al., 2006; World Health Organization, 2011).

According to Walton et al. (2006), the NPSEF is used across various quality and safety initiatives, such as the development of medical curricula, the development of curricula for professional training, the development of safety and quality modules, the implementation of performance elements into training within vocational education for support personnel, and by various organizations to support education in quality and safety. Despite its broad contribution, King and Anderson (2012) note that its utility is more apparent among health professionals in clinical environments than within educational institutions. Based on this, the WHO developed the Patient Safety Curriculum Guide for Medical Schools (World Health Organization, 2009), which also underpins its updated edition (World Health Organization, 2011).

WHO Patient Safety Curriculum Guide

The WHO published the Patient Safety Curriculum Guide for Medical Schools in 2009 (World Health Organization, 2009) and updated it in 2011 as the Patient Safety Curriculum Guide: Multiprofessional Edition. The International Council of Nurses was among the partners involved in its publication. It was highlighted that the new version could raise awareness of the need to integrate patient safety into the curricula of all health professionals, including nurses. The guide draws on the Australian NPSEF and therefore includes all 22 competencies (seven educational areas). Additionally, within the final educational area—Specific Issues—it introduced a competency related to infection prevention and control. The guide's core principles are the development of student competencies in patient safety, flexibility, transparent and accessible language, availability, and support for the learning environment (World Health Organization, 2011). Patient safety is defined as *"the reduction of risk of unnecessary harm associated with health care to an acceptable minimum"* (World Health Organization, 2011, p. 81).

The first part of the guide is intended for educators and summarizes how topics were selected, the guide's learning objectives and principles, and approaches for embedding patient safety teaching into curricula. It also presents fundamental principles for delivering safety education, activities to support topic comprehension, options for assessing patient safety learning and curricula, a range of web resources, and approaches to supporting international efforts in patient safety education. The second part elaborates on the teaching topics, reflecting NPSEF's competencies. The official eleven teaching topics (module titles) are:

- What Is Patient Safety?
- Why Applying Human Factors Is Important for Patient Safety
- Understanding Systems and the Effect of Complexity on Patient Care
- Being an Effective Team Player
- Learning from Errors to Prevent Harm
- Understanding and Managing Clinical Risk/Harm
- Using Quality-Improvement Methods to Improve Care
- Engaging with Patients and Carers
- Infection Prevention and Control
- Patient Safety and Invasive Procedures
- Improving Medication Safety (World Health Organization, 2011).

Each teaching category defines the required performance and knowledge to be demonstrated upon qualification. Each area also includes key aspects, learning objectives, teaching strategies, and examples of teaching methods, such as case studies (World Health Organization, 2009; World Health Organization, 2011).

In evaluating the WHO guide, Mansour et al. (2015) reported that, although it does not prescribe detailed instructions on how patient safety should be taught, its effectiveness—through raising awareness and improving preparedness for safe practice—was highly rated by students and educators. According to the authors, the WHO guide offers a more explicit understanding of human factors and the impact of systems on patient safety than other educational frameworks, while also adequately addressing students' instrumental skills (Mansour, 2012; Mansour et al., 2015). It is therefore commended both for its adaptability across countries, cultures, and systems, and for its impact on human factors and a systems approach to patient safety. However, an assessment of patient safety within the EU found that the guide's topics are more often integrated across curricula rather than addressed as stand-alone thematic blocks (Kirwan et al., 2019).

Safety Competencies Framework (SCF)

Following the publication of the Australian national framework, the Canadian Patient Safety Institute (CPSI) developed the Safety Competencies Framework in 2008. The project's primary goal was to define the requirements for delivering safe healthcare. The SCF thus comprises interprofessional safety competencies for health professionals, developed based on the internationally recognized CanMEDS framework of the Royal College and the methodology used to formulate professional competencies for physicians. Initially, 23 key competencies were specified and organized into six domains. The SCF was launched as "The Safety Competencies: Enhancing Patient Safety across the Health Professions" and was designed to serve as a guide for educational institutions across various health professional groups (Frank & Brien, 2008). The framework adopted a definition of patient safety as *"the reduction and mitigation of unsafe acts within the healthcare system, as well as the use of best practices shown to lead to optimal patient outcomes."* (Davies et al., 2003, p. 11). The SCF's key principles include the interpretation of knowledge, skills, and attitudes related to patient safety competencies for all health professionals, as well as simplicity, flexibility, and clarity with broad applicability (Frank & Brien, 2008). Following publication, many countries incorporated the framework into their national standards or utilized it to develop educational materials for clinical practice. In 2016, CPSI released the Report on the Integration of the Safety Competencies Framework into Health Professions Education Programs in Canada, stating that educational organizations primarily use the SCF to enhance learning outcomes and to review students' competencies before clinical placements. Testimonials in the Report documented the framework's effectiveness and growing popularity, as well as opportunities for improvement (Canadian Patient Safety Institute [CPSI], 2016).

Subsequently, CPSI, together with Patients for Patient Safety Canada, revised the initial edition with expert input to support ongoing interprofessional education and collaboration in patient safety. The structure was retained and, in 2020, CPSI published the updated Safety Competencies Framework – 2020, which articulates 26 key competencies across these six official domain names:

- Patient Safety Culture

- Teamwork
- Communication
- Safety, Risk, and Quality Improvement
- Optimize Human and System Factors
- Recognize, Respond to, and Disclose Patient Safety Incidents

Each domain includes definitions and descriptions of key competencies, permeated by enabling knowledge, skills, and attitudes to support implementation in practice (CPSI 2020). King and Anderson (2012) note that building and transforming a culture of patient safety requires integrating patient safety competencies into the education of health professionals. According to CPSI, utilizing the SCF can accelerate the development of safety-related curricula, integrate safety and improvement methods across all educational levels, and support continuing professional development throughout the continuum of care (CPSI, 2020).

European Network for Patient Safety *(*EUNetPaS*)*

The European Network for Patient Safety project was officially launched in 2008. It was supported by the European Commission under the 2007 Public Health Programme to establish an umbrella network for all 27 EU Member States to initiate and strengthen patient safety initiatives. Within an integrated approach, the project focused on four key areas: fostering a patient safety culture, supporting education and training in patient safety, implementing a reporting and learning system for adverse events, and improving medication safety (European Union Network for Patient Safety [EUNetPaS], 2010). The European Federation of Nurses, as an associate partner of EUNetPaS, was involved in selected working groups on culture, education, and training in patient safety, medication safety, and overall project evaluation (EFNA, 2015). The principal output in the education and training area was the General Guide for Education and Training in Patient Safety. It presents general guidance for educating students in patient safety, covering what is meant by patient safety, who is involved in ensuring it, and how education and training in patient safety should be addressed (EUNetPaS, 2010). Patient safety is defined as the *"freedom of a patient from unnecessary or potential harm associated with health care"* (EUNetPaS, 2010, p. 36).

In the guide's introductory section, European collaboration on patient safety and requirements for education and training are presented. It emphasizes students' knowledge, skills, and attitudes that are key to understanding essential aspects of patient safety, including: creating a safety culture, identifying and assessing risk areas, analyzing the causes of adverse events and near misses, strategies for managing such events, and preventing errors and adverse events. The guide articulates fundamental principles—patient-centeredness, applicability across all care environments, safety as everyone's responsibility, team orientation, multidimensionality, content specificity, and continuous professional activity—and groups professional competencies under six educational areas as follows:

- Basic Knowledge, Skills, and Behaviour for Patient Safety
- Ensuring Patient Safety
- Adopting a Systems-Based Profession
- Creating a Patient Safety Culture
- Setting the Direction for Quality and Safe Health Care
- Implementation Guidance for Education and Training (EUNetPaS, 2010)

For each area, learning objectives are specified. The guide also outlines options for organizing safety education and training, and describes a curriculum design process that encompasses needs analysis, preparation of interventions, delivery, verification of understanding, and evaluation of outcomes. Recognizing the need to embed a culture of patient safety already during training, EUNetPaS also developed a web platform to support implementation (EUNetPaS, 2010; Zikos et al., 2010).

Table 1. Overview of educational areas covering healthcare professionals' competencies relating to patient safety based on general educational frameworks

NPSEF (Australian Commission on Safety and Quality in Health Care, 2005)	**SCF (Canadian Patient Safety Institute, 2020)**	**EUNetPaS (European Union Network for Patient Safety, 2010)**
Effective communication: engaging patients and caregivers as partners in health care; communicating risks; open disclosure with patients after an adverse event; obtaining informed consent; respecting cultures and ensuring awareness. Use of evidence and information: applying best available evidence-based practice; using information technology to enhance safety. Identification, prevention, and management of adverse events and errors: recognizing, reporting, and managing adverse events and near misses; managing risks; understanding adverse events in health care; handling complaints. Safe work: being a team player and assuming leadership; understanding human factors; understanding organizational complexity; ensuring continuity of care; managing fatigue and stress. Ethical issues: maintaining fitness for work and practice, as well as moral behavior and practice. Continuing education: learning in the workplace; being a workplace teacher. Specific issues include the prevention of wrong-site, wrong-procedure, or wrong-patient errors, as well as medication safety.	Patient safety culture: contributing to the creation and maintenance of a just culture; advocating for improvement of the culture of patient safety; contributing to the continuous improvement of patient safety culture. Teamwork: collaborating with patients and their families, respecting professionalism, understanding family roles and responsibilities in interprofessional collaboration, and recognizing the dynamics of interprofessional collaboration, including shared authority and leadership, as well as respectful communication and effective cooperation with all team members. Communication: effective verbal and non-verbal communication; adequate clinical documentation; communication for risk prevention; using communication technology to support safety. Safety, risk, and quality improvement: anticipating, identifying, and reducing adverse events; quality improvement; sustaining quality and safety practices. Optimization of human and system factors: identifying factors that influence performance; critical thinking to enhance decision-making; understanding the impact of human factors and technology; and recognizing the importance of human factors. Recognition, response, and disclosure of adverse events: recognizing adverse events; collaborating with patients and families; disclosing adverse events; learning from adverse events; emotional coping; supporting patients, families, and health care providers.	Core knowledge, skills, and behaviours for patient safety: appreciating the systemic nature of risk; knowledge in key safety areas; fundamentals of patient safety culture and interpersonal skills; the need for proactive planning to prevent errors. Ensuring patient safety: learning from errors and near misses, collaboration and sharing experiences with others, supporting innovation among colleagues, and promoting individual personal development. Adopting a systems-based profession: a systems approach to problem-solving; applying improvement principles; using tools and techniques to improve systems; supporting a culture of change. Creating a culture of patient safety: proactive approaches to patient safety; learning from errors and near misses; risk management; recognizing individual and group roles and responsibilities for patient safety. Setting direction for quality and safe health care: identifying opportunities for change and improvement; evidence-based approaches to patient safety; collaboration with internal and external stakeholders; implementing techniques to evaluate the impact of patient safety approaches.

Nursing-Specific Educational Frameworks

Among the educational frameworks explicitly developed for integrating patient safety into nursing curricula are the Quality and Safety Education for Nurses (QSEN), the Patient Safety Competency Framework (PSCF[a]), and the Patient Safety Competency Framework for Nursing Students (PSCF[b]). The specific competency domains derived from these frameworks for nursing students in relation to patient safety are presented in Table 2 for comparative purposes. The following section elaborates on the specific features of these frameworks, which are designed exclusively for the nursing discipline.

Quality and Safety Education for Nurses (QSEN)

The QSEN framework was developed in the United States in 2007. The project emerged in response to the publication of the initial competencies for nurses in providing safe and high-quality care by the American Association of Colleges of Nursing. Its main goal was to equip future nurses with the knowledge, skills, and attitudes required for the continuous improvement of care quality and safety (Cronenwett et al., 2007). In the first phase of the project, based on recommendations of the U.S. Institute of Medicine, six core competency domains were defined:

- Patient-centered care – recognizes the patient or designee as the source of control and a full partner in providing compassionate and coordinated care based on respect for the patient's preferences, values, and needs.
- Teamwork and Collaboration – function effectively within nursing and interprofessional teams, fostering open communication, mutual respect, and shared decision-making.
- Evidence-Based practice – integrate best current evidence with clinical expertise and patient/family preferences and values for the delivery of optimal health care.
- Quality Improvement – use data to monitor outcomes of care and continuously improve the quality and safety of health care systems.
- Informatics – use information and technology to communicate, manage knowledge, mitigate error, and support decision-making.
- Safety – minimize risk of harm to patients and providers through both system effectiveness and individual performance (Cronenwett et al., 2007; Quality and Safety Education for Nurses [QSEN], 2020).

To support understanding, learning objectives were established for each domain, specifying the expected knowledge, skills, and attitudes to be attained during undergraduate nursing education (Sherwood & Barnsteiner, 2012). Within the safety domain, patient safety was defined as *"minimization of risk of harm to patients and providers through both system effectiveness and individual performance"* (Cronenwett et al., 2007, p. 128). Students' knowledge in the domains covers human factors, basic principles of safety design, technologies that improve safety, categories of errors and hazards in care, safety culture, methods for understanding error causation and responsibility allocation, and relevant safety initiatives and regulations. These are complemented by defined skills and attitudes for nursing students (Cronenwett et al., 2007).

In the second phase, selected nursing schools were invited to pilot the integration of competencies into their curricula. A website was launched to provide teaching strategies and educational resources. Later, the American Association of Colleges of Nursing joined the project, contributing teaching materials, standards, and innovative pedagogical approaches (Cronenwett et al., 2007; Quality and Safety Education for Nurses, 2020). By 2009, QSEN had become a national initiative aimed at transforming nursing education through the integration of quality and safety competencies into curricula. Educational objectives were also formulated for postgraduate nursing programs, and the knowledge, skills, and attitudes within each domain were expanded (Cronenwett et al., 2009).

In 2010–2011, regional workshops for nurses were conducted to provide strategies for embedding quality and safety content into programs. Through a "train-the-trainer" approach, QSEN representatives supported faculty in integrating quality and safety education, mentoring students to deliver high-quality, safe care, and training new educators (Barnsteiner et al., 2013). In 2012, the book Quality and Safety in Nursing: A Competency Approach to Improving Outcomes was published, offering a comprehensive overview of nursing competencies and strategies for curricular implementation (Sherwood & Barnsteiner, 2012). The third edition (2022) includes updates on QSEN initiatives, educational and clinical techniques for building a culture of safety and quality, teaching approaches, and case studies, targeting postgraduate nursing students, educators, specialist nurses, administrators, and professionals involved in nursing development (Sherwood & Barnsteiner, 2012).

At present, quality and safety are no longer optional but mandatory subjects in U.S. nursing education (Armstrong & Barton, 2013). QSEN is widely recognized as a framework that allows competency-based student assessment and contributes to enhancing safety culture (Jones, 2013). Its relevance has also been highlighted in doctoral nursing education (Acton et al., 2017). QSEN provides a detailed mapping of each competency domain across knowledge, skills, and attitudes, accompanied by clear explanations (Mansour et al., 2015). Nevertheless, despite its broad adoption, it has been criticized for lacking dedicated components to address safety, particularly in terms of the complexity of human factors (Howard, 2010; Mansour, 2012).

Patient Safety Competency Framework (PSCF[a])

The Patient Safety Competency Framework was developed specifically for nursing in South Korea in 2012 (Lee et al., 2014). It drew upon international patient safety education frameworks, including the Australian National Patient Safety Education Framework, the Canadian Safety Competencies Framework (SCF), the U.S. QSEN framework, as well as WHO recommendations (World Health Organization, 2009; World Health Organization, 2011). The key competency domains for nursing students include:

- Response to and disclosure of adverse events
- Safety risk management
- Communication
- Teamwork and understanding of safety culture
- Informatics/awareness
- Evidence-based practice

Within each domain, students' knowledge, skills, and attitudes are assessed (Lee et al., 2014).

Patient Safety Competency Framework for Nursing Students (PSCF[b])

To further support competency-based patient safety education for nursing students, the Patient Safety Competency Framework for Nursing Students was developed in Australia in 2017 through a Delphi project. Its purpose was to reach consensus on core patient safety competencies for undergraduate nursing programs, as no such standardized framework previously existed in Australia (Levett-Jones et al., 2017).

The framework was grounded in Miller's pyramid of competence (Miller, 1990), which progresses from knowledge ("knows," "knows how") to skills and performance ("shows how," "does"). The competency domains defined in the PSCF[b] include:

- Person-Centered Care
- Therapeutic Communication
- Cultural Competence
- Teamwork and Collaborative Practice
- Clinical Reasoning
- Evidence-Based Practice
- Preventing, Minimizing, and Responding to Adverse Events
- Infection Prevention and Control
- Medication Safety

Each competency domain is described in terms of definitions, required knowledge, and skills (Levett-Jones et al., 2017). In a subsequent study, Levett-Jones et al. (2020) assessed the knowledge of 1,900 final-year nursing students across 23 institutions in Australia and New Zealand using a 45-item online test based on the PSCF[b] framework. The highest scores were recorded in person-centered care and therapeutic communication, while the lowest scores were found in infection prevention and control, as well as safe medication administration.

Table 2. Overview of educational areas concerning nurses' competencies related to patient safety based on specific educational frameworks

QSEN framework (Cronenwett et al., 2007)	Patient Safety Competency Framework (PSCF[a]) (Lee et al., 2014)	Patient Safety Competency Framework for Nursing Students (PSCF[b]) (Levett-Jones et al., 2017)
Patient-centered care	Recognition, response, and disclosure of adverse events	Person-centered care
Teamwork and collaboration	Safety risk management	Therapeutic communication
Evidence-based practice	Communication	Cultural competence
Quality improvement	Teamwork and understanding of safety culture	Teamwork and collaborative practice
Informatics	Informatics/awareness	Clinical reasoning
Safety	Evidence-based practice	Evidence-based practice
		Prevention, minimization, and response to adverse events
		Infection prevention and control
		Medication safety

Instruments for assessing patient safety among nursing students

In response to international recommendations and the development of patient safety education frameworks, nursing research has increasingly focused on measuring patient safety competencies among nursing students (Bedgood & Mellott, 2021). These competencies are most often conceptualized in terms of knowledge, skills, and attitudes, and they are typically assessed through quantitative designs such as structured questionnaires (e.g., Piscotty et al., 2013; Sullivan et al., 2009; Taskiran et al., 2020).

Self-assessment instruments have become particularly prominent in assessing patient safety. Campbell and Mackay (2001) highlighted that self-assessment can serve as a rapid and effective method for both evaluating and reinforcing professional competencies. This may explain why self-report questionnaires dominate the available tools for measuring patient safety learning in nursing education. The first self-assessment instrument explicitly designed for nursing students' patient safety knowledge, skills, and attitudes emerged in 2008, in parallel with the implementation of the QSEN framework (Schnall et al., 2008). Since then, a substantial number of tools have been developed, either directly aligned with nursing-specific frameworks or based on general health professional safety frameworks. Summaries of available instruments have been provided in scoping and systematic reviews, with between 9 and 12 distinct tools identified (Bartoníčková et al., 2023; Mortensen et al., 2022; Taskiran et al., 2020). The following overview of 14 instruments introduces the most frequently cited and psychometrically tested tools. Each is briefly described in terms of its theoretical foundation, intended scope, and basic structure.

INSTRUMENTS BASED ON GENERAL PATIENT SAFETY FRAMEWORKS

Anchored in multiprofessional frameworks (NPSEF, WHO Patient Safety Curriculum Guide, Safety Competencies Framework, EUNetPaS), current instruments rigorously operationalize sociocultural and systems-level safety competencies into psychometrically tested items. By mapping core domains—teamwork, communication, human/system factors, risk management, incident recognition/disclosure, and safety culture—onto learner-level indicators across academic and clinical settings, these tools enable standardized benchmarking, gap detection, and curriculum calibration with methodological fidelity.

Health Professional Education in Patient Safety Survey (H-PEPSS)

Developed in Canada as part of the Safety Competencies Framework (Frank & Brien, 2008), H-PEPSS is one of the most widely applied tools. It was designed to measure sociocultural dimensions of safety, such as teamwork, communication, and human factors, which are often underemphasized compared to clinical or technical safety skills.

- Structure: Originally 37 items, later refined to 16 items. The items are grouped into six domains: *Teamwork with other health professionals, Effective communication, Addressing security risks, Understanding human and environ-*

mental factors, Recognition, response and detection to adverse events and near misses, and Patient safety culture (Ginsburg et al., 2012).

- Unique features: Students respond separately based on what they learned in the *academic setting* versus the *clinical setting*, allowing for a comparison between theoretical education and practical experience.
- Testing and use: Validated across a wide range of countries, including f.e. Italy (Bressan et al., 2016), Turkey (Taskiran et al., 2020), China (Chen et al., 2019), Belgium (Bergs et al., 2021), Canada (VanDenKerkhof et al., 2017), and Australia (Stomski et al., 2018). Multiple confirmatory factor analyses confirmed the six-factor model, and internal consistency values were consistently high across the studies (Cronbach's $\alpha = 0.81–0.85$).

Patient Safety in Nursing Education Questionnaire (PaSNEQ)

Originating from the EUNetPaS project (2010) and WHO guidelines (World Health Organization, 2011), PaSNEQ was designed to capture students' perceptions of patient safety learning across academic and clinical environments.

- Structure: 57 items across three main areas: *Academic Environment, Clinical Environment, and Patient Safety Competencies*. Each area includes three dimensions (Langari et al., 2017; Tella et al., 2015).
- Testing and use: Validated in Finland and the UK, with factor analyses confirming nine dimensions overall. Internal consistency values were generally high ($\alpha = 0.78–0.85$), except for the error reporting subscale ($\alpha = 0.43$).

Safety Attitudes Questionnaire (SAQ)

Initially developed by Sexton et al. (2006) to evaluate healthcare workers' safety attitudes, the SAQ was later applied to nursing students in China.

- Structure: 31 items in six domains: *Teamwork climate, Safety climate, Perception of management, Job satisfaction, Working conditions, Stress recognition* (Guo & Zhou, 2010; Kong et al., 2019).
- Testing and use: High reliability when tested with nursing students ($\alpha = 0.93$). Strong positive correlations were found between safety-related behaviors (e.g., error reporting, aseptic technique) and attitudes in most domains, except stress recognition (Kong et al., 2019).

Hospital Survey on Patient Safety Culture – Nursing Student version (HSOPS-NS)

Based on the Agency for Healthcare Research and Quality HSOPS instrument (Nieva & Sorra, 2003) and adapted for use in Spain (Gascón-Cánovas et al., 2005), the HSOPS-NS evaluates nursing students' perceptions of patient safety culture.

- Structure: 54 items divided into 13 dimensions, such as *Frequency of events reported, Supervisor/Manager expectations & actions promoting patient safety, Organizational learning, continuous improvement, Teamwork within unit, Communication openness, Feedback & communication about error, Nonpunitive responses to errors, Staffing, Management support for patient safety, Teamwork across units, Handoffs & Transitions, Indicators of good practice, and Overall perception of patient safety* (Ortiz de Elguea et al., 2019).
- Testing and use: Validated on 654 nursing students in Spain. Factor analyses identified five higher-order factors, and internal consistency was acceptable ($\alpha = 0.74$–0.77). Confirmed in Slovakia (Kalánková et al., 2021) and Spain again (De Miguel et al., 2023).

Just Culture Assessment Tool for Nursing Education (JCAT-NE)

Adapted from the original JCAT (Petschonek et al., 2013), this instrument emphasizes the concept of "just culture"—balancing accountability and learning from error.

- Structure: 27 items across six domains: *Balance, Trust, Openness of communication, Quality of reporting processes, Feedback, and Continuous improvement* (Walker et al., 2019).
- Testing and use: Initially validated in the U.S., achieving acceptable reliability ($\alpha = 0.75$; Walker et al., 2019). Later studies refined the factor structure and highlighted fear of reporting and the importance of continuous improvement as critical (Walker et al., 2021).

Patient Safety Culture Scale (PSCS)

Initially developed for healthcare workers (Türkmen et al., 2011), the PSCS was applied to nursing students in Turkey.

- Structure: 51 items across five domains: *Management and leadership, Staff behavior, Error reporting, Staff training, and Environmental care.*
- Testing and use: Applied to 299 students, with excellent internal consistency ($\alpha = 0.97$; Çiftcioğlu et al., 2022).

Attitudes to Patient Safety Questionnaire (APS)

Derived from APSQ-III (Carruthers et al., 2009), APS was adapted for Spanish nursing students.

- The finale comprises two across-items in six domains: *Responsibility, Organizational communication, Teamwork, Clinical practice, Error reporting, and Awareness* (Cervera-Gash et al., 2021).
- Testing and use: Validated in Spain and re-tested in Turkey (Karaman & Alan, 2022) and Estonia (Sepp, 2024), showing acceptable reliability ($\alpha = 0.67–0.81$).

Patient Safety Survey (PSS)

A recent Egyptian development based on WHO guidelines.

- Structure: 20 items grouped into three areas: *Overall safety evaluation, Clinical aspects of safety, and Error reporting* (Khider et al., 2024).
- Testing and use: Content validated by experts, pilot tested with 27 students, with good reliability ($\alpha = 0.89$).

INSTRUMENTS BASED ON NURSING-SPECIFIC FRAMEWORKS

Drawing primarily on nursing-focused frameworks such as QSEN and the Patient Safety Competency Framework (PSCF[a]), a range of instruments has been developed to directly assess nursing students' knowledge, skills, and attitudes related to patient safety. Unlike general tools, these measures explicitly align with nursing curricula, operationalizing core QSEN domains and PSCF[a] competencies into structured scales. Through psychometrically validated subdimensions—encompassing error detection, safety culture, communication, professional accountability, and system-based practice—these instruments facilitate the systematic evaluation of nursing-specific educational outcomes, offering targeted insights for curriculum refinement and competency-based training.

Patient Safety Attitudes, Skills and Knowledge Scale (PS-ASK)

Developed in the U.S. in connection with the QSEN framework (Cronenwett et al., 2007), PS-ASK was the first instrument explicitly designed for nursing students' learning about patient safety.

- Structure: 26 items in three domains: *Attitudes, Skills, and Knowledge*. Subfactors include *Error detection, Time investment, Safety culture creation, Threats to patient safety, Error analysis, and Technological support* (Schnall et al., 2008).
- Testing and use: Reliability varied across subscales ($\alpha = 0.49–0.86$).

Student Perceptions of Safety and Quality Knowledge, Skills, and Attitudes Questionnaire

Developed in the U.S. to evaluate QSEN competencies (Miller & LaFramboise, 2009).

- Structure: 10 items mapped to QSEN competencies.
- Testing and use: Reliability is modest ($\alpha = 0.58–0.65$).

QSEN Student Evaluation Survey (QSEN SES)

Created to assess students' perceptions of QSEN competencies (Sullivan et al., 2009).

- Structure: 41 items across *knowledge, skills, and attitudes*. Skills and attitudes are rated separately in terms of preparedness and importance.
- Testing and use: Adequate psychometric properties confirmed in the U.S., Italy (Marcomini et al., 2022), and Brazil (Freitas et al., 2022).

Health Care Professionals Patient Safety Assessment Curriculum Survey (HPPSACS)

Based on QSEN and developed in the U.S. (Chenot & Daniel, 2010).

- Structure: 34 items in four domains: *Comfort, Error reporting, Denial, Safety culture*.
- Testing and use: Adequate psychometrics confirmed in both the U.S. and the UK (Mansour et al., 2015).

Nursing Quality and Safety Self-Inventory (NQSSI)

Developed in the U.S. as part of QSEN evaluation (Piscotty et al., 2013).

- Structure: 18 items (three questions per QSEN domain).
- Testing and use: Internal consistency excellent ($\alpha = 0.93$). Follow-up study identified a four-factor structure (Letourneau et al., 2019).

Patient Safety Competency Self-Evaluation Tool (PSCSE)

Developed in Korea based on the PSCF[a] framework (Lee et al., 2014).

- Structure: 45 items across *Knowledge, Skills, and Attitudes*, with 12 subdimensions (e.g., *Error reporting, Infection prevention, Handover communication, Professional accountability*).
- Testing and use: Strong psychometric results in Korea, Turkey (Eskici et al., 2021), and Cyprus (Firat Kılıç & Cevheroglu, 2023). Internal consistency ranged from $\alpha = 0.79$ to $\alpha = 0.91$.

Summary of Educational Frameworks and Instruments for Patient Safety in Nursing Education

In recent years, increasing attention has been given to the issue of patient safety in the context of nursing education (Kirwan et al., 2019; Mansour et al., 2018), as it represents a critical indicator of the quality of health care (Morello et al., 2013; Nieva & Sorra, 2003). To facilitate both the understanding of this topic and the integration of patient safety into nursing curricula, several educational frameworks have been developed. These frameworks have been categorized as either general or nursing-specific, depending on whether they addressed patient safety across multiple health professions or were designed exclusively for nursing.

The first educational framework was created in 2005: the National Patient Safety Education Framework (NPSEF), a general framework that later notified the development of the WHO Multi-professional Patient Safety Curriculum Guide, prepared in collaboration with the International Council of Nurses. Another internationally influential framework is the Quality and Safety Education for Nurses (QSEN) initiative, developed in 2007 and categorized as a nursing-specific framework. Two additional frameworks, both general, were introduced in 2008: the Safety Competencies Framework (Frank & Brien, 2008; SCF, 2008) in Canada, and the European Network for Patient Safety framework (EUNetPaS, 2010), developed in collaboration with the European Federation of Nurses. The most recent frameworks, explicitly designed for nursing, are the Patient Safety Competency Framework (Lee et al., 2014; PSCF[a]), developed in South Korea in 2012, and the Patient Safety Competency Framework for Nursing Students (Levett-Jones et al., 2017; PSCF[b]), developed in Australia in 2017. Notably, since 2008, the inclusion of a "*patient safety culture*" has become a standard domain across these frameworks.

Although the frameworks apply different definitions of patient safety (Table 3), they share a common feature: the specification of educational domains and competencies essential for ensuring safe care, which nursing students should acquire before qualifying. The detailed lists of competencies for both general and nursing-specific frameworks are presented in Tables 1 and 2. These competencies were further analyzed and synthesized into overarching domains: Safety, Patient Safety Culture, Teamwork, Communication, Evidence-Based Practice, Patient-Centered Care, Adverse Events, Human and System Factors, Informatics, Quality of Care, Specific Issues, and Other Domains (Figure 1). Geographically, two frameworks originated in the United States (QSEN), one in Canada (SCF), two in Australia (NPSEF and PSCF[b]), one in South Korea (PSCF[a]), and one in Europe (EUNetPaS). These frameworks frequently serve as theoretical foundations for empirical research in nursing education. In countries where no national framework has been established, international frameworks such as QSEN, PSCF[a], PSCF[b], or the WHO Curriculum Guide are often used as guiding references for developing recommendations and integrating patient safety education into nursing curricula.

Complementing these frameworks, an assessment instrument has emerged to evaluate nursing students' knowledge, skills, and attitudes (KSAs) in patient safety, as well as their perceptions of safety culture. Early tools aligned with QSEN include the PS-ASK (Schnall et al., 2008), the Student Perceptions of Safety & Quality KSA Questionnaire (Miller & LaFramboise, 2009), the QSEN SES (Sullivan et al., 2009), HPPSACS (Chenot & Daniel, 2010), and the NQSSI (Piscotty et al., 2013). Instruments grounded in general frameworks comprise the widely used H-PEPSS derived from SCF (Ginsburg et al., 2012), the PaSNEQ based on EUNetPaS and WHO guidance (Tella et al., 2015), and culture-focused measures adapted for students such as HSOPS-NS (Ortiz de Elguea et al., 2019), C-SAQ/SAQ (Kong et al., 2019), JCAT-NE (Walker et al., 2019), PSCS (Çiftcioğlu et al., 2022), APS (Cervera-Gash et al., 2021), and the recent PSS (Khider et al., 2024). Tools linked to PSCF[a]/PSCF[b] include the PSCSE (Lee et al., 2014). Review studies confirm the proliferation of such instruments and their growing use in nursing education research (Figure 2; Bedgood & Mellott, 2021; Mortensen et al., 2022; Taskiran et al., 2020).

Across studies, the instruments are predominantly self-report, employ Likert-type scales, and vary in length from ~10 to 57 items, with dimensionality ranging from brief attitudinal screens to multi-domain competency or culture measures. Some tools—most notably H-PEPSS—have been repeatedly validated across countries and languages, often distinguishing learning in academic versus clinical settings (Bergs et al., 2021; Bressan et al., 2016; Ginsburg et al., 2012; Chen et al., 2019; Stomski et al., 2018; Taskiran et al., 2020; VanDenKerkhof et al., 2017). Since ~2019, there has been a discernible shift toward culture-centric instruments (e.g., JCAT-NE, PSCS, HSOPS-NS, APS), reflecting the centrality of patient safety culture and just culture in contemporary safety science (Cervera-Gash et al., 2021; Çiftcioğlu et al., 2022; Ortiz de Elguea et al., 2019; Walker et al., 2019). At the same time, compact tools such as PSS suggest renewed interest in practice-proximal competence during clinical placements (Khider et al., 2024).

In sum, frameworks provide the conceptual map, while instruments operationalize patient safety learning for evaluation and program improvement. Together, they underpin curriculum design, enable international comparison, and help identify priority domains—whether competency-focused KSA (e.g., QSEN-aligned tools, PSCSE) or culture-focused perceptions (e.g., H-PEPSS, HSOPS-NS, JCAT-NE). Future research studies should continue to triangulate self-report with performance-based evidence and revalidate instruments across contexts, ensuring that assessments keep pace with evolving definitions and expectations of patient safety in nursing education (Mortensen et al., 2022; Taskiran et al., 2020).

REFERENCES

Acton, C., Farus-Brown, S., Alexander, C., Morrow, L., Ossege, J., & Tovar, E. (2017). Quality and Safety Education for Nurses competencies in Doctor of Nursing Practice education: Exemplars from education and practice. *Nurse Educator, 42*(5S Suppl 1), S44–S48. https://doi.org/.DOI: 10.1097/NNE.0000000000000426

American Association of College of Nursing. (2006). Hallmarks of quality and patient safety: Recommended baccalaureate competencies and curricular guidelines to ensure high-quality and safe patient care. *Journal of Professional Nursing*, *22*(6), 329–330. DOI: 10.1016/j.profnurs.2006.10.005 PMID: 17141715

Armstrong, G., & Barton, A. (2013). Fundamentally updating fundamentals: A cross-sectional study. *Journal of Professional Nursing*, *29*(2), 82–87. DOI: 10.1016/j.profnurs.2012.12.006 PMID: 23566453

Attree, M., Cooke, H., & Wakefield, A. (2008). Patient safety in an English pre-registration nursing curriculum. *Nurse Education in Practice*, *8*(4), 239–248. DOI: 10.1016/j.nepr.2007.09.003 PMID: 17945535

Australian Commission on Safety and Quality in Health Care. (2005). *National patient safety education framework.* Commonwealth of Australia. https://www.safetyandquality.gov.au/sites/default/files/migrated/framework0705.pdf

Barnsteiner, J., Disch, J., Johnson, J., McGuinn, K., Chappel, K., & Swartwout, E. (2013). Diffusing QSEN competencies across schools of nursing: The AACN/RWJF faculty development institutes. *Journal of Professional Nursing*, *29*(2), 68–74. DOI: 10.1016/j.profnurs.2012.12.003 PMID: 23566451

Bartoníčková, D., Kohanová, D., & Žiaková, K. (2023). Vzdelávacie rámce a oblasti kompetencií študentov ošetrovateľstva súvisiace s bezpečnosťou pacientov: Integratívny prehľad. *Health and Caring*, *2*(2). Advance online publication. DOI: 10.46585/hc.2023.2.2441

Bedgood, A. L., & Mellott, S. (2021). The role of education in developing a culture of safety through the perceptions of undergraduate nursing students: An integrative literature review. *Journal of Patient Safety*, *17*(8), e1530–e1536. DOI: 10.1097/PTS.0000000000000548 PMID: 30383621

Bergs, J., Peeters, K., Kortleven, I., Creemers, S., Ulenaers, D., Desmedt, M., & Schrooten, W. (2021). Translation and validation of the Dutch version of the Health Professional Education in Patient Safety Survey amongst nursing students in Belgium: A psychometric analysis. *PLoS One*, *16*(3), e0247869. DOI: 10.1371/journal.pone.0247869 PMID: 33657156

Boucaut, R., & Cusack, L. (2016). 'Sometimes your safety goes a bit by the wayside' … exploring occupational health and safety (OHS) with student nurses. *Nurse Education in Practice*, *20*, 93–98. DOI: 10.1016/j.nepr.2016.07.005 PMID: 27525567

Bressan, V., Stevanin, S., Bulfone, G., Zanini, A., Dante, A., & Palese, A. (2016). Measuring patient safety knowledge and competences as perceived by nursing students: An Italian validation study. *Nurse Education in Practice*, *16*(1), 209–216. DOI: 10.1016/j.nepr.2015.08.006 PMID: 26344616

Campbell, B., & Mackay, G. (2001). Continuing competence: An Ontario nursing regulatory program that supports nurses and employers. *Nursing Administration Quarterly*, *25*(2), 22–30. DOI: 10.1097/00006216-200101000-00006 PMID: 18188891

Canadian Patient Safety Institute. (2016). *Report on the integration of the safety competencies framework into health professions education programs in Canada.* Canadian Patient Safety Institute. https://www.patientsafetyinstitute.ca/en/toolsResources/IntegrationofSafetyCompetenciesFramework/Documents/Report%20on%20the%20Integration%20of%20the%20Safety%20Competencies%20Framework.pdf

Canadian Patient Safety Institute. (2020). *The safety competencies: Enhancing patient safety across the health professions* (2nd ed.). Canadian Patient Safety Institute. https://www.patientsafetyinstitute.ca/en/toolsResources/safetyCompetencies/Documents/CPSI-SafetyCompetencies_EN_Digital.pdf

Carruthers, S., Lawton, R., Sandars, J., Howe, A., & Perry, M. (2009). Attitudes to patient safety amongst medical students and tutors: Developing a reliable scale. *Medical Teacher*, *31*(8), e370–e376. DOI: 10.1080/01421590802650142 PMID: 19811201

Cervera-Gasch, Á., González-Chordá, V. M., Manrique-Abril, F. G., Andreu-Pejo, L., Valero-Chillerón, M. J., & Mena-Tudela, D. (2021). Validation of the attitudes to patient safety questionnaire for nursing students in the Spanish context. *BMC Nursing*, *20*(1), 101. DOI: 10.1186/s12912-021-00634-y PMID: 34144691

Chen, L., Huang, F., Yuan, X., Song, J., & Chen, L. (2019). An assessment of the reliability and factorial validity of the Chinese version of the Health Professional Education in Patient Safety Survey (H-PEPSS). *Frontiers in Psychology*, *10*, 2183. DOI: 10.3389/fpsyg.2019.02183 PMID: 31607997

Chenot, T. M., & Daniel, L. G. (2010). Frameworks for patient safety in the nursing curriculum. *The Journal of Nursing Education*, *49*(10), 559–568. DOI: 10.3928/01484834-20100730-02 PMID: 20669876

Çiftcioğlu, Ş., Apaydın Cırık, V., & Efe, E. (2022). Student nurses' perceptions of a patient safety culture: A descriptive and cross-sectional study. *Perspectives in Psychiatric Care*, *58*(2), 658–663. DOI: 10.1111/ppc.12830 PMID: 33931872

Cronenwett, L., Sherwood, G., Barnsteiner, J., Disch, J., Johnson, J., Mitchell, P., Sullivan, D. T., & Warren, J. (2007). Quality and safety education for nurses. *Nursing Outlook*, *55*(3), 122–131. DOI: 10.1016/j.outlook.2007.02.006 PMID: 17524799

Cronenwett, L., Sherwood, G., Pohl, J., Barnsteiner, J., Moore, S., Sullivan, D. T., Ward, D., & Warren, J. (2009). Quality and safety education for advanced nursing practice. *Nursing Outlook*, *57*(6), 338–348. DOI: 10.1016/j.outlook.2009.07.009 PMID: 19942035

Davies, J. M., Hebert, P., & Hoffman, A. (2003). *The Canadian patient safety dictionary*. The Royal College of Physicians and Surgeons of Canada.

De Miguel, M. S., de Elguea, J. O., Gómez-Gastiasoro, A., Urcola, F., Cid-Expósito, M. G., Torres-Enamorado, D., & Orkaizagirre-Gomara, A. (2023). Patient safety and its relationship with specific self-efficacy, competence, and resilience among nursing students: A quantitative study. *Nurse Education Today*, *121*, 105701. DOI: 10.1016/j.nedt.2022.105701 PMID: 36563588

Eskici, G. T., Kanig, M., Ugur, E., & Seren, A. K. H. (2021). The Turkish version of the Patient Safety Competency Self-Evaluation Tool: A validity and reliability study. *Nurse Education in Practice*, *57*, 103229. DOI: 10.1016/j.nepr.2021.103229 PMID: 34673387

European Federation of Nurses Associations. (2015). *EFN guideline for the implementation of Article 31 of the Mutual Recognition of Professional Qualifications Directive 2005/36/EC, amended by Directive 2013/55/EU*. http://www.efnweb.be/wpcontent/uploads/EFNCompetencyFramework19052015

European Union Network for Patient Safety. (2010). *General guide for education and training in patient safety*. https://www.eupatient.eu/globalassets/projects/eunetpas/guidelines_final_22-06-2010.pdf

Fırat Kılıç, H., & Cevheroğlu, S. (2023). Patient safety competencies of nursing students. *Nurse Education Today*, *121*, 105666. DOI: 10.1016/j.nedt.2022.105666 PMID: 36463791

Frank, J. R., & Brien, S. (2008). *The safety competencies: Enhancing patient safety across the health professions*. Canadian Patient Safety Institute. https://simulation.mcmaster.ca/documents/Safety_Competencies.pdf

Freitas, J. S., Sousa, M. R. G., Dolansky, M. A., & Silva, A. E. B. C. (2022). Quality and Safety Education for Nurses Student Evaluation Survey: Adaptation and Psychometric Evaluation of the Brazilian Version. *Journal of Nursing Measurement, 30*(3), 496–507. DOI: 10.1891/JNM-D-20-00114 PMID: 34518404

Gascón-Cánovas, J. J., Saturno-Hernandéz, P. J., Pérez-Fernandéz, P., Vincente-Lópéz, I., Conzáles-Vicente, A., Martínez-Mas, J., & Saura, M. M. (2005). *Spanish version of the Hospital Survey on Patient Safety*. Madrid: Ministerio de Sanidad y Consumo. https://www.sanidad.gob.es/en/organizacion/sns/planCalidadSNS/docs/CuestionarioSeguridadPacientes1.pdf

Ginsburg, L., Castel, E., Tregunno, D., & Norton, P. G. (2012). The H-PEPSS: An instrument to measure health professionals' perceptions of patient safety competence at entry into practice. *BMJ Quality & Safety, 21*(8), 676–684. DOI: 10.1136/bmjqs-2011-000601 PMID: 22562876

Guo, X., & Zhou, W. (2010). Revision of Safety Attitudes Questionnaire and evaluation. *Chinese Journal of Nursing Education, 7*(4), 151–154. DOI: 10.3761/j.issn.1672-9234.2010.04.002

Howard, J. N. (2010). The missing link: Dedicated patient safety education within top-ranked U.S. nursing school curricula. *Journal of Patient Safety, 6*(3), 165–171. DOI: 10.1097/PTS.0b013e3181eee2ab PMID: 21491791

Institute of Medicine (U.S.) Committee on the Health Professions Education Summit. (2003). *Health professions education: A bridge to quality*. National Academies Press. https://www.ncbi.nlm.nih.gov/books/NBK221528/

International Council of Nurses. (2022). *Position statement: Patient safety*. https://www.icn.ch/sites/default/files/inline-files/D05_Patient_Safety_0.pdf

Jones, A. D. (2013). The impact of integrating Quality and Safety Education for Nurses' safety competency in first-year associate degree nursing students. *Teaching and Learning in Nursing, 8*(4), 140–146. DOI: 10.1016/j.teln.2013.06.001

Kalánková, D., Bartoníčková, D., Gurková, E., Žiaková, K., & Kurucová, R. (2021). A validation study of the Slovak version of the Hospital Survey on Patient Safety Culture (with Slovak nurses). *Central European Journal of Nursing and Midwifery, 12*(2), 353–365. DOI: 10.15452/cejnm.2021.12.0010

Karaman, F., & Alan, H. (2022). Turkish Adaptation of the Scale of the Attitudes to Patient Safety: Nursing Student Sample. *Bezmialem Science, 10*(4), 426–433. DOI: 10.14235/bas.galenos.2021.5350

Khider, Y. I. A., Allam, S. M. E., Zoromba, M. A., & Elhapashy, H. M. M. (2024). Nursing students' perspectives on patients' safety competencies: A cross-sectional survey. *BMC Nursing*, *23*(1), 323. DOI: 10.1186/s12912-024-01966-1 PMID: 38735958

King, J., & Anderson, C. M. (2012). The Canadian interprofessional patient safety competencies: Their role in healthcare professionals' education. *Journal of Patient Safety*, *8*(1), 30–35. DOI: 10.1097/PTS.0b013e3182468138 PMID: 22343801

Kirwan, M., Riklikiene, O., Gotlib, J., Fuster, P., & Borta, M. (2019). Regulation and current status of patient safety content in pre-registration nurse education in 27 countries: Findings from the Rationing - Missed nursing care (RANCARE) COST Action project. *Nurse Education in Practice*, *37*, 132–140. DOI: 10.1016/j.nepr.2019.04.013 PMID: 31153130

Kong, L. N., Zhu, W. F., He, S., Chen, S. Z., Yang, L., Qi, L., & Peng, X. (2019). Attitudes towards patient safety culture among postgraduate nursing students in China: A cross-sectional study. *Nurse Education in Practice*, *38*, 1–6. DOI: 10.1016/j.nepr.2019.05.014 PMID: 31163311

Langari, M. N. M., Tella, S., Smith, N.-J., Ma, H., & Turunen, H. (2017). Self-assessment of patient safety competence: A questionnaire survey of final year British and Finnish pre-registration nursing students. *International Journal of Caring Sciences*, *10*(3), 1212–1224. https://internationaljournalofcaringsciences.org/docs/11_lagari_original_10_3.pdf

Lee, N. J., An, J. Y., Song, T. M., Jang, H., & Park, S. Y. (2014). Psychometric evaluation of a patient safety competency self-evaluation tool for nursing students. *The Journal of Nursing Education*, *53*(10), 550–562. DOI: 10.3928/01484834-20140922-01 PMID: 25275988

Lee, S. E., Dathinten, V. S., & Do, H. (2020). Patient safety education in pre-registration nursing programmes in South Korea. *International Nursing Review*, *67*(4), 512–518. DOI: 10.1111/inr.12630 PMID: 33006174

Leotsakos, A., Zheng, H., Croteau, R., Loeb, J. M., Sherman, H., Hoffman, C., Morganstein, L., O'Leary, D., Bruneau, C., Lee, P., Duguid, M., Thomeczek, C., Schrieck-De Loos, E., & Munier, B. (2014). Standardization in patient safety: The WHO High 5s project. *International Journal for Quality in Health Care : Journal of the International Society for Quality in Health Care*, *26*(2), 109–116. DOI: 10.1093/intqhc/mzu010 PMID: 24713313

Letourneau, R. M., & McCurry, M. K. (2019). Testing the Nursing Quality and Safety Self-Inventory. *Journal for Nurses in Professional Development, 35*(5), 275–280. DOI: 10.1097/NND.0000000000000556 PMID: 31157672

Levett-Jones, T., Andersen, P., Bogossian, F., Cooper, S., Guinea, S., Hopmans, R., McKenna, L., Pich, J., Reid-Searl, K., & Seaton, P. (2020). A cross-sectional survey of nursing students' patient safety knowledge. *Nurse Education Today, 88*, 104372. DOI: 10.1016/j.nedt.2020.104372 PMID: 32143174

Levett-Jones, T., Dwyer, T., Reid-Searl, K., Heaton, L., Flenady, T., Applegarth, J., Guinea, S., & Andersen, P. (2017). *Patient safety competency framework (PSCF) for nursing students.* http://psframework.wpengine.com/wpcontent/uploads/2018/01/PSCF_Brochure_UTS-version_FA2-Screen.pdf

Lukewich, J., Edge, D. S., Tranmer, J., Raymond, J., Miron, J., Ginsburg, L., & Van-DenKerkhof, E. (2015). Undergraduate baccalaureate nursing students' self-reported confidence in learning about patient safety in the classroom and clinical settings: An annual cross-sectional study (2010–2013). *International Journal of Nursing Studies, 52*(5), 930–938. DOI: 10.1016/j.ijnurstu.2015.01.010 PMID: 25698119

Mansour, M. (2012). Current assessment of patient safety education. *British Journal of Nursing (Mark Allen Publishing), 21*(9), 536–543. DOI: 10.12968/bjon.2012.21.9.536 PMID: 22585267

Mansour, M., Skull, A., & Parker, M. (2015). Evaluation of World Health Organization multi-professional patient safety curriculum topics in nursing education: Pre-test, post-test, none-experimental study. *Journal of Professional Nursing, 31*(5), 432–439. DOI: 10.1016/j.profnurs.2015.03.002 PMID: 26428349

Mansour, M. J., Al Shadafan, S. F., Abu-Sneineh, F. T., & Alamer, M. M. (2018). Integrating patient safety education in the undergraduate nursing curriculum: A discussion paper. *The Open Nursing Journal, 12*(1), 125–132. DOI: 10.2174/1874434601812010125 PMID: 30069269

Marcomini, I., Destrebecq, A., Rosa, D., & Terzoni, S. (2021). Self-reported skills for ensuring patient safety and quality of care among Italian nursing students: A descriptive cross-sectional study. *International Journal of Health Promotion and Education, 60*(2), 67–78. DOI: 10.1080/14635240.2021.1944270

Miller, C. L., & LaFramboise, L. (2009). Student Learning Outcomes After Integration of Quality and Safety Education Competencies into a Senior-Level Critical Care Course. *The Journal of Nursing Education, 48*(12), 678–685. DOI: 10.3928/01484834-20091113-07 PMID: 20000249

Miller, G. E. (1990). The assessment of clinical skills/competence/performance. *Academic Medicine*, *65*(9, Suppl), S63–S67. DOI: 10.1097/00001888-199009000-00045 PMID: 2400509

Morello, R. T., Lowthian, J. A., Barker, A. L., McGinnes, R., Dunt, D., & Brand, C. (2013). Strategies for improving patient safety culture in hospitals: A systematic review. *BMJ Quality & Safety*, *22*(1), 11–18. DOI: 10.1136/bmjqs-2011-000582 PMID: 22849965

Mortensen, M., Naustdal, K. I., Uibu, E., Mägi, L., Kangasniemi, M., Põlluste, K., & Moi, A. L. (2022). Instruments for measuring patient safety competencies in nursing: A scoping review. *BMJ Open Quality*, *11*(2), e001751. DOI: 10.1136/bmjoq-2021-001751 PMID: 35379672

Nieva, V. F., & Sorra, J. (2003). Safety culture assessment: A tool for improving patient safety in healthcare organizations. *BMJ Quality & Safety*, *12*(90002, Suppl 2), ii17–ii23. DOI: 10.1136/qhc.12.suppl_2.ii17 PMID: 14645891

Ortiz de Elguea, J., Orkaizagirre-Gómara, A., Sánchez de Miguel, M., Urcola-Pardo, F., Germín-Bes, C., & Lizaso-Elgarresta, I. (2019). Adapting and validating the Hospital Survey on Patient Safety Culture (HSOPS) for nursing students (HSOPS-NS): A new measure of patient safety climate. *Nurse Education Today*, *75*, 95–103. DOI: 10.1016/j.nedt.2019.01.008 PMID: 30738365

Petschonek, S., Burlison, J., Cross, C., Martin, K., Laver, J., Landis, R. S., & Hoffman, J. M. (2013). Development of the just culture assessment tool: Measuring the perceptions of healthcare professionals in hospitals. *Journal of Patient Safety*, *9*(4), 190–197. DOI: 10.1097/PTS.0b013e31828fff34 PMID: 24263549

Piscotty, R., Grobbel, C., & Abele, C. (2013). Initial psychometric evaluation of the nursing quality and safety self-inventory. *The Journal of Nursing Education*, *52*(5), 269–274. DOI: 10.3928/01484834-20130412-03 PMID: 23586354

Quality and Safety Education for Nurses. (2020). *Quality and safety education for nurses (QSEN).* Case Western Reserve University. https://qsen.org/about-qsen/

Schnall, R., Stone, P., Currie, L., Desjardins, K., John, R. M., & Bakken, S. (2008). Development of a self-report instrument to measure patient safety attitudes, skills, and knowledge. *Journal of Nursing Scholarship*, *40*(4), 391–394. DOI: 10.1111/j.1547-5069.2008.00256.x PMID: 19094156

Sepp, K. (2024). Advancing patient safety competencies in nursing education: An examination of student attitudes. *Agronomy Research (Tartu)*, *22*(S1), 537–553. DOI: 10.15159/AR.24.018

Sexton, J. B., Helmreich, R. L., Neilands, T. B., Rowan, K., Vella, K., Boyden, J., Roberts, P. R., & Thomas, E. J. (2006). The Safety Attitudes Questionnaire: Psychometric properties, benchmarking data, and emerging research. *BMC Health Services Research*, *6*(1), 44. DOI: 10.1186/1472-6963-6-44 PMID: 16584553

Sherwood, G., & Barnsteiner, J. (Eds.). (2012). *Quality and safety in nursing: A competency approach to improving outcomes*. Wiley-Blackwell.

Stomski, N., Gluyas, H., Andrus, P., Williams, A., Hopkins, M., Walters, J., Sandy, M., & Morrison, P. (2018). The influence of situation awareness training on nurses' confidence about patient safety skills: A prospective cohort study. *Nurse Education Today*, *63*, 24–28. DOI: 10.1016/j.nedt.2018.01.019 PMID: 29407256

Sullivan, D. T., Hirst, D., & Cronenwett, L. (2009). Assessing quality and safety competencies of graduating prelicensure nursing students. *Nursing Outlook*, *57*(6), 323–331. DOI: 10.1016/j.outlook.2009.08.004 PMID: 19942033

Taskiran, G., Eskin Bacaksiz, F., & Harmanci Seren, A. K. (2020). Psychometric testing of the Turkish version of the Health Professional Education in Patient Safety Survey: H-PEPSS-TR. *Nurse Education in Practice*, *42*, 102640. DOI: 10.1016/j.nepr.2019.102640 PMID: 31756625

Tella, S., Smith, N.-J., Partanen, P., Jamookeeah, D., Lamidi, M. J., & Turnen, H. (2015). Learning to ensure patient safety in clinical settings: Comparing Finnish and British nursing students' perceptions. *Journal of Clinical Nursing*, *24*(19–20), 2954–2964. DOI: 10.1111/jocn.12914 PMID: 26216053

Türkmen, E., Altuntaş, S., Baykal, Ü., & Seren, Ş. (2011). Hasta güvenliği kültürü ölçeğinin geliştirilmesi [Development of patient safety culture scale]. *Anadolu Hemsirelik ve Saglik Bilimleri Dergisi*, *14*(4), 38–46.

VanDenKerkhof, E., Sears, N., Edge, D. S., Tregunno, D., & Ginsburg, L. (2017). Patient safety in practical nurses' education: A cross-sectional survey of newly registered practical nurses in Canada. *Nurse Education Today*, *51*, 48–56. DOI: 10.1016/j.nedt.2017.01.003 PMID: 28126688

Walker, D., Altmiller, G., Barkell, N., Hromadik, L., & Toothaker, R. (2019). Development and Validation of the Just Culture Assessment Tool for Nursing Education. *Nurse Educator*, *44*(5), 261–264. DOI: 10.1097/NNE.0000000000000705 PMID: 31305358

Walker, D., Hromadik, L., Altmiller, G., Barkell, N., Toothaker, R., & Powell, K. (2021). Exploratory factor analysis of the Just Culture Assessment Tool for nursing education. *Journal of Research in Nursing : JRN*, *26*(1-2), 49–59. DOI: 10.1177/1744987120951589 PMID: 35251224

Walton, M. M., Shaw, T., Barnet, S., & Ross, J. (2006). Developing a national patient safety education framework for Australia. *Quality & Safety in Health Care*, *15*(6), 437–442. DOI: 10.1136/qshc.2006.019216 PMID: 17142595

World Health Organization. (2009). *Patient safety curriculum guide for medical schools.* World Health Organization. https://apps.who.int/iris/handle/10665/44091

World Health Organization. (2011). *Patient safety curriculum guide: Multi-professional edition.* World Health Organization. https://www.who.int/publications/i/item/9789241501958

Zikos, D., Diomidous, M., & Mantas, J. (2010). A framework for the development of patient safety education and training guidelines. *Studies in Health Technology and Informatics*, *155*, 189–195. DOI: 10.3233/978-1-60750-563-1-189 PMID: 20543328

APPENDIX

Table 3. Definitions of patient safety used in educational frameworks

Educational framework	Patient safety —definition
Australian National Patient Safety Education Framework (NPSEF)	*"The prevention of harm caused by errors of commission and omission. The process by which an organisation makes patient care safer. This process should involve: risk assessment; the identification, reporting and analysis of incidents; the ability to learn from incidents, to follow them up and to implement solutions to minimize the risk of recurrence."* (Australian Commission in Safety and Quality in Health Care, 2005, p. 199).
Institute of Medicine (IOM)	*"Prevention of patient harm."* (Institute of Medicine (U.S.) Committee on the Health Professions Education Summit, 2003).
Institute of Medicine (IOM)	*"Avoiding injuries to patients from the care that is intended to help them."* (Institute of Medicine (U.S.) Committee on the Health Professions Education Summit, 2003).
Canadian Safety Competencies Framework (SCF)	*"The reduction and mitigation of unsafe acts within the health care system, as well as the use of best practices shown to lead to optimal patient outcomes."* (Davies, Hebert, Hoffman, 2003, p. 11).
European Network for Patient Safety (EUNetPaS)	*"Freedom for a patient from unnecessary harm or potential harm associated with health care."* (European Union Network for Patient Safety, 2010, p. 36).
Quality and Safety Education for Nurses (QSEN)	*"Minimization of risk of harm to patients and providers through both system effectiveness and individual performance."* (Cronenwett et al., 2007, p. 128).
World Health Organization (WHO)	*"A framework of organized activities that creates cultures, processes, procedures, behaviours, technologies and environments in health care that consistently and sustainably lower risks, reduce the occurrence of avoidable harm, make error less likely and reduce its impact when it does occur."* (World Health Organization, 2021, Executive summary V).

Figure 1. Overarching educational areas of patient safety in nursing

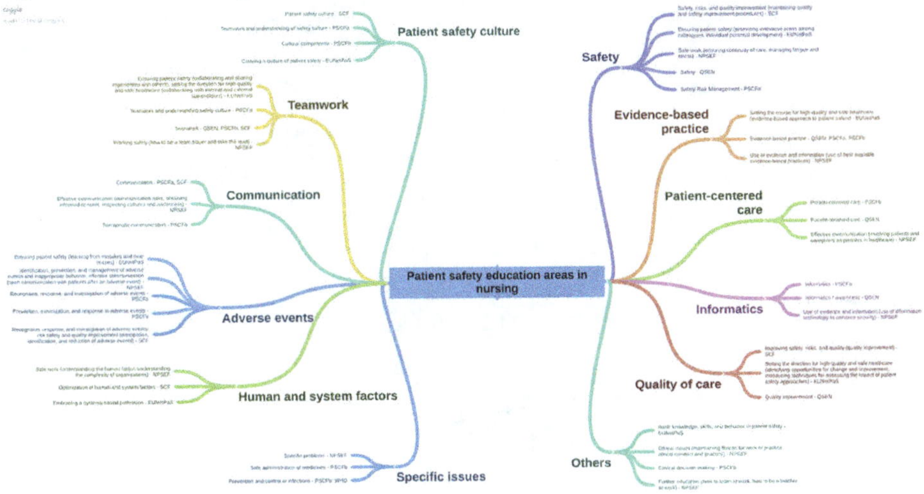

Figure 2. Instruments for measuring patient safety in nursing education

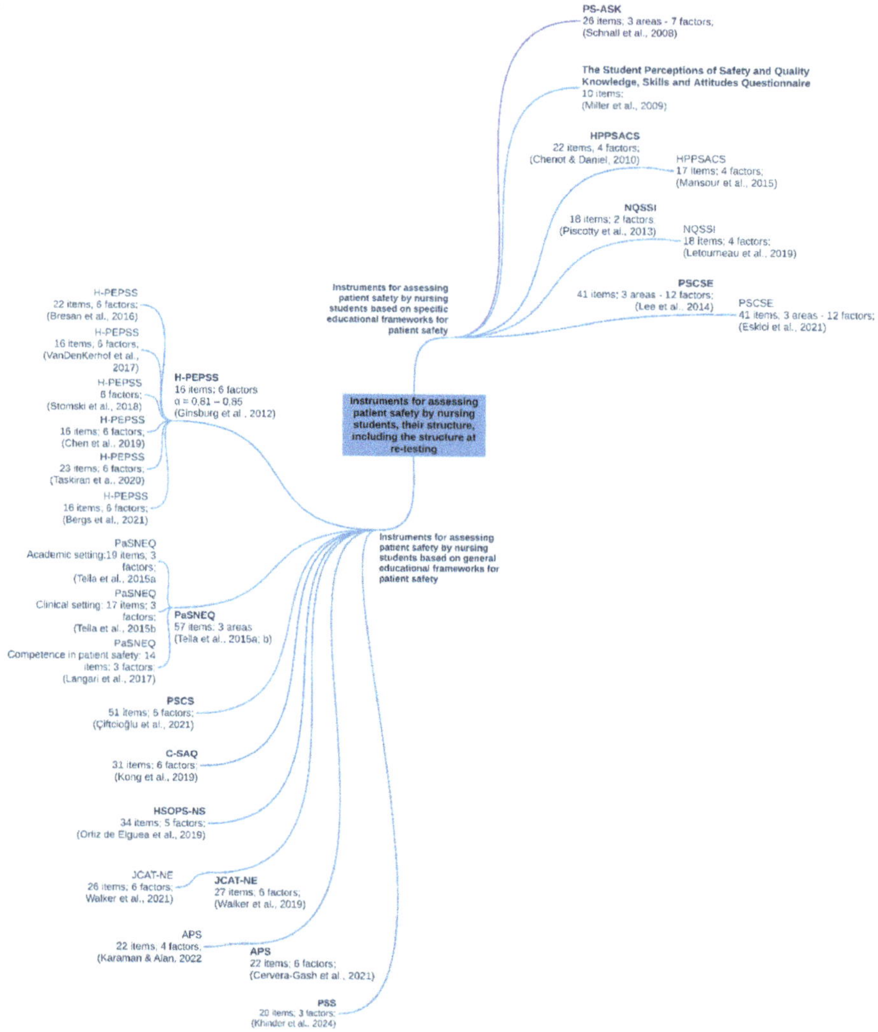

Chapter 8

Creativity as a Sociological Category and a Factor of Mental Health

Dmitry Petrovich Gavra
https://orcid.org/0000-0002-6536-9277
St. Petersburg State University, Russia

Julia Paulevna Bayer
https://orcid.org/0000-0002-1866-3633
Russian Academy of National Economy and Public Administration, Russia

ABSTRACT

Creativity is considered one of the most complex human competences/abilities or behaviors. As sociologists, we consider creativity as a considerable factor in humanity's welfare, in terms of sense of fulfilment and happiness. We believe that social well-being, going hand in hand with the creative realization of one's purpose, is a two-way process. So, there are two factors that influence the enrichment of life: firstly, the state and conditions for creativity, which determines the feeling of inner satisfaction, and; secondly, the individual realization of one's own destiny and the socialization of an inner 'gift', i.e. abilities and talent. In this chapter we dive into the basic definitions of creativity and its theories, social conditions and beneficial, as well as hindering factors.The authors consider the ability of being creative as one of the main mental health conditions factors, as well as the opportunity to contact with art in all the ways during time of being disabled in the hospital as beneficial factor for mental health.The authors consider that environment can be supportive to creativity and suppressive and that each organization (hospitals included) can help the creative potential to unfold, creating a proper environment – the authors

DOI: 10.4018/979-8-3373-5931-1.ch008

call them socially harmonious (laminar, favorable) conditions for creativity, or suppress it by social rules and norms, we call them socialization unfavorable (conflict, turbulent) factors of creativity.

INTRODUCTION

The field of sociology concerns itself with, among other topics, society, human behavior, and aspects of everyday life. One area where sociological research can be applied are the social factors of the mental well-being and psychological comfort of individuals. As sociologists, we consider creativity to be an important factor in the mental well-being of individuals and humanity as a whole in terms of reproducing a sense of fulfillment and happiness. Thus, we see it as our duty to delve deeper into what creativity is and to disseminate our findings among the professional community and the general public. Professionals and public might be interested in what factors motivate humanity to be creative, or the social conditions that bolster creativity's effects on unlocking our best selves. In this chapter we will consider the healing effects of creative state of mind in general and especially when we consider patients of the hospital before and after the surgery, in the period of physical limitation and, consequently, increased psychological stress. Also, we will consider how consuming art in all its forms can enhance the recovery period. This chapter plans to do just that.

Currently, discussions continue to be held around the concepts of creativity and nature as well as the social conditions for being creative. Demand for creativity as a professional competence has significantly increased in the 21st century. This was detailed in our earlier publication defining the creative social potential of the digital society, the features of its formation, the social factors influencing it, and we proposed a typology of creativity and ways of its social regulation (Gavra, Bajer 2021).

Creativity is considered one of the most complex human competences/abilities or behaviors. Opinions about the origins of creativity vary, and none of them fully explains the genesis and dynamics of the creative process at the individual, organizational or societal level. Creativity is seen as: a divine quality, random activity, 'planned luck' and 'method' (Cook, 1998).

The problem of a sociologically operational definition of creativity as a characteristic of a social subject, a social process or a product of social activity is not fully resolved in modern sociology. One thing remains certain and confirmed through the empirical studies, is that creative state of mind is correlated with the higher brain waves. This state Dr. Joe Dispenza describes as "getting beyond the analytical mind" and he names these states of mind ***delta*** (the highest,) and ***alpha*** (it goes before the delta state) (Dispenza, 2017). Creating is like meditation, it is always getting beyond the analytical mind and it means that the creative person reaches the delta brainwaves that are considered as healing (Dispenza, 2017). That is also one of the reasons that creativity is strongly correlated with happiness. Being creative is an internal state that doesn't depend on external circumstances. Like for meditation a person just needs a place to seat, for creativity a person only needs usually simple tools to create. Even in prison, even out of civilization – creative person will create, because he/she is being driven by the internal forces to fulfill his/her potential.

Because, as we have mentioned earlier, creative state of mind is strongly correlated with healing beta brainwaves, we go further and can state that being creative contributes to the state of being happy and that is – strongly correlates with mental health and lowers depression and anxiety. This is one of the main reasons why we recommend to implement opportunities of being creative to the patients in the hospitals as well as giving them option to "consume" art in forms of reading books, listening to music, watching the classy masterpieces in movies or drawings on the screen.

In a Maslow's hierarchy pyramid, where he describes the five levels of human needs, from basic survival to self-fulfillment and self-realization, being creative is the highest in the hierarchy. We can counter this approach with the thesis that the need for creativity does not necessarily have to be satisfied after all other basic needs have been satisfied (food, water, sexual needs, safety, love and belonging, self-esteem and acknowledgement). History knows many examples, when creators produce their art being in prison, being psychologically deviant, not being loved and acknowledged by society) and still producing to the world the masterpieces of literature, paintings, music and so on.

Creative characteristics as a personality trait of social subjects have become relevant both in their own right (participation in and winning competitions, creative products and cultural artifacts such as books, hits, and paintings), and in the service of advertising, blue ocean marketing strategies, science, and so on.

The location of creative act becomes not important. From the global lockdown we learned that place of creating a masterpiece can be from home sofa to remote corner in nature. Thus, we will take the assumption that creativity as social activity can be (and should be) encouraged to be realized in the hospitals as well.

We can assert that both the public demand for creativity and the supply of this characteristic are undergoing significant changes in modern society. Creativity has now become a sought-after skill, capable of generating high income for its possessors. So, if we consider the time of the patients in the hospital as time to re-consider their life, to pause and open up through creating their potential, the "sick list" time will be perceived in public opinion as time to recover not only physically, but also spiritually.

Unleashing the potential of creativity in social exchanges facilitates the creation, retention, and growth of social capital in the context of the expansion of digital communications.

The digital communications have no boundaries and are not attached neither are dependent on any geolocation. Every patient in the hospital can transmit his/her creative product to the whole world by just publishing it on Instagram, YouTube or any other social media platform. Nowadays we cannot deny the influence of opinion leaders such as bloggers, on society. Bloggers act as opinion leaders, shaping their followers' attitudes toward events in politics, culture, and everyday life. Bloggers, and now TikTokers, are role models in lifestyle, fashion style, choice of phone brand, car, and so on. Interestingly, in terms of pure professional competences, bloggers seem extremely vulnerable. They, in most cases, lack professional training in the subject matter they write about. And they write about virtually everything that catches the attention of their audiences. This means that in a digital platform society, the nature of social capital is changing. But its functions remain the same.

The legitimacy of the social influence of digital opinion leaders as concentrators of the attention is ensured by thousands, even millions, of devoted followers. Thanks to public support, these traffic monopolists receive carte blanche for creativity, freedom of expression (only the legal boundaries), and financial independence (again, thanks to their followers, bloggers earn money from advertising). Thus, they can devote their free time to produce new, creative products and creativity as social force in general.

Let's now consider that every patient in the hospital can actually have public feedback and, what is very important for the socially isolated (or limited in communications) patients, have communication with hundreds, thousands and even millions people in different parts of the world through his/her creative product / piece of art in whatever form it may be and whatever shape this piece of art might take. So, for us as sociologists, it is very important to consider the fact that in digital era there is almost no option **not to** become famous if you have talent and have any devise with access to the internet. Patients can become bloggers, using time being in bed to upgrade their skills, discover talents that in usual life could not be fulfilled (main work, routine, family obligations).

We believe that creativity and artistic expression become social phenomena only through the process of social acceptance by various social groups—that is, more broadly, when a creative product is incorporated into a system of social exchanges. Therefore, manuscripts "put in the drawer," "in the fire" (outstanding Russian writer N. Gogol, who burned his manuscript, is a great example) as well as other creative products that never see the light of day, cannot be considered creative products.

That is why we insist here that sharing\communicating the products of creativity is essential final stage of creative act and especially it is necessary for the isolated creators, that is, in our example, those, who can't share with the society directly, patients in the hospital.

So, the conditional social isolation of the patients in the hospital becomes their conscious choice. If they want – they limit it to the level of semi-solitude, communicating only with the nurse, doctor and family members, but if they don't want to be/feel isolated – they always have access to the bigger audience.

So, let's return to the question posed above about the dual nature of creativity. We tend to think that one complements the other. Of course, if talent and an inclination toward creativity are clearly expressed, and the circumstances of place and time are favorable, then society, in most cases, is unable to "retain" this talent within the creator (we know of many examples of this). And the creators, in turn, are unable to retain it within themselves, since there is social demand for this creative product. At the same time, we will never know about those talents that have not manifested themselves due to societal limitations and the creator's lack of personal courage.

We understand the complex nature of creativity as an integral part of an individual's innate, biological, and genetically determined characteristics, as well as social characteristics, primarily those of socialization. We also believe that creativity, as a social phenomenon and, we would add, an economic phenomenon, emerges only through the process of social exchange.

Despite the wide range of works on the general and social theory of creativity, both classical (Guilford 1950; Parnes 1972; Parnes, Noller 1972; Amabile 1982; Amabile 1983; Baer 1988; Csikszentmihalyi 1988; Csikszentmihalyi 1996; Torrance 1996) and new (Sternberg 1999; Sternberg, Kaufman, Pretz 2001; Kaufman, Baer 2005), some methodologically important problems remain unclear.

We view the basic ability to be creative in a society or social group as an important component of quality of life and wellbeing. We believe that without the opportunity to be creative, the life of a modern person will be incomplete. In this chapter we invite you to dive into the new definitions, new understandings and typologies of creativity.

Indeed, when a person is at least somewhat able to rise above daily worries such as food and safety, ordinary life emotions and fears, and has the time to freely create, his life acquires an important intrinsic meaning that enriches everyday routine with purpose.

We believe that social well-being, going hand in hand with the creative realization of one's purpose, is a two-way process. So, there are two factors that influence the enrichment of life: firstly, the state and its society create conditions for creativity, which determines the feeling of inner satisfaction, and secondly, the individual realization of one's own destiny and the socialization of an inner 'gift', i.e. abilities and talent.

We believe that ontologically, creativity can be considered in two statuses:

1. *The first – basic – is the modus vivendi of any social actor.* We consider the basic ability to be creative as an important component of the quality of life. Without this possibility, at least in some limited subject period, the life of a modern person will not be of full value. That's why we propose that hospitals develop programs to encourage patients to engage in creative practices during their recovery period, using creative practices as social technologies for ensuring comprehensive rehabilitation. This opportunity can become the impetus for changing a patient's life or achieving a breakthrough.
2. *The second ontological status of creativity* is associated with the transition of this characteristic into the sphere of professional self-realization of the social actor. In this status, creativity is already a professional characteristic, quoted on the social exchange market. It is a sought-after soft skill for almost any information professional and is also utilized by those who implement routine services. Encountering examples such as cleaning the floor and singing, or making coffee while drawing a sketch on a paper cup are creative practices where we are nicely surprised and uplifted us through these interactions. At the same time, it's clear that no additional creative market value is generated that would increase the subject's social capital. A floor washed in silence is no different to an employer than one washed while singing a cheerful song.

In the postmodern era of information and technology the concept of creativity has become especially in demand. When quoting and replicas or even AI products have become commonplace in creativity; when cultural actors recognize that it is difficult to create something new.

Thus, we can assert that both the public demand for creativity and the supply for this characteristic are undergoing noticeable changes in modern society. Creativity has now become a sought-after competency that can bring high income to its owners.

THEORIES/PARADIGMS

Based on the research of P. Sorokin, K. Neigus, M. Pickering, T. Adorno and others, we will consider creativity to be the ability of an individual, using his/her imagination, abilities and sociocultural experience, to create an innovative, original product in any field life of society. *At the same time, this innovative creative product has two characteristics. First, it has a market value in the system of social exchanges. Secondly, it increases the social capital of the creative subject.*

We highlight the main sociological paradigms in the study of creativity in modern science:

1. *Transcendental paradigm* (key categories: muse, divine providence, higher power). Creativity is regarded as a response to an internal need, to a higher power and to creative self-expression.

World-famous sociologist, Pitirim Sorokin, who studied the nature of true masterpieces, in his works cites great scientists, writers, artists, musicians, where everyone conveys in different words the same essence of creativity, "I am just a channel, I am like a medium." (Sorokin, 1962). Thus, due to the fact that we are obviously dealing with the transcendental nature of true inspiration, this is how it has become common to call it creativity. Moreover, understanding and acceptance of this nature of creativity has led to the return of mediation, a 'technique' for bridging the mind-body gap, into the lives of Western world.

Creativity as a state of mind helped many famous people to keep their mental health during limitations that they were enduring being in prison as well as in hospital, being limited in movements as well as possibilities of communication. So, we can state here that the decision and state of mind of being creative comes from within the person and anyone can fulfil it no matter how the external circumstances are unfolding. Viktor Frankl is one of the greatest examples of the creative scientist being in prison and not only creating, but also supporting others not to give up.

Researchers and common people have recorded/noticed the rapidly growing popularity of various mentors, books on development, retreat practices, yoga and meditation. Even employers (in Silicon Valley, for example) are introducing meditation into daily work practices in order to increase the productivity and creativity of their employees. Within this paradigm, it is generally accepted that meditation, unlike drugs and alcohol, is the most reliable way to establish contact with the 'muse'.

The modern American scientist, Dr. Joe Dispenza, has proven the benefits of meditation in overcoming the analytical mind and revealing creative abilities (Dispenza, 2012).

2. *Market, externally determined paradigm* (key category: market, demand). Creativity as a response to an external, market request, i.e. creativity is forced, creativity makes order. Depending on the level of professionalism by the subject, it can be performed in an original way, with novelty in form and content, and therefore is also considered creative.

In this case, the manufactured product cannot always be considered creative, but only if it contains innovative potential, which is revealed in further social practices of consuming this product. Figuratively speaking, this happens when the creator's muse is ready to fulfill the technical task or whim of the customer and, moreover, to comply with the dead-line - just like the executor of orders for creativity. If the muse is capricious, the creator still fulfils the order, based on skill and craft experience, and the result is a craft product with a creative component that is insufficient to be recognized as a truly creative product. Let's designate it as **a craft** or **para-creative product**. And we will designate the subject's activity itself in this format as **paracreative**. There is undoubtedly a creative component in it, the creator always has it, but this component is subordinate, secondary.

3. *Introspective paradigm* (key categories: internal motive, liberation, psychotrauma). Creativity as a response to personal problems is a creative 'purge' of psychological traumas, fears and complexes. It may be of interest due to the brightness and originality of the presentation and the openness of the individual themselves. For example, the famous artist, Frida Kahlo, is a striking example of personal creativity, whose psychotraumas and fears, creatively presented on canvas, became a message to society, received worldwide resonance and even contributed to the development of feminism in Latin America.

We also believe that ***creativity*** becomes a social phenomenon only in the process of perception by society, by various social groups. To put it more broadly, when a creative product is included in the system of social exchanges. Thus, such manuscripts that are created, put into the fire, as well as other results of creativity that did not have time to 'be published', cannot be considered a creative product.

We understand the complex nature of creativity as integral to the biologically innate, genetically predetermined characteristics of the individual, and social characteristics, primarily in the realm of society. We also believe *that creativity as a social phenomenon and, we would add, an economic phenomenon, is born only in the process of social exchanges.*

We would like to introduce another dichotomous dimension of creativity. *Creativity can be individual and collective.* Likewise, a creative product can be a product of individual or collective creativity. For example, a painting or a piece of music are basically individual creative products. However, an opera based on this piece or a film is already a collectively creative product.

We believe that creativity cannot be elevated to some kind of absolute. Creativity is important for growth and development, creating new products and services, creating new *blue ocean markets. Conformity and creativity are equally important in the development of society.* Creativity and conformity are not genius and villainy. Society must change, must develop, and at the same time consolidate and reproduce characteristics that ensure positive social inheritance.

Conformity is responsible for stability, predictability, calm and comfort. For stable and progressive development, carriers of conformal identity are no less important.

In addition, it can be assumed that creative and conformist principles can coexist within the same personality.

The combination of creative individuals (leaders) and followers provides a kind of balance. From both a biological and a sociological point of view, society does not need only bright, explosively creative individuals, but rational, conformative and thus predictable humans as well, in order to provide stability inside the social institutions.

Now let's move on to the concept of creative products. Indeed, in the modern market of goods and services, where creativity is a highly paid quality, it is important to determine the main characteristics by which we will determine the degree of creativity of products, and therefore their market value.

The authors of the article believe that creative products:

- Firstly, have market value in the system of social exchanges;
- Secondly, establish the status of a social subject as a subject of creative practices;
- Thirdly, contribute to the direct and social capitalization of this entity.

To construct a typology of creativity, we have distinguished two types of grounds:

1. The *first group of grounds* is designated as *socialization.*

On the foundations of socialization related to creativity, we understand a set of social factors that promote or hinder the process of socialization of an individual as a subject of creative practices.

Let's call this process *creative socialization.* Using the example of Van Gogh and Mozart, we can talk about socialization factors that promote and hinder the realization of creative potential and, accordingly, about *socialization harmony* (laminar, favorable - the socialization of Mozart as a historical case) and *socialization conflict* (turbulent, unfavorable, opposing - the socialization of Van Gogh) creativity. In our subsequent studies, we will consider which social factors contribute to the development of talent and creativity, and which ones suppress it and prevent it from happening.

2. The *second group of grounds* for the typology of creativity consists of factors in the *socio-political environment external to the creative subject.*

To establish this, we use the different attitudes towards creativity evident in ancient Athens and Sparta. In doing so, we come to two types of social conditions in the realization of creative potential and designate them as *societally favorable* (the historical example of the ancient state of Athens, that was encouraging arts and sciences in its highest state at 5-th century BC) and *societally unfavorable* (the historical example of the state of Sparta with its dictatorship suppressive attitude towards its citizens). In this case, society, its norms and values, and the style of government have been proven to influence the flourishing or decline in creative productivity. In a totalitarian regime, it is difficult to expect the flourishing of science, art and the creative, carefree, bold manifestations of individuals. However, in some cases, harsh state repression can give rise to an internal creative response. This can be compared to the internal immune response of the spirits to have the ability to create open for them no matter what. As an example, consider underground fine art and rock music in the Soviet Union in the 1960s and 1970s.

We stated earlier that creativity is as important in society as conformity. They form a dialectical pair. Nevertheless, it is creativity that makes a person's life more fulfilling and therefore happier, and thus should take place in the lives of individuals, regardless of the field of activity, which they are engaged in. That is why, since happiness is a common denominator of creativity and freedom, we suggest here to introduce this state of mind to the patients, also because creativity eliminates or just reduces fear, anxiety and thus – hormone cortisol. Low level of cortisol enhances the strength of the immune system.

Within the context of large-scale communications campaigns with a creative component, the very nature of creativity is largely determined by the type of communications strategy chosen. This establishes a fundamental premise that determines the nature of strategic creativity.

This premise stems from the need for strategic coherence in each major communications campaign, which implies a kind of strategic "Russian matryoshka" logic, whereby the organization's overall strategy provides a framework for developing a communications strategy, which, in turn, defines the framework for the marketing strategy, within which the communications strategy is integrated.

This communicative strategy can be implemented in any business, governmental, medical or educational organization.

Strategy (both corporate and marketing) determines the nature and extent of creativity in content development, channel selection, message packaging, and, ultimately, the communicator's image and demeanor, as well as the artifacts and visual aids that accompany this communication. Imagine, that if a medical hospital will position itself on the market that not only that it provides its patients with high quality surgery implementing and medical assistance, but also with the equipment and possibilities for creative practices on the recovery period in order to make the recovery smoother, faster and preventing the depressive syndrome. Abilities of helping and supporting creative state of mind is being a crucial factor of helping hospital patients to be happier and path through tough times easier and without traumas.

Thus, successful creative communication at the corporate level is an effectively implemented set of communications practices for the creation and application of creative products, aimed at implementing a communications strategy as an integral part of the corporate strategy. Creative communication in case of hospitals will mostly occur between nurses and patients, but also the doctors can advise their patients to try being creative in different ways as well as consume art, poetry, literature while recovering.

From well-known strategy typologies we will take the *blue ocean theory* of R. Mauborgne and K. Chan, which is relevant to our objectives. Its authors distinguish two main scenarios of market behavior: red and blue ocean strategies.

Red/blood ocean strategy: a social actor focuses on competing with other actors within a market niche. Time and effort are spent monitoring the market and competitors' communication strategies. "Companies stuck in a red ocean followed a traditional approach, striving to defeat competitors and trying to achieve a defensible position within the established industry order" (Kim & Mauborgne, 2014).

Blue ocean strategy presupposes a high level of creativity, courage, and confidence in success. "Blue ocean strategy aims to encourage companies to break out of the red ocean of competition by creating a market niche where they can avoid competition" (Kim & Mauborgne, 2014).

This dichotomy represents a potential divergence in the conditions for realizing the creative potential inherent in each market player. Under equal competitive conditions and relatively equal creative potential, it is the choice of strategy along this parameter that determines the success of unlocking creative potential.

Personnel employed by a company that has chosen a red ocean strategy are constrained in their creative communications by the rules, stereotypes, and norms of red ocean markets. The hospitals, for example, working in the red ocean strategies, don't suggest their patients the opportunities to create.

Thus, continuing and developing the ideas we have expressed above, we can say that the strategic context of red oceans is characterized by socially unfavorable (conflictual, turbulent) factors for creativity. We define the choice and implementation of such a strategy as a factor that hinders the realization of creative potential. In such conditions, employees will most often choose a strategy of responding to market challenges, remaining within a given, and therefore limited, market labyrinth.

A company that has discovered a blue ocean strategy, creates socially harmonious (laminar, favorable) conditions for creativity. We define such a strategy as a strategy of communicative motivation of creativity. Thus, the strategy chosen by management of whatever organization (governmental, business, medical, educational etc.) determines the possibilities for implementing creative practices.

In the context of a blue ocean communication strategy, employee/client/patient creativity will have the opportunity to reach new levels of innovation and non-conformity. Moreover, a blue ocean strategy will require well-developed creative environment that will facilitate the development of talent.

This is what should be provided in case of maintaining mental health along with physical health among patients in any medical hospital. If hospital will not only acknowledge that mental health and opportunities to create has direct correlation with physical health, but also will educate the personnel (from doctors to nurses) to implement communication with the patients the way that it provides the opportunities and environment for the patients to maintain mental health by being creative. This can go even further. If we consider the illness as a "wake up call", the opportunity of opening up the creative potential during "sick list time" can be considered not only as a method of maintaining mental health, but also as a leap in personal growth. Thus, each illness can be perceived by the culture of a healthcare organization as a time for the patient to slow down, to rethink what aspects of the previous lifestyle and social factors led to the illness, and at the same time, as an opportunity to use targeted communication with works of art, literature, music, etc., as well as to create artistic products and thereby act as a factor in the healing process. And the blue ocean strategy will be very appropriate for such healthcare institutions.

The profile parameter in relation to creativity has two dimensions and highlights core and non-core creative potential.

First, we propose distinguishing *creative and non-creative profiles* in each area of social practice. With a profile for creative potential of either an individual or group, we understand the potential that is realized from the main profile of their professional activity. Accordingly, non-core potential is realized either in leisure practices or in professional practices not related to the main profile of the subject's professional activity.

Based on the nature of innovation criterion contained in a creative product, we propose a typological division into *conformal* and *non-conformal/radical creativity.*

Conformal creativity generates a creative product within the framework set by existing norms for the subject of creative practice. These can be norms of different types: norms of culture, aesthetics, technological processes, engineering and so forth. Examples of this can be seen in the generally accepted standards of beauty in painting, or classical canons in poetry, drama, and design. While preserving all the attributes of creativity, conformal creativity ensures laminar dynamics of the sphere in which it is realized. This type of creativity functionally supports social continuity.

Non-conformal/radical creativity, on the contrary, is responsible for social variability, so its dynamics are turbulent. Innovations contained in a non-conforming/radical creative product do not rely on existing norms, they break them, and if successful, set new norms. Such creativity is a breakthrough into new frameworks and boundaries that have not yet been established, so it is difficult for consumers of non-conforming creativity to accept it. Legitimacy and internalization of a radical creative product is a complex social process that requires, in addition to its own creative subject, a subject of a different type. Let's call this subject a creative mediator. As a rule, this is the holder of a high expert status in the relevant field, based on competencies and social/cultural capital. The mediator's task is to ensure the internalization of the new norm generated by a radical creative product.

WHAT IS CREATIVITY?

Our position is as follows:

Creativity is the competence of an individual, using his/her imagination, abilities and sociocultural experience, to create an innovative, original socially demanded product in any sphere of society.

Social demand can be immediate or deferred, projected into the future. This is how so-called "unrecognized geniuses" function, those ahead of their time.

At the same time, this innovative creative product has two characteristics.

- First, it has a market value in the system of social exchanges;
- Secondly, it increases the personal social capital of the creative subject.

As previously stated, creativity is a soft skill that is very highly valued in the labor market. It is the quality of any product, which therefore, due to their unique creativity, are sold very expensively. As well, this content delivers intellectual and/ or aesthetic pleasure, which is why visiting theater productions, film premieres and art exhibitions are so highly valued.

Furthermore, as always happens in the market, where there is an original, there is also a copy, or even, a fake. In the market paradigm, along with a creative product, a *paracreative product* can function.

Let's understand how creative products are manufactured when they have a customer. A creative product is created, figuratively speaking, when the creator's muse is ready to fulfill the technical task or whim of the customer, precisely as the muse also follows the dead-line. This process results in a *Creative Product.*

However, inspiration may not come, and the muse may be capricious but the creator still fulfills the order, based on skill and craft experience, and the output is a craft product with a creative component. None the less we still have to acknowledge that it is insufficient to recognize this product as fully creative, though containing creative component. There is still an old saying: "Everything that the hand of a master touches becomes a masterpiece."

Let's designate it as a craft or para-creative product. Here we will designate the subject's activity itself in this format as *paracreative*. There is undoubtedly a creative component in it, the creator always has it, but this component is subordinate, secondary. The difficulty also lies in the fact *that creative and paracreative products can often be distinguished only by an expert* or, in controversial cases, a creative mediator, who, as we wrote above, legitimizes and internalizes the creative product in society. The reason, according to formal criteria, is that a 'product' enters the market, and only a specialist can confidently evaluate its creative or para-creative characteristics, which often even an inexperienced customer will not see.

In a society built on the principle of freedom of self-expression and the encouragement of this self-expression, the emancipation and outrageousness of the average person would not be surprising. It is these qualities that are often passed off as creativity, while, in fact, they are *paracreative.*

True talent in any field will be unmistakably noticeable to a specialist. Moreover, excellent social conditions will be created for the development of this talent. In this case, the fundamental difference between the subjects of creativity and paracreativity will be obvious. But in other cases, this divergence is practically indistinguishable. Even a great maestro has successes and failures, outstanding masterpieces and run-of-the-mill commissioned works, but because they bear the stamp of his name and individuality, experts and society more often than not classify these failures as genuinely creative products. The logic here is that "if it's made by an entity socially legitimized as creative, then it's a creative product."

By creative social practices we mean practices that result in the creation of creative products.

We define a *creative product* as *a product of human activity, functioning in the field of social exchanges, the consumer value of which is the satisfaction of a certain set of higher needs, in particular, aesthetic, symbolic, the need for belonging, etc. It is the creative component that determines the exchange value of a creative product as a commodity.*

Thus, creative products, *firstly*, have market value in the system of social exchange; *secondly*, establish the status of a social subject as a subject of creative practice and *thirdly*, contribute to the direct and social capitalization of this subject.

To more accurately characterize a creative product in the context of the criterion of non-conventionality, *we propose to introduce three dimensions:*

1. novelty/unconventionality of the idea/product;
2. novelty/unconventional situation of using the product;
3. novelty/unconventional way of using the product.

Each of these characteristics can be present in a creative product, stand-alone, or any combination.

The criterion of market relevance retains its role. As a result, *we propose to distinguish three types of creative products with characteristics of market relevance:*

- based on subject (product) creativity;
- based on situational creativity;
- based on application (that is, usefulness) creativity.

From our point of view, there are three ontological dimensions of creativity: *product, subjective and activity.*

The *starting point* is the *subject (product) dimension.* In this regard, creativity is a characteristic of a product, giving it a special quality - the quality of a creative product.

Two more related ontological dimensions are subjective and activity.

In the subjective understanding, creativity is a characteristic of the subject who creates a creative product. Such a subject can be designated as a creative subject, a creator.

The second dimension is *activity-based*, emphasizing that *creativity is a characteristic of the type of activity, nature of performance of certain productive functions while producing a product recognized as creative. Accordingly, creativity in society exists and is realized as a special type of activity.*

Let's add to this that *the use value of a creative product can have both a rational and an emotional dimension.*

On the one hand, *in a rational dimension*, a creative product allows social subject to solve problems and satisfy his\her needs of in a more effective way than similar products without a creative component. Furthermore, this difference in the efficiency of use/consumption is the grain of rational use value and the basis for rational pricing of a creative product.

In the *emotional dimension*, the use value of a creative product has a fundamentally different nature. Here, the first place comes from the pleasure of consumption, positive emotions, associated effects on different sensory systems such as vision, hearing, smell, taste, joy and pride in ownership, etc. In the case of emotional use value, a kind of goodwill is formed.

Let's now move on to consider the *communicative nature of a creative product and its legitimization in a sociological sense.* This kind of understanding of the nature of a creative product brings to the conclusion about its communicative nature. Let us venture to formulate an important thesis: that the ontology of creativity, as well as the nature of the creative product, is linked to the category of communication. *A creative subject puts a certain message into their product - pragmatic, aesthetic, emotional. This message is sent to the relevant target audiences of the creative product, its potential consumers.* Only by decoding the meanings embedded in a given product message, related to novelty/unconventionality and practical usefulness/market relevance, does target audiences give this product the status of creative.

Considering *the social functioning of a creative product,* let us turn to the study of this creative product in the process of its social functioning, and note that *it has two components: internal content and form of presentation.* Each of these components is capable of having creative characteristics that together generate the power of influence of the creative product on target audiences.

Internal content is the meaning, the idea conveyed by a creative product. The meaning and idea can be new and revolutionary. The creators of computers, cars, airplanes, mobile phones, of course, were distinguished by one thing - they saw and believed in a radically new, conventionally speaking, creative product. A fundamentally new innovative idea, a 'blue ocean' in which there are no competitors.

The creative internal content of an idea may or may not be combined with the same innovative form of its presentation.

There may be situations when *only the form of presentation is creative.* It, the form of presentation, is fundamentally important in cases where the idea is 'as old as time' - themes of love, the beauty of nature, life dramas, etc. Each generation of writers, artists, directors present it in its own, unique and artistic way.

If we rely on the introduced two-dimensional understanding of creativity, we can assume the possibility of the existence of *three forms of social existence of creative products:*

- creative in internal content + creative in presentation form;
- creative in internal content + ordinary in presentation form;
- ordinary in content + creative in presentation form.

As a result, we can conclude that creativity in the sociological dimension is not only a characteristic of a social subject or product of activity, it is always a social-communicative relationship within the triad of production-exchange-consumption of some special value contained in a creative product.

Society and its power institutions, by creating and supporting social norms aimed at developing internal freedom and creativity, contributes to the formation of a happier society in a broad sense, where each participant in social interaction has the conditions created for the disclosure and realization of his/her own creative potential.

Digital reality creates new conditions for the social scaling of creative practices and creative products, since, if desired, each creator can tell the whole world about him/herself and set the communicative, and therefore social, scale of his/her creative practices independently.

In the 21st century, in the era of artificial intelligence and neural networks, where not only people, but also technology compete to create a new, original creative product, it is extremely important for sociologists to highlight what distinguishes a creative product, what are the main social factors that influence the formation of creativity as a universally *sought-after soft skill*, and how creativity can be measured in society for the purpose of maximum disclosure. In our further research, we will propose methods for sociological measurement of creativity.

We advance the hypothesis that the opportunity to be creative, to discover talents and one's purpose makes each individual in society more subjectively happy, and therefore increases the index of social wellbeing in society as a whole. Of course, this is not the only factor, but we are convinced that it is one of the fundamental ones. We believe that the opportunity for self-realization through the opportunity to be creative in a profession or hobby has a direct impact on life satisfaction.

Thus, creativity is not only a sought-after soft skill of our age, but also a social function that, if successfully managed, will create healthy, satisfied social groups and societies.

We would like to change the paradigm of illnesses and condition of people being sick that their life is being put on hold. On the contrary, we think that *hospitals should provide their patients with supportive environment to create and consume art,* and use the time of being sick as a time to make a leap in their spiritual growth which will make them happier and more fulfilled by the time that they recover. Hospitals, who provide these, *societally favorable factors*, for their patients, will definitely create a blue ocean market and will win not only economically, but also reputationally among the grateful patients and their parents.

REFERENCES

Amabile, T. (1982). Social psychology of creativity: A consensual assessment technique. *Journal of Personality and Social Psychology*, *43*(5), 997–1013. DOI: 10.1037/0022-3514.43.5.997

Amabile, T. (1983). *The social psychology of creativity*. SpringerVerlag. DOI: 10.1007/978-1-4612-5533-8

Baer, J.Jr. (1988). Long-term effects of creativity training with middle school students. *The Journal of Early Adolescence*, *8*(8), 183–193. DOI: 10.1177/0272431688082006

Cook, P. (1998). *Best practice creativity*. Gower Publishing Limited.

Csikszentmihalyi, M. (1988). Society, culture, and person: A systems view of creativity. In Sternberg, R. J. (Ed.), *The nature of creativity* (pp. 325–339). Cambridge University Press.

Csikszentmihalyi, M. (1996). *Creativity: Flow and the psychology of discovery and invention*. HarperCollins.

Dispenza, J. (2012). *Breaking the habit of being yourself: How to lose your mind and create a new one*. Hay House, Inc.

Dispenza, J. (2017). *Becoming supernatural: How common people are doing the uncommon*. Hay House, Inc.

Gavra, D., & Bajer, Y. (2021) Creative social potential of digital society. *Administrative Consulting*. Vol. 154. No. 10. P. 54-61. . (In Russ.).DOI: 10.22394/1726-1139-2021-10-54-61

Kim, W. C., & Mauborgne, R. A. (2014). *Blue ocean strategy, expanded edition: How to create uncontested market space and make the competition irrelevant*. Harvard business review Press.

Sorokin, P. A. (1962). *Social and Cultural Dynamics* (Vol. 3).

Chapter 9
Global Health Literacy and Nursing's Role in Health Promotion Across Borders

G. SudhaAnanthi
https://orcid.org/0009-0001-5062-5311
Winners Academy, India

T. C. Manjunath
https://orcid.org/0000-0003-2545-9160
Rajarajeswari College of Engineering, Bengaluru, India

ABSTRACT

Global health literacy represents a fundamental pillar in promoting equitable health outcomes, reducing disease burden, and fostering informed decision-making across diverse populations. At its core, health literacy encompasses the ability of individuals and communities to access, comprehend, evaluate, and utilize health-related information to make informed decisions regarding their physical, mental, and social well-being. In an increasingly interconnected world, where health challenges transcend national boundaries, understanding global health literacy is crucial not only for individual empowerment but also for shaping resilient healthcare systems and sustainable public health strategies. Despite its recognized importance, global health literacy is unevenly distributed, reflecting and perpetuating existing socio-economic disparities. Populations in low- and middle-income countries (LMICs), marginalized communities, and vulnerable demographic groups.

DOI: 10.4018/979-8-3373-5931-1.ch009

INTRODUCTION

Global health literacy represents a fundamental pillar in promoting equitable health outcomes, reducing disease burden, and fostering informed decision-making across diverse populations. At its core, health literacy encompasses the ability of individuals and communities to access, comprehend, evaluate, and utilize health-related information to make informed decisions regarding their physical, mental, and social well-being. In an increasingly interconnected world, where health challenges transcend national boundaries, understanding global health literacy is crucial not only for individual empowerment but also for shaping resilient healthcare systems and sustainable public health strategies. Despite its recognized importance, global health literacy is unevenly distributed, reflecting and perpetuating existing socio-economic disparities. Populations in low- and middle-income countries (LMICs), marginalized communities, and vulnerable demographic groups often face significant barriers, including limited educational resources, inadequate healthcare infrastructure, linguistic and cultural differences, and systemic inequities. Such disparities undermine their capacity to engage in proactive health management, contributing to delayed diagnosis, poor adherence to treatment, and heightened susceptibility to preventable diseases. Conversely, in high-income regions, although healthcare accessibility may be greater, challenges persist in the form of health misinformation, complex medical terminologies, and varying levels of digital literacy, all of which can hinder effective decision-making and risk comprehension.

The rapidly evolving global health landscape has further amplified the significance of health literacy. Epidemics, pandemics, and emerging infectious diseases demand that populations are equipped with timely and accurate knowledge to adopt preventive measures, comply with public health directives, and counteract the proliferation of misinformation. The COVID-19 pandemic, in particular, underscored the consequences of low health literacy, where misinformation about disease transmission, vaccine efficacy, and treatment protocols propagated rapidly, exacerbating morbidity and mortality. Such experiences highlight that global health literacy is not merely an individual competence but a collective societal resource, with implications for policy-making, health system resilience, and international cooperation. Integrating health literacy into broader educational curricula, community-based programs, and digital health platforms can serve as powerful interventions. Programs that contextualize information culturally, linguistically, and socially demonstrate enhanced uptake, as individuals are more likely to internalize and act upon health guidance that resonates with their lived experiences and belief systems. Additionally, participatory approaches that involve communities in co-creating health content ensure relevance, trust, and sustainability, thereby strengthening health literacy from a grassroots level. Technological advancements present both opportunities and challenges in this domain. The proliferation of digital health tools, mobile applications, telemedicine, and online health information platforms provides unprecedented access to health resources, potentially bridging gaps in regions with limited physical healthcare infrastructure.

However, the digital divide poses a critical challenge, as those with limited access to technology, digital skills, or internet connectivity may remain excluded from these advancements, further widening disparities. Moreover, the sheer volume of information available online, coupled with inconsistent quality and credibility, necessitates the cultivation of critical appraisal skills. Health literacy in the digital era thus extends beyond comprehension to encompass the ability to discern trustworthy sources, interpret data accurately, and apply information appropriately. This shift emphasizes the need for integrated interventions that combine traditional health education with digital literacy, ensuring populations are not only informed but also capable of navigating and utilizing information responsibly. Policy frameworks and international initiatives play an instrumental role in advancing global health literacy. The World Health Organization (WHO) and other multilateral organizations recognize health literacy as a determinant of health equity and advocate for systemic interventions that prioritize education, communication, and community engagement (Barry et al. 2012). Cross-sectoral collaboration, involving governments, educational institutions, healthcare providers, non-governmental organizations, and media outlets, is essential to create environments conducive to informed health choices. For example, embedding health literacy into primary and secondary school curricula equips younger generations with foundational skills, while community health worker programs can address adult literacy gaps in underserved populations.

THE ROLE OF NURSING IN GLOBAL HEALTH PROMOTION

Nursing, as a profession grounded in patient-centered care, advocacy, and health education, plays a pivotal role in promoting global health and addressing the complex challenges associated with contemporary health systems. Nurses represent the largest segment of the healthcare workforce worldwide, serving at the frontlines in hospitals, clinics, community settings, and emergency response units. Their unique position enables them to influence individual health behaviors, shape community health practices, and contribute to population-level health outcomes, making nursing indispensable in global health promotion. The scope of nursing extends beyond direct patient care; it encompasses health education, preventive strategies, policy advocacy, research, and leadership roles that collectively contribute to the advancement of public health objectives. Nurses are often the primary interface between health systems and communities, particularly in resource-limited and marginalized settings, where they provide critical care, disseminate evidence-based health information, and facilitate access to essential health services. Through these interventions, nurses actively address health disparities, promote equitable care, and empower communities to participate in their own health management, highlighting the profession's intrinsic connection to health promotion and disease prevention at a global scale. A central aspect of nursing in global health promotion is health education.

The educational role of nursing extends to health promotion campaigns addressing infectious diseases, sexual and reproductive health, mental health awareness, and substance abuse prevention, among other priorities. By acting as both educators and advocates, nurses bridge the gap between medical knowledge and practical implementation, ensuring that populations are informed, motivated, and equipped to make healthier choices. Nurses also serve as advocates for systemic change and policy development, influencing health determinants beyond the individual level. They contribute to the formulation of policies that promote equitable access to care, strengthen public health infrastructure, and prioritize preventive measures. Globally, nurses participate in international health organizations, governmental advisory boards, and non-governmental organizations (NGOs), shaping interventions that address health inequities, emergency preparedness, and health system resilience. For instance, nursing involvement in vaccination campaigns, disaster response, and pandemic preparedness demonstrates the profession's ability to operationalize health promotion strategies in large-scale, coordinated efforts. Additionally, nurses engage in community mobilization and partnership-building, collaborating with stakeholders to design interventions that respect cultural norms while promoting evidence-based practices. Through these advocacy and leadership roles, nursing extends its influence from the bedside to the broader health ecosystem, ensuring that health promotion is integrated into policy, planning, and resource allocation at local, national, and global levels.

Research and evidence-based practice form another cornerstone of nursing's contribution to global health promotion. Nurses conduct studies, collect data, and evaluate interventions to identify best practices that optimize health outcomes. By integrating research findings into clinical practice and public health initiatives, nurses facilitate continuous improvement in health promotion strategies, enhancing efficacy, efficiency, and sustainability. For example, community-based participatory research led by nurses has been instrumental in understanding disease patterns, social determinants of health, and barriers to care in diverse populations. Such research informs interventions that are culturally sensitive, contextually relevant, and adaptable to evolving health challenges. Moreover, nurses serve as educators and mentors within academic and professional training programs, equipping future healthcare professionals with the skills, knowledge, and ethical frameworks necessary to advance global health promotion. In this capacity, nursing simultaneously addresses immediate health needs and cultivates a workforce capable of sustaining long-term public health improvements. Technological innovation and digital health also present opportunities for nurses to enhance global health promotion (Greenhalgh et al. 2020). Telehealth, mobile health applications, electronic health records, and online education platforms allow nurses to reach broader populations, particularly in remote or underserved regions. Nurses utilize these tools to provide virtual consultations, deliver educational content, monitor chronic conditions, and facilitate remote disease surveillance, thereby extending the reach and impact of health promotion initiatives. However, integrating technology into nursing practice requires attention to issues such as digital literacy, data privacy, accessibility, and equity, ensuring that technological solutions enhance, rather than exacerbate, health disparities. Nurses' role in guiding populations through digital health tools reinforces their position as essential mediators between emerging technologies and effective, human-centered health promotion strategies. Global health challenges, including emerging infectious diseases, climate change, migration, and socio-economic inequalities, underscore the critical importance of nursing in shaping health promotion agendas.

Nurses address these complex determinants of health through preventive care, early intervention, and community engagement, mitigating risk factors and promoting resilience. For instance, in regions affected by natural disasters or conflict, nurses provide not only immediate medical care but also education on hygiene, nutrition, mental health support, and disease prevention, exemplifying the multifaceted nature of health promotion. Furthermore, nurses' cultural competence, ethical awareness, and empathetic communication strengthen trust within communities, enhancing receptivity to health interventions and reinforcing the sustainability of health promotion efforts. By integrating clinical expertise with public health principles, nurses contribute to the development of holistic approaches that address physical, psychological, and social dimensions of health, advancing the vision of health for all. Recognizing and supporting the multifaceted contributions of nursing is therefore essential for achieving sustainable global health objectives, strengthening healthcare systems, and fostering resilient, healthy societies across diverse socio-economic and geographic contexts. The role of nursing in global health promotion is not merely supportive or auxiliary; it is central, transformative, and indispensable, offering a pathway toward improved health outcomes, reduced disparities, and the realization of global public health goals (Koparde et al. 2026).

ASSESSING HEALTH LITERACY IN DIVERSE POPULATIONS

Health literacy, broadly defined as the capacity to obtain, process, and understand basic health information and services necessary to make appropriate health decisions, is a critical determinant of individual and population health outcomes. Accurate assessment of health literacy is essential to identify disparities, guide interventions, and tailor health communication strategies to meet the needs of diverse populations. However, assessing health literacy across heterogeneous groups presents significant methodological, cultural, and contextual challenges. Populations vary widely in terms of education, socioeconomic status, linguistic proficiency, cultural norms, and exposure to healthcare systems, all of which influence the comprehension, interpretation, and application of health information. For instance, individuals from marginalized communities may have limited formal education, restricted access to healthcare resources, or face systemic barriers such as discrimination and poverty, which can hinder their ability to engage with health information effectively. Conversely, populations in high-resource settings may encounter challenges related to health information overload, medical jargon, and conflicting guidance from multiple sources, demonstrating that health literacy is not merely a function of knowledge but also of context, accessibility, and cognitive and social capacity.

Standardized instruments have been developed to assess health literacy, including tools such as the Test of Functional Health Literacy in Adults (TOFHLA), Rapid Estimate of Adult Literacy in Medicine (REALM), and the Newest Vital Sign (NVS). These instruments evaluate reading comprehension, numeracy, and understanding of medical terminology, providing quantitative metrics that can inform intervention planning. While valuable, these tools have limitations when applied to diverse populations. Many standardized instruments were developed and validated in specific demographic contexts, often in high-income countries with predominantly English-speaking populations. As a result, they may fail to capture nuances in health comprehension for populations with different languages, dialects, or cultural conceptualizations of health and illness. Moreover, such tools may not adequately assess digital health literacy, a growing concern as healthcare increasingly relies on online information, telemedicine, and mobile health technologies. Digital health literacy encompasses the ability to seek, evaluate, and apply health information obtained via digital platforms, and disparities in access to technology, internet connectivity, and digital skills can exacerbate inequities in understanding and engagement with health resources. Therefore, assessment methods must be adapted to the linguistic, cultural, and technological contexts of diverse populations to ensure validity and relevance. Culturally sensitive approaches are critical in assessing health literacy effectively.

Cultural beliefs, health practices, and social norms shape how individuals perceive disease, treatment, and prevention, influencing both the interpretation of health information and willingness to act upon it. For example, in some communities, traditional medicine, spiritual beliefs, or communal decision-making may guide health behaviors more strongly than biomedical recommendations. Standard health literacy assessments that do not account for these factors risk misrepresenting an individual's true capacity to manage health effectively. To address this, qualitative methods such as structured interviews, focus groups, and participatory research approaches are increasingly employed alongside quantitative assessments. These methods provide deeper insights into how individuals navigate health information, interpret messages, and make health-related decisions within their socio-cultural contexts. Incorporating community perspectives in the design and validation of assessment tools ensures that instruments are culturally congruent, linguistically appropriate, and sensitive to the lived experiences of the target populations, thereby enhancing the accuracy and utility of health literacy evaluation. Socioeconomic determinants further complicate the assessment of health literacy in diverse populations. Poverty, educational inequities, geographic isolation, and limited access to healthcare services create structural barriers that influence individuals' ability to acquire, understand, and utilize health information. For example, individuals in rural or underserved urban areas may face limited availability of healthcare providers, educational programs, or culturally relevant health materials, which constrains opportunities to develop functional health literacy. Language barriers, including limited proficiency in the dominant language of healthcare communication, compound these challenges, leading to misinterpretation of medical instructions, nonadherence to treatment, and suboptimal health outcomes. Assessing health literacy in these contexts necessitates not only evaluation of individual competencies but also consideration of systemic factors that impact health understanding. Health literacy assessment frameworks that integrate both individual and environmental determinants enable a more comprehensive understanding of disparities and inform interventions designed to reduce inequities (Kupcu et al. 2024). Capacity-building among healthcare professionals in health literacy assessment, cultural competence, and communication strategies is equally critical, ensuring that assessments translate into meaningful, actionable interventions. In conclusion, assessing health literacy in diverse populations is a complex but essential endeavor, requiring multidimensional approaches that account for cultural, linguistic, socioeconomic, and technological factors (Maia et al. 2024).

NURSING STRATEGIES FOR PROMOTING HEALTH LITERACY

Nurses play a central role in promoting health literacy, a critical determinant of individual and population health outcomes. Health literacy encompasses the knowledge, skills, and confidence necessary for individuals to access, understand, evaluate, and apply health information effectively. In their multifaceted roles as educators, advocates, communicators, and care coordinators, nurses are uniquely positioned to implement strategies that enhance health literacy across diverse populations, ultimately contributing to improved health behaviors, treatment adherence, and health equity. Promoting health literacy requires a proactive, systematic, and patient-centered approach, encompassing interventions at the individual, community, organizational, and policy levels. Effective nursing strategies integrate clear communication, culturally sensitive education, patient engagement, digital health integration, and interprofessional collaboration, reflecting the complex interplay of cognitive, social, cultural, and structural factors that influence an individual's ability to navigate health information and services. Community health nursing approaches leverage local knowledge, cultural norms, and social networks to deliver education that resonates with community members. For example, nurses can collaborate with local leaders, schools, and faith-based organizations to disseminate information on vaccination, nutrition, hygiene, chronic disease prevention, and mental health. Group-based educational sessions, peer-led programs, and participatory activities encourage active learning, facilitate discussion, and reinforce key health messages. By engaging the community as partners rather than passive recipients, nurses foster ownership of health information, empower individuals to apply knowledge in everyday decision-making, and create sustainable changes in health behaviours (Medina et al. 2022).

Nurses also promote health literacy through the integration of technology and digital tools, particularly in an era of rapid digital transformation in healthcare. Telehealth platforms, mobile applications, patient portals, online educational resources, and social media campaigns extend the reach of health information, enabling individuals to access guidance, monitor conditions, and communicate with healthcare providers remotely. Digital health literacy initiatives involve guiding patients to credible online sources, demonstrating the use of digital tools, and providing support for navigating electronic health records or teleconsultations. Nurses must assess patients' digital competencies and address barriers related to access, connectivity, or technical skills to ensure equitable engagement with digital health resources. By bridging the gap between technology and patient understanding, nurses enhance information accessibility, encourage proactive health management, and empower patients to participate in their care in increasingly complex healthcare environments. Interprofessional collaboration is another critical strategy for promoting health literacy. Nurses work alongside physicians, pharmacists, dietitians, social workers, and educators to deliver coordinated, consistent, and evidence-based health information. By influencing policy and organizational practices, nurses extend the impact of health literacy interventions beyond individual encounters, creating systemic changes that facilitate informed decision-making, improve health outcomes, and reduce disparities at a population level. Evaluation and continuous improvement are integral to nursing strategies for promoting health literacy. Nurses utilize assessment tools, patient feedback, and outcome measures to identify literacy gaps, monitor intervention effectiveness, and refine educational approaches. Tools such as the Rapid Estimate of Adult Literacy in Medicine (REALM), Test of Functional Health

Literacy in Adults (TOFHLA), and patient-reported understanding assessments enable nurses to evaluate comprehension, identify barriers, and tailor strategies accordingly. Continuous professional development, research, and evidence-based practice further strengthen nurses' capacity to implement effective, innovative, and culturally appropriate interventions. By systematically assessing and addressing health literacy needs, nurses contribute to more effective patient education, improved adherence to treatment regimens, reduced hospital readmissions, and enhanced overall quality of care (Mishra et al. 2025).

CULTURAL COMPETENCE IN GLOBAL HEALTH NURSING

Cultural competence is a foundational element of effective global health nursing, encompassing the ability of healthcare professionals to deliver care that is respectful of, responsive to, and aligned with the diverse cultural values, beliefs, and practices of the populations they serve. In the context of global health, where nurses often interact with patients from heterogeneous sociocultural, linguistic, and religious backgrounds, cultural competence is essential for promoting equitable care, enhancing patient outcomes, and reducing disparities. It involves not only awareness and understanding of cultural differences but also the integration of cultural knowledge into clinical decision-making, communication, health education, and advocacy. Nurses who are culturally competent recognize the profound impact that culture has on health behaviors, perceptions of illness, adherence to treatment, and engagement with healthcare systems. They employ strategies that respect individual identities, accommodate cultural norms, and bridge gaps between biomedical models of care and traditional or community-based health practices. By doing so, culturally competent nurses foster trust, facilitate patient-centered care, and empower communities to actively participate in their health management. The development of cultural competence in global health nursing involves several interrelated components, including cultural awareness, knowledge, skill, encounters, and desire.

For instance, understanding dietary restrictions, traditional healing methods, religious practices, family dynamics, and community hierarchies enables nurses to tailor interventions that are culturally appropriate and effective. Cultural skill refers to the ability to conduct culturally sensitive assessments, communicate effectively across cultural boundaries, and develop care plans that integrate both biomedical and culturally relevant approaches. Cultural encounters, through direct interaction with diverse populations, allow nurses to apply their knowledge and skills in real-world contexts, fostering adaptability, empathy, and cross-cultural problem-solving. Finally, cultural desire reflects a genuine motivation to engage respectfully with different cultures, seek continuous learning, and prioritize patient-centered care that honors cultural identity. Collectively, these elements provide a framework for nurses to deliver competent and ethical care in global health settings. In practical terms, cultural competence shapes multiple aspects of nursing practice, including assessment, communication, health education, care planning, and advocacy. During patient assessment, culturally competent nurses elicit information about beliefs, practices, and social contexts that may influence health behaviors, recognizing that conventional biomedical assessments may not capture the full picture of a patient's needs. In communication, nurses employ culturally sensitive strategies, including language translation services, plain-language explanations, nonverbal cues, and negotiation of culturally appropriate care approaches. Health education interventions are tailored to accommodate literacy levels, linguistic diversity, and culturally influenced learning preferences, ensuring that patients comprehend, retain, and act upon essential health information. Such approaches underscore that cultural competence is not an optional skill but a professional and ethical imperative in global health nursing, ensuring that care is both respectful and effective across diverse contexts (Nirupama et al. 2025).

The integration of cultural competence into global health nursing also has profound implications for education, training, and professional development. Nursing curricula increasingly emphasize cultural competence, providing students with theoretical frameworks, experiential learning opportunities, simulation exercises, and community engagement experiences that foster awareness, knowledge, and practical skills. As the global health landscape becomes increasingly complex and diverse, the ability of nurses to provide culturally competent care is central to achieving equitable, patient-centered, and sustainable health outcomes worldwide. Nurses, through their professional expertise, ethical commitment, and cultural sensitivity, serve as pivotal agents in bridging cultural divides, empowering communities, and advancing the overarching goals of global health.

GLOBAL HEALTH INITIATIVES AND NURSING'S CONTRIBUTION

Global health initiatives are structured efforts undertaken by international organizations, governments, non-governmental organizations (NGOs), and professional associations to improve health outcomes, reduce disparities, and strengthen healthcare systems worldwide. These initiatives address pressing health challenges, including infectious diseases, maternal and child health, non-communicable diseases, mental health, environmental health, and health system resilience. Nurses, as the largest and most accessible group of healthcare professionals globally, play a pivotal role in the design, implementation, and evaluation of these initiatives. Their contributions extend beyond bedside care, encompassing health education, advocacy, leadership, research, policy development, and community engagement. The unique position of nurses allows them to bridge global health priorities with local contexts, ensuring that initiatives are culturally sensitive, accessible, and effective in achieving sustainable outcomes. By integrating clinical expertise with public health principles, nurses contribute to advancing the objectives of global health initiatives while promoting equity, capacity-building, and community empowerment. One of the primary areas where nursing significantly contributes is in infectious disease control and prevention. Global health initiatives such as the World Health Organization's (WHO) "End TB Strategy," the Global Polio Eradication Initiative, and immunization campaigns against measles, influenza, and COVID-19 rely heavily on the active participation of nurses. Through these interventions, nurses not only improve immediate health outcomes but also foster long-term behavioral changes and strengthen community resilience, demonstrating the integral role of nursing in achieving the Sustainable Development Goals (SDGs) related to maternal and child health (Pelikan et al. 2022).

Nurses also play a crucial role in combating non-communicable diseases (NCDs), which represent a growing global health burden. Initiatives targeting diabetes, cardiovascular diseases, cancer, obesity, and mental health rely on nurses for education, screening, lifestyle counseling, chronic disease management, and support for medication adherence. Nurses implement evidence-based interventions to promote healthy behaviors, monitor patient outcomes, and coordinate care across multidisciplinary teams. They educate communities about risk factors, prevention strategies, and early detection, emphasizing the importance of self-management and informed decision-making. In international organizations and professional associations, nurses participate in advisory boards, working groups, and committees that guide program implementation and evaluation. Leadership in nursing also includes mentoring and capacity-building for local healthcare professionals, fostering a skilled workforce capable of sustaining global health efforts over time. Through advocacy, nurses amplify the voices of marginalized populations, ensuring that global health initiatives are inclusive, responsive, and ethically grounded. Research and evidence-based practice further enhance nursing contributions to global health initiatives. Nurses conduct community-based participatory research, clinical studies, and program evaluations that inform best practices, measure outcomes, and guide continuous improvement.

Figure 1. The framework for the role of the nurse

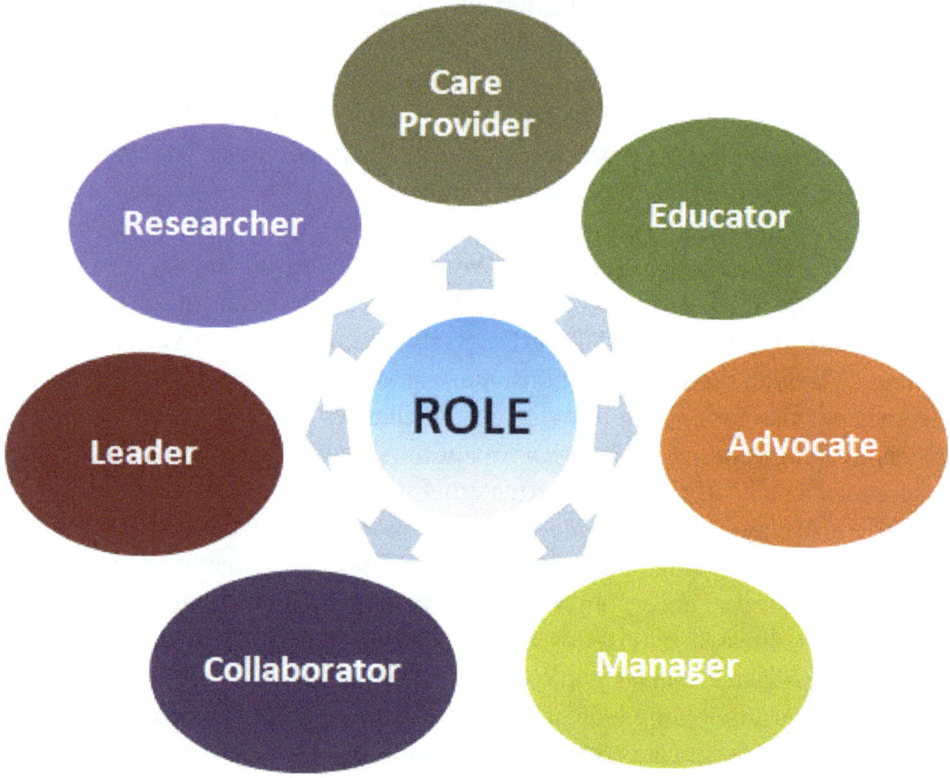

Global health challenges, including pandemics, climate change, migration, and conflicts, underscore the indispensable role of nursing in international health initiatives. Nurses respond to emergencies, provide essential care in humanitarian crises, and participate in disaster preparedness and recovery efforts. Their frontline experience, clinical expertise, and community engagement capacities enable rapid assessment, triage, and intervention in complex and resource-constrained environments. Furthermore, nurses advocate for vulnerable populations affected by crises, ensuring access to care, psychosocial support, and continuity of health services. These contributions highlight the adaptability, resilience, and leadership of nurses in addressing both acute and long-term global health challenges, reinforcing their centrality to the success of global health initiatives. In conclusion, nurses are integral to the design, implementation, evaluation, and sustainability of global health initiatives. Through roles encompassing direct patient care, health education, community engagement, policy advocacy, research, leadership, and technological integration, nurses bridge the gap between global objectives and local realities.

INTERNATIONAL COLLABORATION IN HEALTH PROMOTION

International collaboration in health promotion is increasingly recognized as a critical mechanism for addressing global health challenges, reducing disparities, and advancing equitable access to healthcare resources across borders. In a world characterized by interconnected populations, global travel, environmental changes, and the rapid spread of infectious diseases, health issues in one region can quickly impact populations worldwide. Collaborative efforts between nations, international organizations, non-governmental organizations (NGOs), academic institutions, and professional networks are essential to share expertise, coordinate strategies, mobilize resources, and implement evidence-based interventions. These partnerships enable the pooling of knowledge, technological innovations, and financial support to address complex health issues that no single country can manage in isolation. International collaboration in health promotion encompasses joint initiatives in disease prevention, health education, policy development, capacity building, research, and emergency preparedness, emphasizing the importance of cooperation, mutual learning, and culturally sensitive approaches in achieving sustainable health outcomes on a global scale. One of the primary drivers of international collaboration is the need to combat communicable diseases that cross national borders, such as tuberculosis, malaria, HIV/AIDS, and emerging infectious diseases like COVID-19 and Ebola.

Global initiatives, including the World Health Organization's (WHO) Global Health Security Agenda, the Global Fund to Fight AIDS, Tuberculosis and Malaria, and regional disease surveillance networks, rely on collaboration among countries to share epidemiological data, coordinate vaccination campaigns, standardize treatment protocols, and mobilize rapid response teams. Nurses, public health professionals, epidemiologists, and community health workers contribute to these initiatives by implementing interventions on the ground, educating communities, monitoring disease trends, and evaluating program effectiveness. Cross-border collaboration ensures that knowledge and resources are distributed equitably, outbreaks are contained efficiently, and best practices are disseminated internationally, strengthening global health security and population resilience. Policy development and advocacy are also central to effective international collaboration in health promotion. Multilateral organizations, national governments, and professional associations work together to establish policies, standards, and regulations that promote equitable health access, improve public health outcomes, and address social determinants of health globally.

Collaborative policy initiatives, such as the Framework Convention on Tobacco Control, global strategies on non-communicable diseases, and international mental health action plans, exemplify how countries can coordinate approaches to complex, transnational health challenges. Nurses and public health professionals contribute to these processes by providing evidence-based recommendations, highlighting community needs, and advocating for culturally sensitive interventions that consider the diversity of health systems and populations. By participating in policy dialogues, health professionals help shape international frameworks that guide resource allocation, program design, and evaluation, ensuring that global health promotion strategies are contextually relevant, ethically sound, and sustainable (Sivanand & Selvakumar, 2025). Research collaboration is a further dimension of international health promotion. Multicountry studies, cross-national surveillance projects, and international trials provide robust data that inform evidence-based interventions and program design. Challenges in international collaboration include linguistic and cultural differences, disparities in healthcare infrastructure, variations in political and regulatory environments, and resource limitations. Effective collaboration requires cultural competence, adaptability, mutual respect, transparent communication, and shared accountability among all stakeholders. Nurses, with their frontline experience and community engagement skills, serve as mediators who translate international strategies into locally appropriate interventions, advocate for community needs, and build trust between populations and global health organizations. By addressing these challenges proactively, international collaborations can achieve measurable improvements in health literacy, preventive behaviors, disease control, and overall population health outcomes.

In conclusion, international collaboration in health promotion is a multidimensional endeavor that integrates disease prevention, health education, capacity building, policy development, research, and digital health innovation. Nurses play an indispensable role in these collaborations, bridging global priorities and local realities, delivering culturally competent care, educating communities, participating in research, and influencing policy. Through their expertise, leadership, and commitment to equity, nurses facilitate effective implementation of global initiatives, ensuring that health promotion efforts reach diverse populations, reduce disparities, and achieve sustainable impact. As health challenges continue to transcend national borders, fostering and strengthening international collaboration—with nurses as central contributors—remains essential to achieving global health goals, enhancing population resilience, and promoting equitable access to healthcare worldwide. Nurses, through their integration of clinical knowledge, public health principles, and cultural sensitivity, serve as pivotal agents in translating global strategies into tangible improvements in the health and well-being of communities around the world (Raman et al. 2025).

NURSING'S ROLE IN DISASTER RESPONSE AND GLOBAL HEALTH

Nurses play a critical and multifaceted role in disaster response and global health, serving as essential frontline responders, coordinators, educators, and advocates in times of crisis. Disasters—whether natural, such as earthquakes, floods, hurricanes, and tsunamis, or man-made, such as armed conflicts, industrial accidents, and pandemics—pose significant threats to population health, often overwhelming healthcare systems and disrupting essential services. The frequency, intensity, and complexity of disasters have increased in recent decades due to factors including climate change, urbanization, population displacement, and global interconnectedness. Within this context, nurses are uniquely positioned to respond effectively due to their clinical expertise, adaptability, leadership skills, and holistic approach to care. Their contributions span the entire disaster management continuum, including preparedness, mitigation, response, and recovery, integrating principles of emergency care, public health, community engagement, and health system resilience. By leveraging their knowledge and skills, nurses help to minimize morbidity and mortality, protect vulnerable populations, and promote rapid recovery and sustainable health outcomes in affected communities. In the preparedness phase, nurses contribute significantly to disaster readiness by assessing risks, developing emergency plans, and participating in training programs and simulations.

During the acute response phase, nurses are central to delivering life-saving care in high-pressure, resource-constrained environments. They provide triage, emergency medical treatment, wound care, infection control, and critical care interventions to victims of disasters. In mass casualty events, nurses assess patient priorities, allocate scarce resources, and coordinate care with multidisciplinary teams, demonstrating adaptability, rapid decision-making, and clinical expertise under challenging circumstances. Nurses also address the psychosocial and mental health needs of survivors, offering emotional support, counseling, and referrals to mental health services to mitigate trauma and promote psychological resilience. Their culturally sensitive approach ensures that care is delivered with respect for local beliefs, practices, and community norms, fostering trust and facilitating engagement during chaotic situations. By combining technical proficiency with compassionate care, nurses enhance both immediate survival and longer-term recovery outcomes (Saito & Creedy 2021). Public health nursing strategies are particularly crucial in disaster response and global health. Nurses implement disease surveillance, monitor environmental hazards, and provide preventive interventions such as vaccination, sanitation, and vector control to reduce the risk of outbreaks in disaster-affected populations. Furthermore, nurses contribute to policy development, emergency protocols, and standard operating procedures that guide disaster preparedness and response at local, national, and international levels, ensuring that lessons learned from previous crises inform future interventions.

Technology and digital health play an increasingly significant role in nursing contributions to disaster response and global health. Telemedicine, mobile health applications, geographic information systems (GIS), electronic health records, and online training platforms enable nurses to coordinate care, monitor health indicators, and deliver education remotely. In areas affected by natural disasters or conflict, digital tools facilitate communication, patient tracking, and dissemination of critical health information to both healthcare providers and communities. Nurses leverage these technologies to overcome geographic barriers, optimize resource allocation, and enhance the effectiveness of interventions, particularly in low-resource or hard-to-reach settings. The integration of digital health into disaster response enhances the scalability, accessibility, and efficiency of nursing interventions, contributing to improved health outcomes and population resilience on a global scale (Suka et al. 2020). Education and capacity building are central to sustaining nursing contributions in disaster response and global health. Nurses train community health workers, volunteers, and local healthcare providers in emergency preparedness, first aid, triage, infection control, and psychosocial support. International collaboration through exchange programs, workshops, and simulation exercises equips nurses with the competencies needed to respond to diverse disaster scenarios while fostering knowledge transfer across countries. By building local capacity, nurses ensure that communities are better prepared to respond to future emergencies, thereby promoting sustainable health outcomes and resilience. In addition, ongoing professional development in disaster nursing equips nurses with the skills to adapt to evolving challenges such as climate change, pandemics, and complex humanitarian emergencies. Challenges in disaster response and global health nursing include resource constraints, safety risks, cultural and language barriers, emotional strain, and logistical complexities.

INTEGRATING GLOBAL HEALTH INTO NURSING EDUCATION

Integrating global health into nursing education is essential to prepare nurses for practice in an increasingly interconnected, complex, and culturally diverse healthcare environment. Global health encompasses the health of populations worldwide, transcending national boundaries and emphasizing equity, social determinants of health, disease prevention, health promotion, and health system strengthening. As global health challenges—including pandemics, non-communicable disease epidemics, climate change, migration, and humanitarian crises—become more prominent, nursing education must evolve to equip future nurses with the knowledge, skills, and competencies required to respond effectively and ethically. Incorporating global health into nursing curricula ensures that nurses understand the interconnectedness of health systems, recognize health disparities, appreciate cultural diversity, and are prepared to contribute to international health initiatives and sustainable development goals (SDGs). It also fosters critical thinking, advocacy, leadership, and collaborative skills necessary for addressing complex global health issues.One key aspect of integrating global health into nursing education is developing curricula that encompass theoretical and practical components, including epidemiology, public health, global disease burden, social determinants of health, health policy, ethics, and cultural competence. Courses in global health enable students to understand the distribution and determinants of health and disease, analyze disparities, and explore strategies for health promotion and disease prevention at local, national, and international levels.

Emphasis on cultural competence and health equity equips nursing students to provide care that is respectful of and responsive to diverse populations, integrating cultural values, beliefs, and practices into clinical decision-making. Furthermore, incorporating global health ethics helps students navigate complex moral dilemmas encountered in international practice, such as resource allocation, care prioritization, and engagement with vulnerable populations, ensuring that future nurses uphold professional integrity while advocating for equity and social justice. Experiential learning is a critical component of global health education in nursing, bridging theoretical knowledge with practical application. International clinical placements, exchange programs, service-learning opportunities, and community-based projects expose students to diverse healthcare systems, populations, and health challenges. Through immersion in different cultural and clinical contexts, nursing students develop adaptability, cross-cultural communication skills, and an understanding of the structural and social determinants of health. These experiences also foster empathy, resilience, and problem-solving abilities, enabling nurses to deliver patient-centered care that is both culturally sensitive and evidence-based. Service-learning projects, in particular, allow students to collaborate with local communities to identify needs, implement interventions, and evaluate outcomes, promoting both global awareness and social responsibility. By participating in hands-on experiences, students gain firsthand insights into the complexities of global health, preparing them for professional practice in diverse and resource-constrained settings. Interprofessional education (IPE) is another vital strategy for integrating global health into nursing education. Collaborative learning with students from medicine, public health, social work, nutrition, and other disciplines enables nursing students to understand the roles, expertise, and perspectives of different healthcare professionals in addressing complex global health challenges.

IPE enhances teamwork, communication, and collaborative problem-solving, which are critical for effective participation in international health initiatives, disaster response, and population-level interventions. Nurses trained in interprofessional settings are better equipped to contribute to multidisciplinary efforts in disease prevention, health promotion, policy development, and emergency response, ensuring that global health interventions are comprehensive, coordinated, and contextually appropriate. Digital health education also plays a growing role in integrating global health into nursing programs. Online learning platforms, virtual simulations, telehealth modules, and international webinars enable students to explore global health topics, connect with experts, and engage in remote collaborative projects. Digital tools expand access to educational resources, facilitate cross-cultural exchange, and provide exposure to innovative health technologies used worldwide. For instance, telemedicine simulations help students understand remote care delivery, patient monitoring, and digital health literacy, while virtual global health conferences allow engagement with international research, policy discussions, and evidence-based interventions. By leveraging digital education, nursing programs can provide flexible, scalable, and interactive learning experiences that prepare students for practice in digitally connected and resource-diverse global health contexts. Research and evidence-based practice are fundamental to integrating global health into nursing education.

Nursing students must be trained to critically appraise global health research, analyze data on disease patterns, health disparities, and intervention outcomes, and apply findings to clinical and community-based practice. Research skills also enable students to contribute to global health knowledge generation, participate in international studies, and implement evidence-informed interventions that are culturally and contextually relevant. Exposure to research promotes analytical thinking, continuous learning, and professional development, preparing nurses to assess population needs, design effective health programs, and evaluate the impact of interventions on health outcomes across diverse settings. Moreover, engagement in global health research fosters collaboration with international partners, enhances cultural competence, and strengthens students' capacity to address complex health challenges in practice. Integrating global health into nursing education also requires a focus on policy, leadership, and advocacy. Nurses educated in global health are equipped to engage in policy development, influence health system strengthening, and advocate for health equity at local, national, and international levels.

Education in global health governance, international regulations, and sustainable development frameworks enables students to understand the role of multilateral organizations such as the World Health Organization, United Nations agencies, and global health coalitions in shaping health outcomes. Leadership and advocacy training empowers nursing graduates to serve as agents of change, championing initiatives that address social determinants of health, reduce disparities, and promote community resilience. By understanding the interplay between policy, practice, and population health, nurses can effectively contribute to global health strategies that prioritize equitable, sustainable, and culturally sensitive interventions. Challenges in integrating global health into nursing education include limited resources, curriculum overcrowding, insufficient faculty expertise, logistical barriers to international placements, and the need for culturally and contextually appropriate educational content. Addressing these challenges requires institutional commitment, faculty development, strategic partnerships with global health organizations, and innovative teaching methods. Collaborative initiatives between nursing schools, NGOs, international agencies, and community organizations facilitate the exchange of expertise, provide access to experiential learning opportunities, and support the development of culturally relevant curricula. Faculty trained in global health can mentor students, guide research projects, and facilitate cross-border collaborations, enhancing the quality and impact of education. By overcoming these barriers, nursing programs can ensure that graduates are competent, culturally sensitive, and prepared to address global health challenges effectively.

In conclusion, integrating global health into nursing education is vital for preparing a workforce capable of responding to the complex, interconnected, and evolving health challenges of the twenty-first century. By incorporating theoretical knowledge, experiential learning, interprofessional collaboration, digital health, research, policy education, leadership, and advocacy into nursing curricula, educational institutions equip students with the competencies necessary to provide culturally sensitive, evidence-based, and equitable care in diverse global contexts. Nurses educated in global health are not only prepared to deliver high-quality clinical care but also to contribute to population health initiatives, participate in international collaborations, and influence policy and practice for sustainable impact. Through a comprehensive and integrated approach to global health education, nursing programs foster the development of adaptable, culturally competent, and socially responsible practitioners who are capable of advancing health equity, strengthening health systems, and improving the health and well-being of communities worldwide. By embedding global health into nursing education, the profession ensures that future nurses are prepared to serve as effective leaders, educators, and advocates in a world where health challenges are increasingly transnational and complex.

PREPARING NURSES FOR GLOBAL HEALTH CHALLENGES

Preparing nurses for global health challenges is an essential component of modern healthcare education and professional development, reflecting the growing complexity and interconnectedness of health issues worldwide. Global health challenges encompass a wide range of concerns, including emerging infectious diseases, pandemics, non-communicable disease epidemics, climate-related health crises, migration, health inequities, humanitarian emergencies, and the effects of social determinants on population health. These challenges transcend national boundaries, requiring nurses to possess not only clinical expertise but also cultural competence, public health knowledge, leadership, advocacy skills, and the ability to engage in interprofessional and international collaborations. Preparing nurses to address these complex and dynamic challenges involves a multifaceted approach that integrates education, training, experiential learning, policy understanding, technological literacy, and research engagement. By equipping nurses with the knowledge, skills, and attitudes necessary for global health practice, healthcare systems can enhance resilience, equity, and responsiveness in the face of both acute crises and long-term health threats. Education forms the foundation of preparing nurses for global health challenges, beginning with the integration of global health concepts into nursing curricula(Zhang et al. 2024). Core topics include epidemiology, infectious and non-communicable diseases, health systems, environmental health, disaster preparedness, health promotion, health disparities, social determinants of health, and health policy. Nursing programs emphasize critical thinking, evidence-based practice, and ethical decision-making, enabling students to analyze complex health problems, design effective interventions, and advocate for populations in diverse cultural and resource contexts.

Cultural competence is a central element of global health education, equipping nurses to provide care that is respectful, contextually appropriate, and responsive to the beliefs, values, and practices of different populations. Understanding global health frameworks, international organizations such as the World Health Organization (WHO), and global health governance mechanisms also prepares nurses to navigate transnational health issues, align interventions with international guidelines, and participate in policy development or advocacy efforts that promote equity and access to care (Wit et al. 2023). Experiential learning is critical for translating theoretical knowledge into practical competence in global health. Clinical placements, community-based service projects, international exchange programs, and simulation exercises expose nursing students to real-world health challenges, including resource-limited settings, disaster-affected areas, refugee camps, and multicultural populations. These experiences cultivate adaptability, problem-solving, communication skills, and cultural sensitivity. For instance, nursing students may engage in maternal and child health programs in low-resource countries, participate in vaccination campaigns, implement public health education initiatives, or assist in emergency preparedness exercises (Tørris & Nortvedt 2024). Through these immersive experiences, nurses gain firsthand understanding of the logistical, ethical, and clinical complexities of global health, preparing them to respond effectively to crises and deliver patient-centered care across diverse environments.

CONCLUSION

Interprofessional practice also strengthens the ability of nurses to participate in international collaborations, global health research, and policy development, ensuring that initiatives are holistic, evidence-based, and culturally appropriate. Disaster preparedness and emergency response are central to the training of nurses for global health challenges. Nurses are educated in triage, emergency care, mass casualty management, infection control, mental health support, and resource allocation in crisis settings. Simulations, workshops, and drills enable nurses to practice rapid decision-making, crisis communication, and leadership under pressure, enhancing their capacity to respond effectively during natural disasters, pandemics, conflicts, or other emergencies. Nurses also learn to address the psychosocial and mental health needs of affected populations, integrating trauma-informed care, community engagement, and culturally sensitive interventions into their practice. Training in disaster preparedness equips nurses to anticipate risks, mobilize resources, and deliver timely, efficient, and equitable care in complex and resource-constrained environments. Technology and digital health literacy are increasingly important components of preparing nurses for global health challenges. Nurses must be proficient in telehealth, electronic health records, mobile health applications, geographic information systems (GIS), and data analytics to facilitate remote care, monitor population health, and support evidence-based decision-making. Digital tools enable nurses to deliver education, track disease trends, communicate across distances, and implement interventions efficiently in both routine and crisis contexts.Moreover, digital literacy supports participation in global health research, international collaboration, and continuous professional development, ensuring that nurses remain responsive to emerging health challenges and capable of leveraging innovation to improve outcomes. Research and evidence-based practice are essential to global health preparedness for nurses. Nursing education emphasizes the ability to critically appraise research, design studies, evaluate interventions, and translate evidence into practice. Nurses contribute to the generation of knowledge in areas such as disease surveillance, outbreak response, maternal and child health, vaccination strategies, non-communicable disease management, and health system strengthening. Participation in global health research equips nurses to assess population needs, identify effective interventions, and adapt strategies to diverse cultural, social, and environmental contexts. Evidence-based practice ensures that nursing interventions are effective, efficient, and ethically sound, enhancing both patient outcomes and the impact of global health initiatives. Policy, leadership, and advocacy are also integral to preparing nurses for global health challenges. Nurses educated in global health are equipped to engage in policy development, participate in health system strengthening initiatives, and advocate for health equity and social justice. Understanding international health regulations, sustainable development frameworks, and the roles of global health organizations empowers nurses to influence decision-making, align local interventions with international standards, and promote the rights of vulnerable populations. Leadership training enables nurses to coordinate multidisciplinary teams, mobilize resources, and guide public health programs, ensuring that global health initiatives are effectively implemented, monitored, and adapted to changing needs. Advocacy skills allow nurses to champion equitable access to healthcare, address disparities, and amplify the voices of marginalized populations in local and global health agendas. Preparing nurses for global health challenges also requires attention to resilience, adaptability, and emotional intelligence. Nurses often work in high-stress, unpredictable, and resource-limited environments where emotional strain, ethical dilemmas, and complex social dynamics are prevalent. Education and training programs that foster resilience, stress management, reflective practice, and professional self-care enable nurses to maintain well-being, sustain performance, and deliver compassionate, patient-centered care in challenging circumstances. Emotional intelligence enhances nurses' ability to communicate effectively, build trust, and respond to the psychological and social needs of individuals and communities affected by global health crises. In conclusion, preparing nurses for global health challenges is a multifaceted endeavor that requires comprehensive education, experiential learning, interprofessional collaboration, disaster preparedness, digital health proficiency, research engagement, leadership, advocacy, and resilience-building. By equipping nurses with the knowledge, skills, and attitudes necessary to navigate complex global health landscapes, healthcare systems ensure that practitioners are capable of responding to emerging threats, addressing health disparities, and promoting population health across diverse cultural and socioeconomic contexts. Nurses prepared for global health challenges serve as critical agents of change, integrating clinical expertise with public health principles, cultural competence, and ethical practice to improve outcomes, strengthen health systems, and contribute to global efforts in health promotion, disease prevention, and sustainable development. By investing in comprehensive training and professional development, the nursing profession can ensure a workforce that is adaptable, competent, and empowered to meet the evolving demands of global health in the twenty-first century.

REFERENCES

Barry, M. M., Battel-Kirk, B., & Dempsey, C. (2012). The CompHP Core Competencies for Health Promotion in Europe: Developing the workforce for effective public health and cross-border health promotion (nursing workforce implications). *Health Education Research, 27*(1), 149–160. DOI: 10.1093/her/cyr077

Greenhalgh, T., Wherton, J., Shaw, S., & Morrison, C. (2020). Video consultations for COVID-19 — Implications for cross-border telehealth and nursing health-promotion roles. *BMJ (Clinical Research Ed.), 368*, m998. DOI: 10.1136/bmj.m998 PMID: 32165352

Koparde, S. A., Selvakumar, P., Jha, R. P., Deepthi Reddy, K., Kuchipudi, J. D., Manjunath, T. C., & Sharma, M. (2026). Generative AI in Predicting and Preventing Foodborne Illnesses. In Madaan, G., Singh, A., Chahal, B., David, A., & Singh, G. (Eds.), *Generative AI in Food Systems: Predictive Demand, Smart Supply Chains, and Sustainable Service Futures* (pp. 205–232). IGI Global Scientific Publishing., DOI: 10.4018/979-8-3373-5182-7.ch010

Kupcu, C., Bodur, G., Kucukkaya, A., & Goktaş, P. (2024). Assessing nursing students' e-health literacy and foresights to global health challenges during COVID-19 restrictions: A cross-sectional study with a machine learning approach. *Nurse Education in Practice, 81*, 104179. DOI: 10.1016/j.nepr.2024.104179 PMID: 39520839

Maia, A. C., Marques, M. J., Goes, A. R., Gama, A., Osborne, R., & Dias, S. (2024). Health literacy strengths and needs among migrant communities from Portuguese-speaking African countries in Portugal: A cross-sectional study. *Frontiers in Public Health, 12*, 1415588. Advance online publication. DOI: 10.3389/fpubh.2024.1415588 PMID: 39022410

Medina, M., Maia, A. C., & Costa, A. (2022). Health literacy in migrant communities: A primary health care unit study in Portugal. *Frontiers in Public Health, 9*, 798222. DOI: 10.3389/fpubh.2021.798222 PMID: 35141189

Mishra, B. R., Selvakumar, P., Kaur, R., Kalshetti, P., Mishra, K. K., Sharma, M., & Manjunath, T. C. (2025). Innovation and Digital Transformation in the Public Sector Entities. In Santos Ferreira, A., & Lourenço dos Santos, C. (Eds.), *Enhancing Public Sector Accountability and Services Through Digital Innovation* (pp. 409–436). IGI Global Scientific Publishing., DOI: 10.4018/979-8-3693-9251-5.ch013

Nirupama, E., Seenivasan, S., Bhardwaj, K., Karunakaran, N. B., & Basava Aradhya, S. G., Selvakumar, P., & Manjunath, T. C. (2025). Transforming Digital Supply Chains With Gamification and Metaverse Integration. In G. Malik, D. Singh, & R. Bansal (Eds.), *Addressing Practical Problems Through the Metaverse and Game-Inspired Mechanics* (pp. 123-152). IGI Global Scientific Publishing. https://doi.org/ DOI: 10.4018/979-8-3693-8886-0.ch006

Pelikan, J. M., Ganahl, K., & Röthlin, F. (2022). Measuring health literacy in general populations — The HLS19 instrument and its cross-national applications relevant to nursing and global health promotion. *International Journal of Environmental Research and Public Health*, *19*(2), 1008. DOI: 10.3390/ijerph19021008 PMID: 35055825

Raman, M. S., Koppa, K. B., Chithambar Gupta, V., Bhat, V. A., Guru Basava Aradhya, S., & Selvakumar, P. (2025). Digital Transformation and Sustainability Artificial Intelligence and Sustainable Development. In Yıldırım, D., Yıldırım, S., & Kandpal, V. (Eds.), *Effects of Digitalization and Circular Economy on Sustainable Policy and Climate Change Prevention* (pp. 69–96). IGI Global Scientific Publishing., DOI: 10.4018/979-8-3693-9909-5.ch003

Saito, A. S., & Creedy, D. K. (2021). Determining mental health literacy of undergraduate nursing students to inform learning and teaching strategies. *International Journal of Mental Health Nursing*, *30*(5), 1117–1126. DOI: 10.1111/inm.12862 PMID: 33760328

Sivanand, R., & Selvakumar, P. (2025). Navneet Sharma, Nanotechnology Applications in Cancer Drug Delivery Systems: A Review. *Journal of Environmental Nanotechnology*, *14*(2), 458–470. DOI: 10.13074/jent.2025.06.2511221

Suka, M., Yamauchi, T., & Hashimoto, H. (2020). Relationship between health literacy, self-rated health, and mortality in Japan: Findings and implications for nursing and health promotion. *BMC Public Health*, *20*, 1182. DOI: 10.1186/s12889-020-09202-8

Tørris, C., & Nortvedt, L. (2024). Health literacy and self-care among adult immigrants with type 2 diabetes: A scoping review. *BMC Public Health*, *24*(1), 3248. DOI: 10.1186/s12889-024-20749-6 PMID: 39578821

Wit, R. F., de Veer, A. J. E., Batenburg, R. S., & Francke, A. L. (2023). International comparison of professional competency frameworks for nurses: Addressing health promotion and e-health across borders. *BMC Nursing*, *22*, 343. DOI: 10.1186/s12912-023-01514-3 PMID: 37770894

Zhang, S., Wang, W., Wu, S., Ye, H., Dong, L., Wang, J., Ning, X., & Cui, H. (2024). Analysis of the mediating effect between ehealth literacy and health self-management of undergraduate nursing students' mental health literacy. *BMC Nursing*, *23*(1), 264. DOI: 10.1186/s12912-024-01920-1 PMID: 38654311

Chapter 10
An Interdisciplinary Partnership of Nursing Education and Instructional Technology in Türkiye

Alev Ateş-Çobanoğlu
https://orcid.org/0000-0002-8319-9822
Faculty of Education, Ege University, Turkey

Fatma Orgun
Ege University, Turkey

Nilay Özkütük
https://orcid.org/0000-0003-1405-4600
Ege University, Turkey

Duygu Ceren Güngör
http://orcid.org/0000-0002-3614-7835
Ege University, Turkey

Devrim Özge Yılmaz
Izmir Katip Çelebi University, Turkey

Cennet Kayhan
https://orcid.org/0009-0003-3386-3988
Ege University, Turkey

Onur Mustafa Güneş
Yaşar University, Turkey

ABSTRACT

The present chapter explores the significance of interdisciplinary study in the fields of nursing education and educational technology, with a particular emphasis on the integration of blended learning methodologies within nursing education. The chapter covers the role of nursing education in healthcare, the Turkish nursing education system, the legal and institutional framework of nursing education, the philosophy of nursing education and blended learning, the impact of paradigms

DOI: 10.4018/979-8-3373-5931-1.ch010

on nursing education and blended learning, the role of educational technology in nursing education, the characteristics of nursing education. The necessity for an interdisciplinary partnership between nursing education and instructional technology is underscored. The authors posit that the integration of blended learning is conducive to effective learning and teaching opportunities across a wide range of disciplines in higher education, including nursing education. An interdisciplinary approach is considered essential for designing effective learning experiences in nursing education.

INTRODUCTION

In a rapidly evolving technology and health care landscape, it is imperative to integrate nursing education and instructional technology through an interdisciplinary partnership. This partnership has a great potential to enhance knowledge and skill levels, foster collaborative learning environments, align theoretical concepts with practical applications, and optimize healthcare quality. It is posited that the contemporary healthcare environment is characterized by its complexity and diversity. Moreover, the training of nurses who are both effective and innovative in their practices necessitates interdisciplinary approaches and technological innovations. The integration of instructional technologies into nursing education has been demonstrated to enhance academic achievement and equip graduates with the skills necessary to effectively contribute to the next generation of health systems. Also, the needs of nursing education stakeholders should be taken into account for effective technology integration. Since that integration directly contributes to essential professional qualities such as strong communication, leadership, critical thinking, and continuous learning.

The literature shows that interdisciplinary collaboration enhances nursing students' competencies in receiving and interpreting information from different fields. By integrating methods from different disciplines (e.g. technology, educational sciences), students develop a well-rounded knowledge base. Utilizing instructional technologies facilitates the integration of theoretical and clinical knowledge and strengthens students' adaptation to innovations (Dauchess, 2025; Gause et al., 2022; Yang et al., 2024). Consequently, it is the authors' conviction that the present chapter exemplifies a compelling collaboration of nursing education experts and instructional technologists, in conjunction with their research assistants, concerning the formulation of innovative teaching methodologies through the utilization of educational technology.

BACKGROUND

The role of nursing education in healthcare

Nursing education is a healthcare discipline that aims to stabilise and improve the health of society, families and individuals; to restore health when it is compromised in any way; and to restore human life functions. The aging population and rapid global changes in our era necessitate changes to nursing education within the healthcare system (Goldberg & Burhenn, 2018; Yüceyurt & Şenyuva, 2023). The changes that are being experienced in nursing and nursing education are the result of a number of factors. These include technological expansion, the demand for quality care, cost pressures, shorter hospital stays, disease processes and increased patient sensitivity. To respond to these changes and developments, education systems must adapt. And in order to achieve this alignment, it is imperative to continuously examine, evaluate, update, and improve nursing education (Kaya & Şendir, 2021). In this context, institutions and organisations involved in nursing and nursing education are under an obligation to produce dynamic and high-quality work on nursing education in order to provide qualified nursing care. It is imperative that nurses and nursing educators recognise the significance of nursing education and assume an active role in these processes (Yüceyurt & Şenyuva, 2023). Furthermore, concerted efforts should be made to create opportunities to emphasise the critical importance of nursing education, its relationship with the quality of health for individuals and societies globally, and how educational research can enhance the quality of nurses' professional practice (Sharpnack, 2025).

A glimpse at the Turkish nursing education system

Nursing had existed for many years as a community service in Türkiye before nursing education began. Throughout history, nurses have cared for the sick in communities and hospitals. Modern nursing is considered to have begun during the Crimean War (1820-1910), led by Florence Nightingale. When considering the seminal figures in the development of modern nursing in the United States, the name Safiye Hüseyin Elbi emerges with distinction. Elbi's decision to continue her nursing profession during wartime is a testament to her dedication and selflessness. During the war, Safiye Hüseyin Elbi persisted in her practice, which encompassed a wide range of effective health maintenance strategies, including sanitation, anesthesia, shock intervention, blood transfusion, nasogastric tube insertion, wound care and debridement, intensive care services, and psychological support. In addition, she assumed the responsibility of providing nursing care to wounded soldiers (Aydemir & Öztekin, 2024).

The evolution of nursing education can be traced back to a historical pursuit to advance human health and provide care in a professional capacity (Ergöl, 2011). Prior to the establishment of nursing as a formal educational discipline in Türkiye, notable contributions included the publication of the seminal work Hastabakıcılık (Nursing) by Kenan Tevfik and Refik Münir, along with the translation of the French text Anatomy into Turkish by Fatma Zeliha, daughter of Asaf Osman Sadık Paşa. Subsequent to these developments, which contributed to the establishment of nursing education in Türkiye, the inaugural formal nursing education program was initiated in 1911 with the establishment of a volunteer nursing course. The participants in the course received six months of training. Turkish women who successfully completed the training and received their certificates participated in patient care during the Balkan and Gallipoli wars.

These advancements in Turkish nursing have garnered international attention, as evidenced by the observations of Margaret Varley, Nursing Advisor to the Rockefeller Foundation's International Health Division. In her report, Varley noted that "women who volunteered as nurses during the Balkan Wars, despite the cost to their traditional values, laid the foundation for professional nursing and nursing education" (Aydemir & Öztekin, 2024).

The inception of academic nursing education in Türkiye can be traced to 1920, marked by the establishment of the Nursing School under the auspices of Admiral Bristol Hospital. The duration of the nursing school's education program was initially two years and six months, later increased to three years, and in 1957, extended to four years. The program received approval from the Ministry of National Education, thereby attaining vocational high school equivalence. The inaugural nursing school to open during the Republican era was the Red Crescent Nursing School. In 1955, the first university-level college in our country was the Ege University College of Nursing. Contemporary nursing education is characterized by a professional educational process grounded in scientific principles, commencing at the university level. In this setting, professional knowledge and skills are systematically imparted (Ergöl, 2011).

In recent years, there has been a notable proliferation of higher education institutions in Türkiye that have initiated nursing education programs. Nursing education comprises a training programme that encompasses not only knowledge and clinical experience but also fundamental nursing skills and practices. In this nation, the fundamental concepts of nursing education are defined by the attributes of depth, breadth, quality, flexibility, suitability, innovation, and adequacy. Furthermore, it plays a pivotal role in establishing a balance between theoretical knowledge and clinical practice. The provision of education in a university setting in Türkiye has been demonstrated to facilitate the enhancement of nursing students' self-efficacy, concurrently fostering the development of their professional competencies. As of 2016, Türkiye had 114 faculties/colleges providing nursing education, including 28 foundation universities, 86 state universities, 60 faculties, and 54 colleges (Özkütük, 2018). A review of current data reveals that as of 2023, 184 nursing undergraduate programs were operational within 153 universities in Türkiye (Arslan Yürümezoğlu & Kocaman, 2023).

Advancements in nursing education are imperative for the academic and professional advancement of the profession. Consequently, nursing education persists in its role as a catalyst for the advancement of nursing students' knowledge and skills. This paradigm shift fosters specialization in diverse domains of nursing science, facilitates the development of proficient nurses in both academic and clinical domains, and consequently, enhances the quality of healthcare services. (Çamlıca, 2021; Öztürk & Bahçecik, 2021). Concurrently, advancements in the nursing education system in Türkiye are facilitating the adoption of innovative approaches and the integration of technological developments into educational programs. These developments present opportunities to incorporate simulations, e-learning platforms, and interactive education methods into education curricula (& Dağlı, 2022).

The Legal and Institutional Framework of Nursing Education

The profession is characterised by specific functions, which are regulated in accordance with the administrative and legal framework of society. The capacity of a profession to perform its duties and assume responsibility is contingent upon its ability to function independently within the applicable legal framework. The nursing profession has obtained the right to work independently within the legal framework in various respects. The first legal regulations for the nursing profession were established with the enactment of the Nursing Law in 1954 (Açıkgöz & Baykal, 2023; Kıvanç, 2015). The “Law on Amendments to the Nursing Act” is a legislative instrument that incorporates contemporary developments in nursing and retains its relevance in the present day. Revolutions in science and technology have had a profound impact on the nursing profession, including nursing education. It is evident that nurses fulfil their professional roles not only in the field of care, but also in different areas, such as theory creation and participation in professional institutions and organisations. The capacity for a profession to fulfil its duties and act independently is contingent upon the existence of legal regulations pertaining to that profession. Focusing on this aspect of nursing, which can be considered a strength, and raising awareness in these areas plays a key role in the professional autonomy and independence of nursing (Terzioğlu & Uslu Şahan, 2017; Yüceyurt & Şenyuva, 2023). Nevertheless, the augmentation in student numbers, economic inadequacies, and the advent of the digital information age, especially in recent years, have precipitated the globalisation of education. These developments have had a significant impact on the nursing education process. These global trends have underscored the necessity for standardisation in nursing education across nations. It is evident that a number of organisations have been established with the objective of ensuring standardisation in education and to provide guidance for nursing education and practice. The institutions in question include the World Health Organization (WHO, 2019), the National League for Nursing Education (NLNE), the International Council of Nurses (ICN), and the Association for the Evaluation and Accreditation of Nursing Education Programs (HEPDAK) in Türkiye. A common objective shared by these health organisations is the enhancement of educational standards (Açıkgöz & Baykal, 2023; Yüceyurt & Şenyuva, 2023).

The enhancement of the quality of nursing education and the contribution to the development of nursing students' knowledge and skills is contingent on standardisation in education, with adaptation to the age of information and technology being a key element in this process. Blended learning, which incorporates the use of technology, has emerged as an effective method for adapting to this era (Öztürk & Bahçecik, 2021). Blended learning is defined as the integration of online and face-to-face learning environments, leading to the development of e-learning platforms (Aşiroğlu, Nuhoğlu & Sarkın, 2022; Çamlıca, 2021). This approach ensures the incorporation of interactive teaching methods within educational curricula.

The Philosophy of Nursing Education and Blended Learning

Philosophy can be defined as the processes undertaken by an individual who seeks to understand the concept of reality through systematic thinking. Nursing is a scientific health discipline that addresses practice, research, and theory in relation to philosophy. Nursing is a field that requires a body of knowledge, specific values, ethical standards, and a purpose; it has its own philosophy and specific paradigms. The nursing profession serves as a conduit between individuals, families, or communities seeking healthcare or a peaceful death and the field of medical science and treatments. It is at the vanguard of the struggle to provide care and improvement to all segments of society. The presence of nurses who do not adhere to a distinct philosophy of nursing and do not act in accordance with the principle of justice has the potential to impede the advancement of public health and the ongoing provision of care as a set of values based on human dignity (Dubavaya & Tenaglia, 2025). It is submitted that one of the most efficacious methods by which nurses may develop a philosophical perspective and reflect this philosophy in their professional lives is to emphasise the importance of this topic in nursing education. In this context, educators must establish a robust foundation in philosophy and theoretical knowledge to advance the nursing discipline. It is imperative that course content is revised within the adopted philosophy, and nurses need to develop an awareness of their roles and responsibilities (Lippe, Braden, & Gill, 2025; Negarandeh & Khoshkesht, 2022).

In order to implement the philosophy of nursing education, it is essential that students are equipped with critical thinking skills, and that student-centred learning is instilled accordingly. In the context of nursing education, the ability to engage in critical thinking has become a pivotal skill. The Socratic method, a philosophical underpinning of nursing, has the capacity to equip nurses with critical skills in education and to implement student-centred learning. The Socratic method is predicated on ancient Greek philosophy and has emerged as a nursing theorist philosophy in the 21st century. The Socratic method, predicated on critical thinking and student-centred learning, also addresses issues of professional accountability and patient care. The objective of this method is to optimize the efficiency of patient care. Within the domain of nursing education and academia, it has been demonstrated to enhance critical thinking skills while facilitating student-centred learning methodologies. Moreover, this theoretical philosophy plays an instrumental role in the clinical practice of nursing education (Berg & Lepp, 2023; Dikmen et al., 2019).

The role of educators in higher education institutions working in nursing departments is also significant in adopting student-centred learning principles and encouraging students to think critically. A significant body of research has been conducted on the subject, and the results indicate that a considerable number of educators continue to utilise the teacher-centred learning model. It is imperative that educators comprehend and acknowledge the methodologies employed to achieve student-centred learning and the rationale underpinning its implementation.

In order to comprehend student-centred learning and establish it as a discipline, it is imperative to define student-centred learning, augment students' knowledge levels with innovative content courses, and devise diverse teaching platforms to facilitate learning through interaction with peers (Karasu, 2020; Naz & Kausor, 2023). In this approach, nursing students prepare individually before class and use self-assessment to take control of their learning process. Students are required to work collaboratively in groups, with the instructor overseeing their preparation and taking into account the students' needs. The implementation of student-centred learning is predicated on several factors, including the augmentation of theoretical and practical learning, the provision of general competencies such as problem-solving and critical thinking skills, and the strengthening of self-confidence through the empowerment of students to direct their own work (Berg & Lepp, 2023; Naz & Kausor, 2023).

One of the learning approaches developed based on critical thinking and student-centred learning is blended learning, which combines the positive aspects of face-to-face and online learning. Blended learning can be implemented at all stages of the educational process, including planning, implementation, and evaluation, using a variety of learning environments and online tools. It is hypothesised that integrating effective blended teaching with student-centred active learning approaches is more feasible than traditional approaches (Gülbahar, Kalelioğlu & Adanır, 2020). Consequently, the effective implementation of blended learning in nursing education necessitates the planning of effective learning designs in a student-centred manner (Aşiroğlu, Nuhoğlu & Sarkın, 2022). Therefore, the integration of blended learning environments within nursing education has emerged as a pivotal strategy to effectively reflect and uphold the tenets of nursing philosophy.

The Impact of Paradigms on Nursing Education and Blended Learning

The science of nursing has evolved within a series of paradigms, each of which is characterised by specific philosophical assumptions regarding the nature of reality, knowledge, and the methodological approach to its study. One of the ways in which to adapt to the changing conditions of our era and the information age is to create a paradigm that comprehensively addresses all the beliefs, values, and philosophies that nursing education aims to instill. These factors have precipitated a paradigm shift in nursing, thus elevating it to the forefront of the healthcare agenda. Nursing theorists' paradigms address concepts such as the individual, the nurse, health, illness, and the environment, and are based on assumptions that give meaning to these concepts (Güngör, Orgun & Özkütük, 2023; Kara, Akdeniz & Kavaslar, 2022).

The paradigms used in nursing education and science are characterized by ontological, methodological, and epistemological processes. Knowledge specific to the nursing discipline emerges from philosophical views and paradigms embedded within these concepts. It is not possible to guide contemporary nursing care, research, and practice with outdated information. Therefore, in nursing education and its application areas, it is necessary to continuously update the paradigms existing in the philosophy of nursing science in order to implement contemporary nursing education. The most prominent features of our era include the use of technology and the rapid change of societies (Arslan Özkan & Akduran, 2014; Yüksekdağ, 2021). In today's information society, where changes in direction and content are emphasized, it is only possible for people to keep up with these rapid transformations through education.

The integration of education with the values of the information society supports the formation of a model of people who learn how to learn, anticipating rapid technological transformation, continuous change and development, the regular use of information, and the development of individuals as lifelong learners (Akince, Özkütük & Orgun 2022; Özkan & Akduran, 2014). In the contemporary world, where knowledge is constantly multiplying and spreading rapidly, educators must create paradigms that enable students to question knowledge, generate solutions to problems, renew and develop themselves, and make the right decisions through critical thinking. Furthermore, there is a necessity to update curricula and programs within the framework of these paradigms in order to adapt to the requirements of the age.

In the context of nursing education, educators are required to formulate teaching plans that are aligned with these evolving paradigms. Furthermore, it is imperative that they embrace digital transformation in order to create the content of these plans. In the context of nursing education, educators must be cognizant of the need to review digital teaching strategies and materials when planning teaching based on changing paradigms. It is imperative that educators are able to utilize novel learning methods and techniques in education when assessing students. Technological changes and developments in science in the information age have been shown to affect ways of thinking and experiences, which in turn contribute to the formation of paradigms. These emerging paradigms also have an impact on the philosophy of nursing education, forcing changes in its models, theories, and practices (Akince, Özkütük & Orgun 2022; Özkan & Akduran, 2014; Takmak, 2024; Yılmaz & Kuğuoğlu, 2024; Yüksekdağ, 2021).

Certain paradigms influence the nursing profession, and it is known that nursing education has an impact on the formation of these paradigms. The paradigms that influence nursing education and their relationship with blended learning are discussed in the relevant literature (Akince, Özkütük & Orgun 2022; Aşiroğlu, Nuhoğlu, & Sarkın, 2022; Gülbahar, Kalelioğlu & Afacan Adanır, 2020; Kara, Akdeniz & Kavaslar, 2022; Özkan & Akduran, 2014; Takmak, 2024; Yüksekdağ, 2021) is summarized in Table 1.

Table 1. The paradigms affecting nursing education and their relationship with blended learning

The Paradigm	*Relation with Blended Learning*
Paradigm of Discipline and Disciplinary Depth	It deepens theoretical knowledge with online materials.
Research Paradigm	It facilitates research skills through the utilization of digital resources.
Information and Communication Technologies Paradigm	The integration of technology into the learning process is paramount.
Creativity and the Constructivist Paradigm	It encourages active and creative learning of students.
Vocational Education Paradigm	It integrates clinical practice with digital simulation.
Distance Learning Paradigm	It balances online and in-person learning.
Multicultural Education Paradigm	It increases interaction among students from different cultures.

continued on following page

Table 1. Continued

The Paradigm	*Relation with Blended Learning*
Positivist/Rationalist Paradigm	It makes evidence-based knowledge accessible.
Global Education Paradigm	It facilitates the dissemination of international knowledge and expertise.

A multitude of factors influence the selection of the prevailing paradigm in nursing education. Among these factors, technological changes and adaptation to the digital age are at the forefront. The factors previously enumerated have necessitated the employment of varied or multiple paradigms. When nursing education is subject to rigid classification, it can be said that the dominant paradigms are essentially positivist and anti-positivist. The influence of positivism and the efforts to develop the scientific and theoretical foundations of nursing are significant factors underlying this paradigm choice.

Today, while the accumulation of knowledge in all types of nursing models is increasing, there is no single dominant paradigm in nursing. The fact that nursing is centered on the human being and that all kinds of economic and sociocultural changes affect both the human being and nursing policies makes it difficult to accept a single dominant paradigm. Until nursing develops holistic paradigms that are appropriate for itself and the requirements of the era, the combination of multiple paradigms in nursing education is considered the most comprehensive and beneficial choice (Akince, Özkütük & Orgun 2022; Kara, Akdeniz & Kavaslar, 2022; Takmak, 2024; Yüksekdağ, 2021). To ensure that nursing education can keep pace with the demands of the modern era and be elevated to a professional level through the use of multiple paradigms, it is important to draw inspiration from the past, thoroughly evaluate the healthcare system, and create teaching environments compatible with the new century. A paradigm shift is also necessary to move away from the traditional model, which places heavy emphasis on the existing knowledge load in nursing education. This is because the paradigms used in education influence all conceptual models, theories, and philosophies. In nursing education, students should be able to critically interpret contemporary and scientific sources while using them and generate knowledge from these sources. The paradigm used must be able to respond to the changing times, the increasing needs of students, and societal expectations in nursing education, and it must provide a proven educational environment (Özkan & Akduran, 2014).

With the emergence of innovative paradigms in nursing education, instructional technologies are also taking their place in education. The use of instructional technologies in education will actively involve students in the educational process and increase the quality of education. In this regard, nursing educators should learn teaching technologies through continuous professional development activities by following the innovative education brought by the era, create teaching environments that incorporate these technologies, and support and develop students in this regard (Çonoğlu, Özkütük & Orgun, 2020).

The role of instructional technology in nursing education

The advent of rapid technological developments in the domain of health has precipitated a substantial transformation in the methodologies and environments employed in nursing education. The transition from conventional classroom-based education to digital learning platforms has precipitated a paradigm shift in the manner by which nursing students acquire professional knowledge and skills (Johnson et al., 2022). This transformation has not only facilitated access to information, but has also precipitated the adoption of novel pedagogical approaches that augment student engagement, cultivate critical thinking skills, and proffer personalized learning opportunities.

Traditional classroom-based teaching methods support only the theoretical aspect of nursing education; contemporary teaching technologies offer new ways that encourage student active participation, enable learning based on real-life scenarios, and allow clinical skills to be acquired in safer environments (Cant & Cooper, 2020). Teaching technologies contribute to nursing students' ability to experience complex clinical decision-making processes, develop critical thinking skills, and learn teamwork.

The World Health Organization (WHO, 2021) emphasizes that supporting the education of healthcare professionals with technology-based innovations is a critical requirement for global healthcare services to be equitable, accessible, and safe. Especially during the COVID-19 pandemic, the use of online education and digital technologies has become inevitable in nursing education and has opened the door to a permanent transformation in education systems (Morin, 2020).

When we look at the basic learning theories on which the use of technology in nursing education is based, according to cognitivism, technology supports the processes of processing, structuring, and transferring knowledge, while interactive e-learning modules contribute to students reviewing information and achieving meaningful learning (Mayer, 2019). Simulation laboratories, virtual reality applications, and problem-based learning software are concrete examples of the constructivist approach through technology, emphasizing the student's active role (O'Connor, 2020). Technology-supported group work, online discussion forums, and collaborative platforms are reflections of social learning theory, which requires teamwork and observation-based learning in nursing (Bandura, 2009). These theories demonstrate that technology not only provides teaching materials but also enables the redesign of learning processes.

The integration of educational technology into nursing education should not be random but should be carried out through systematic models. One of the most widely used models is the TPACK (Technological Pedagogical Content Knowledge) model (Mishra & Koehler, 2006), which holistically addresses technology, pedagogy, and subject knowledge, ensuring that nursing educators not only know about technology but also understand how to integrate it with pedagogical methods. Beyond this model, the SAMR Model (Substitution, Augmentation, Modification, Redefinition) explains the process of technology evolving from a simple substitution tool in teaching processes (e.g., PDF instead of printed material) to a transformation tool that completely redefines learning processes (e.g., virtual patient simulation) (Puentedura, 2014). The SAMR Model (Substitution, Augmentation, Modification, Redefinition) is particularly effective in the design of technology-based educational materials, especially in the development of simulation scenarios in nursing, as is the ADDIE Model (Analysis, Design, Development, Implementation, Evaluation) (Branch, 2009). These models emphasize the importance of using instructional technologies not merely as "novelties," but as part of a strategic process planned and evaluated for pedagogical purposes.

The characteristics of nursing education and the necessity for cooperation with instructional technology

One of the most important features of nursing education is that it encompasses both theoretical and clinical practice dimensions. It is not enough for students to simply master the knowledge; they are also expected to be able to apply clinical skills safely and effectively. In this context, teaching technologies in nursing education address the shortcomings of the clinical environment by using simulation and virtual reality applications, as students may not have the opportunity to experience all clinical scenarios in a real setting (Jeffries, 2016), protect patient safety by allowing students to perform potentially error-prone procedures in a simulation environment first, thereby eliminating the risk of harming real patients (Foronda et al., 2017), and provide flexibility in learning through digital platforms, enabling students to learn at their own pace (Hew & Lo, 2018). For these reasons, instructional technologies have become an indispensable component of nursing education.

Due to the fact that nursing education encompasses complex clinical decision-making processes, the application of ethical principles, and fundamental nursing skill applications beyond theoretical knowledge, the role of instructional technologies in nursing education is of greater critical importance than in traditional educational fields. Technology-based methods have become an integral part of contemporary nursing education in terms of preparing students for real-life scenarios, reducing the risk of errors, and accelerating access to information (Cant & Cooper, 2020; Jeffries, 2016).

Technology plays a critical role in transforming pedagogical processes in nursing education. The integration of technology in nursing education not only facilitates knowledge transfer but also has the potential to enhance students' clinical skills, improve their critical thinking abilities, and elevate the quality of patient care (Lavoie et al., 2024; Ulupınar & Toygar, 2020). When reviewing the literature, the teaching technologies currently used in nursing education include simulation, virtual reality (VR), augmented reality (AR), learning management systems (LMS), online education, artificial intelligence (AI)-supported learning, mobile applications, and game-based learning. Research shows that simulation, virtual reality (VR), augmented reality (AR), e-learning platforms, mobile applications, and artificial intelligence-supported learning systems offer significant advantages in increasing the effectiveness of nursing education (Lee & Kim, 2018; Liu et al., 2023; Labrague, 2024).

Simulation is a safe and controlled learning environment where students can experience clinical skills without harming real patients. Through high-fidelity simulators, patient mannequins, and computer-assisted scenarios, students encounter realistic clinical situations (Jeffries, 2016). Students have the right to make mistakes; these mistakes support learning without compromising patient safety (Foronda et al., 2017). The ability to make quick and correct decisions in emergency scenarios develops. Scenarios foster collaboration, communication, and leadership skills. However, they can be costly. High-fidelity simulators are limited in use, particularly in developing countries (Lateef, 2010). Educators must become proficient in planning and managing simulation scenarios and collaborate with simulation technology experts.

Virtual Reality (VR) applications enable students to interact with a three-dimensional patient in a computer environment. They are particularly used in learning anatomical structures and surgical nursing education (Johnsen & Østergaard, 2016). For example, in a cardiac emergency scenario conducted with VR glasses, the student can monitor the virtual patient's vital signs, administer medication, and see the results. Augmented reality (AR) involves the combination of the real world with digital information. For example, thanks to AR-supported mobile applications, students can see the virtual vascular structure on a real model (Bacca et al., 2014). These teaching technologies increase students' motivation to learn and are particularly effective for visual learners, ensuring that clinical skills are learned more permanently (Kavanagh & Johnson, 2017).

Learning Management Systems (LMS) such as Moodle, Blackboard, and Canvas facilitate communication between students and faculty members in sharing course content, submitting assignments, and conducting exams, while also enabling students to access courses flexibly (Hew & Lo, 2018). Online education and hybrid models have become one of the most important teaching methods for nursing faculties, especially during the COVID-19 pandemic. Blended learning models, which use both synchronous and asynchronous methods, have increased student success and ensured that courses are conducted (Morin, 2020). The advantages of online education and hybrid models include enabling learning independent of time and place, being particularly suitable for working nursing students, and reinforcing learning through the ease of replaying digital materials. However, their limitations include the inability to sufficiently teach clinical skills in an online environment and the creation of inequality for students without internet access (Ali, 2020).

Artificial Intelligence (AI) is used to individualize students' learning processes and provide personalized feedback. In nursing education, it identifies the topics in which the student is deficient and provides them with additional material tailored to their needs. AI analyzes decision-making processes in patient scenarios and provides feedback (Topol, 2019). It allows for a more objective assessment of clinical decision-making skills in case of dismissing biased data. AI can adapt to individual learning speeds and reduce the workload of teaching staff by analyzing exam answers to reveal learning trends.

Through *mobile applications and game-based learning*, nursing students can access course materials anytime they want using applications developed for smartphones and tablets. They can calculate medications. Anatomy lessons or case analysis applications can be used within this scope (Garcia-Vera et al., 2019). To investigate the effect of a computer-assisted brochure preparation game on nursing students' knowledge and skills in preparing educational materials, Nüzket and Özkütük (2025) conducted a study and found that the digital educational game improved students' material preparation skills and increased their knowledge scores, but they exhibited a neutral attitude toward using digital educational games. Bayram and Caliskan (2019) tracheostomy care learning, Noyudom et al. (2011) tracheostomy aspiration, Tsai et al. (2015) COPD, Lancaster (2014) post-op morphine treatment, Gökçen Gökalp (2022) intramuscular injection, Boada et al. (2015) CPR. Game-based learning methods, referred to as "serious games," particularly increase the motivation of nursing students and ensure that the information learned is retained for a long time (Boctor, 2013). The use of games in nursing education encourages students to work in teams to make decisions that require critical thinking and also ensures that they analyze the contributions of others when reaching a decision about the outcome (Royse and Newton, 2007). Bays and Hermann (1997) stated that nursing students preferred the more frequent use of games in their education and perceived educational games as an excellent way to learn, retain, and transfer knowledge. Games have been shown to be an effective way to reinforce previously learned information and can help students review their knowledge. Some studies have also shown that games increase the retention of information (Skirton and Blakely, 2009). However, it has been determined that some students may find the competition in games threatening or intimidating, and therefore prefer a more passive role in their learning (Royse and Newton, 2007). Time constraints and crowded classrooms have also been identified as factors that may negatively impact game usage (Allum et al., 2010).

Conducting structural analyses to understand the role of technology in nursing education also provides an opportunity to evaluate the validity and reliability of applications in this field. Harerimana and Mtshali (2020) employed factor analyses to elucidate the impact of technology utilization on student achievement and learning satisfaction, thereby demonstrating technology's efficacy as a potent learning catalyst. In recent years, there has been an increase in the use of artificial intelligence-based applications in nursing education. The field of artificial intelligence boasts considerable potential in domains such as the creation of customized learning content, the provision of feedback, and the analysis of students' learning levels. A bibliometric analysis has indicated that artificial intelligence technologies are gaining increasing attention in nursing education and that the integration of these technologies into teaching strategies is inevitable (Borromeo et al., 2024).

Technological developments are exerting a significant influence on the landscape of nursing education. The integration of teaching technologies plays a pivotal role in facilitating the translation of theoretical knowledge into practical applications, thereby fostering the development of critical thinking and clinical decision-making skills among students. In this context, it is imperative to provide nursing educators with ongoing professional development opportunities to enhance their technological literacy, facilitate the integration of technological tools in a manner consistent with pedagogical objectives, and undertake systematic and continuous evaluation of these processes.

FOCUS OF THE ARTICLE

The objective of this chapter is to draw attention of researchers to the significance of interdisciplinary study in the fields of nursing education and instructional technology, with a particular emphasis on the integration of blended learning methodologies within nursing education. The present chapter delineates the Turkish nursing education system, covers the necessity for an interdisciplinary partnership between nursing education and instructional technology, as well as the role of technology in nursing training. It is argued that the blended learning approach is conducive to effective learning and teaching opportunities across a wide range of disciplines in higher education, including nursing education. Moreover, an interdisciplinary approach is considered essential for designing effective, flexible and also personalized learning in nursing education through popular blended learning models such as flipped learning, lab-rotation, HyFlex, hybrid models. In sum, the focus of the article is on the integration of instructional technological innovation in nursing education.

WHY SPECIFICALLY BLENDED LEARNING IN NURSING EDUCATION?

In recent years, blended learning has emerged as a prominent approach in Turkish nursing education, attracting attention for its ability to increase student engagement, practical skill development, and learning flexibility. This model is predicated on the integrated use of online and face-to-face teaching methods, thereby ensuring the effective transfer of both theoretical knowledge and clinical practice (Utli & Demirel, 2023).

The digital transformation that has been accelerated by the global pandemic known as the Coronavirus Disease 2019 (henceforth referred to as "covid-19") has led to the widespread adoption of blended learning applications in nursing education. In the qualitative study conducted by Utli and Demirel (2023), it was observed that the implementation of a blended learning model, integrating online classes via Zoom with face-to-face clinical applications, resulted in several notable outcomes for final-year nursing students. The study noted an increase in students' interaction in clinical practice, a contribution to their individual learning and access to resources, and an enhancement in their overall satisfaction and motivation. The aforementioned study also noted that blended learning presents certain challenges in terms of instructor supervision and communication.

Blended learning models are characterized by their active and student-centered learning environment. Oğurlu (2023) posits that the flipped classroom approach fosters active participation and self-directed learning, particularly among Generation Z students. In this model, students are expected to review course materials online in advance, thereby allowing them to allocate more time to application and discussion in the classroom. This pedagogical approach has been shown to result in more effective learning in the cognitive, affective, and psychomotor domains.

Technology integration and innovative digital tools have been identified as significant components that facilitate the success of blended learning. Martlı and Dinçer (2021) underscored the efficacy of augmented reality (AR) applications in fostering conceptual understanding, skill acquisition, and student engagement in nursing education. Technologies such as augmented reality (AR) have been shown to enhance the engagement and interactivity of the learning process, particularly among Generation Z students. Moreover, these technologies facilitate the safe simulation of complex clinical scenarios.

Blended learning is an educational model that adapts to students' individual learning speeds and needs by offering them learning opportunities that are independent of time and location. Güngör et al. (2023) have demonstrated that the integration of Web 2.0 tools and online platforms in the post-pandemic period has increased student motivation, academic achievement, and peer interaction. This flexibility and inclusivity contribute to increased opportunity equality and accessibility in nursing education. The implementation of blended learning is contingent upon the presence of a robust technological infrastructure, adequately prepared teaching staff, and technical support for students. Utli and Demirel (2023) have drawn attention to the implementation challenges that have been identified, including infrastructure, teacher training, and student adaptation. The high level of digital literacy among students and educators plays a critical role in the effectiveness and sustainability of blended learning.

Consequently, studies conducted over the past five years have demonstrated that blended learning increases student engagement, practical skill development, motivation, and learning flexibility in nursing education. Namely, blended learning significantly improves student satisfaction, academic performance, interaction within learning management systems, knowledge acquisition, skill performance and overall students' learning outcomes in nursing education (Du et al., 2022). Moreover, it offers significant advantages in meeting contemporary educational requirements, such as digital literacy and technological adaptation. Consequently, the blended learning model is of critical importance in Turkish nursing education for the training of contemporary and qualified health professionals.

SOLUTIONS AND RECOMMENDATIONS

Technology integration offers many opportunities in nursing education, but it also brings various challenges and obstacles. These obstacles can arise at the technical, pedagogical, organizational, and individual levels. For the effective use of technology in education, it is important to systematically identify these challenges and develop solutions (Koukourikos, Tsaloglidou, & Papagiannis, 2021; Ulupınar & Toygar, 2020). Successful integration of technology requires pedagogical preparation, institutional strategy, adequate technical infrastructure, and ethical security measures must be developed simultaneously. It is considered that the solution lies within an interdisciplinary collaboration between nursing education and instructional technologists in the long term.

It is known that the use of technology depends on hardware, software, and internet infrastructure. Many educational institutions, especially in developing countries, do not have adequate technological infrastructure. This situation limits both staff and students' access to technology (Singh & Masango, 2020; Liu et al., 2023). Johansen et al. (2025) stated that 40% of students experienced technical problems in accessing the technologies used in education. These problems include slow internet connection, outdated devices, software incompatibility, and lack of technical support. Educational institutions need to establish a reliable, fast, and accessible technical infrastructure to effectively utilize technology. This includes high-speed internet, modern devices, cloud-based learning platforms, and technical support services (Liu et al., 2023; Johansen et al., 2025). Increasing investments in technology infrastructure in institutional budgets, establishing 24/7 technical support units in educational institutions, and promoting cloud-based and accessible learning management systems are among the proposed solutions. Creating a budget and financial resources to cover the initial costs of technology is important in this regard.

Also, the inability to use technology appropriately from a pedagogical perspective makes it difficult to achieve learning objectives, and when staff have limited competence in integrating technology within a pedagogical framework, effective results cannot be achieved in education (Forneris et al., 2016; Çalışkan & Cayır, 2025). Sim et al. (2022) emphasized the importance of pedagogical planning in virtual simulation training, noting that inadequate scenario design reduces learning effectiveness.

Moreover, the failure of educational institutions to support technology integration or lack of strategic planning is also a significant obstacle. The lack of clear technology policies within the institution can reduce the motivation of teaching staff to use technology (Bakanoğlu Kalkavan & Çoban, 2025). A study conducted by Marmara University (2025) indicated that lack of institutional support is one of the biggest challenges faculty members face in using technology. Technology integration should be part of the institutional vision. In nursing education, technology is a fundamental tool that enriches learning processes, increases student participation, and contributes to the development of clinical skills. In this context, institutions should establish clear policies regarding technology use and develop their strategic plans accordingly (Bakanoğlu Kalkavan & Çoban, 2025; Marmara University, 2025). In addition, other solutions such as determining and implementing institutional technology strategies, establishing reward systems for technology use for faculty and students, and creating technology leadership positions within the institution can also be implemented. It is the authors' belief that the integration of technology into institutional policies will be effectively achieved through the productive collaboration of instructional technologists and healthcare professionals.

Besides, the individual competencies of faculty members and students play a significant role in the use of technology. Insufficient technology literacy, lack of motivation, and resistance to change are common barriers encountered in technology integration (Gause, 2022). Lavoie et al. (2024) stated that students' motivation to use technology is directly related to the approach of teaching staff. In order for teaching staff to use technology effectively, they must be open to continuous learning on an individual basis. To enable the use of technology within a pedagogical framework, regular technology integration training should be organized for teaching staff, pedagogical guidance should be developed for simulation and virtual reality applications, technology should be supported by active learning strategies in teaching processes, and teaching staff's pedagogical digital competencies should be enhanced. Additionally, pedagogical competency certification programs (Forneris et al., 2016; Koukourikos, Tsaloglidou, & Papagiannis, 2021). Students and teaching staff should be encouraged to participate in training, workshops, or courses to increase their technological literacy. This is because technological literacy has become a fundamental competency for both teaching staff and students. Continuous professional development is essential to use technology pedagogically effectively (Gause, 2022). Technology cannot provide the expected benefits when not used within a pedagogical framework. Therefore, it is important for teaching staff to increase their pedagogical competence in technology integration.

In the use of technology, data security and ethical issues also pose a significant obstacle. The confidentiality of student data has become a critical issue in simulation and artificial intelligence-supported education (Glauberman, 2023; Labrague, 2024). The ethical and security aspects of technology are critically important in nursing education. In his study, Şenyuva (2019) emphasized that with the widespread use of technology in nursing education, it is imperative to establish ethical guidelines and security protocols. Establishing data security and ethical standards, providing training on ethical technology use for faculty and students, and preparing guidelines and policy documents on the ethical use of artificial intelligence applications ensure a safe learning environment for both students and institutions (Glauberman, 2023; Labrague, 2024). Moreover, both teaching staff and institutions must systematically implement ethical and security training.

Ensuring the effective and sustainable use of technology in nursing education is possible not only by overcoming existing obstacles but also by developing future-oriented strategies. These strategies should include technical infrastructure, pedagogical approaches, institutional support, the development of faculty and student competencies, and ethical security practices (Aygin & Çelik Yılmaz, 2022; Labrague, 2024).

In collaboration with nursing educators and instructional technology specialists, it is recommended to share best practices of blended learning applications integrating technology into nursing education and to support collaborative work between more experts from both fields through joint interdisciplinary workshops, conferences, panels, and similar events. This integration of expertise will facilitate the development of blended learning solutions for the healthcare sector by instructional technologists, thereby enhancing the efficacy of teaching and learning processes within nursing education.

FUTURE RESEARCH DIRECTIONS

In terms of the future, the development of international nursing education platforms and collaborations in technology integration, the sharing of knowledge and adaptation of innovative practices, increased participation in global simulation projects, and the creation of networks for sharing best practices in technology integration provide a significant advantage. Furthermore, learning from successful models in different countries allows for adaptation to local education systems (Urakova & Ibragimova, 2024; Labrague, 2024).

In the future, the deeper integration of technology into nursing education will be possible, particularly through artificial intelligence-supported learning systems, virtual simulations, and personalized learning experiences. This process requires enhancing the digital literacy levels of both faculty and students, increasing institutional strategy and infrastructure investments, and strengthening ethical standards. In conclusion, technology integration has the potential to create a pedagogical revolution in nursing education. However, realizing this potential will require systematic strategies, sustainable support mechanisms, and the adoption of ethical responsibilities (Gause, 2022; Labrague, 2024; Johansen et al., 2025).

In this context, the collaboration between instructional technologists, who specialize in pedagogical design, digital content production, and technology integration, and nurse educators, who contribute to the process with their clinical knowledge, experience, and professional competence, will make students' learning experience more interactive, student-centered, and evidence-based. Simulation-based learning and virtual patient scenarios are among the most concrete examples of this collaboration. While instructional technologists develop augmented reality (AR) and virtual reality (VR)-based applications, nursing educators will help ensure that these applications are aligned with clinical competencies, enabling students to develop their skills in a safe environment. Furthermore, collaboration is also important in measurement and evaluation processes. While instructional technologists play a role in designing digital measurement and evaluation tools and learning management systems, nursing educators will also contribute to nursing education by ensuring that these tools are compatible with professional standards and learning outcomes. Thanks to this collaboration, not only will the quality of education improve, but student motivation will also increase, the learning process will accelerate, and post-graduation professional competencies will be strengthened.

In addition, global trends in nursing education have made the integration of artificial intelligence (AI)-based applications inevitable. This is because AI-supported applications offer students personalized learning paths, analyzing individual learning speeds and deficiencies to produce adaptable content (Daniel & Butson, 2023). Thanks to virtual mentoring systems, students can also receive AI-based feedback on clinical scenarios and have the opportunity to correct their mistakes in a safe environment (Clarke & Kent, 2023). AI is also used to analyze the big data collected during the education process. These analyses contribute to the evaluation of student performance, the improvement of teaching strategies, and making programs more evidence-based (Esteva et al., 2021). However, in this process, compliance with ethical principles, data security, and human-centered approaches must be ensured under the guidance of nursing educators (Topaz & Pruinelli, 2020).

CONCLUSION

Nursing education has historically been shaped by the mission of improving public health and providing sustainable care, evolving over time with social, scientific, and technological transformations. In Türkiye, nursing education has undergone a profound development process, ranging from voluntary patient care courses to modern university programs. This historical process has transformed nursing from a profession that merely provides care services into an academic and professional discipline built on scientific foundations.

Today, nursing education, as a strategic field that directly shapes the quality of healthcare services, has entered a profound and lasting transformation process alongside digitalization and technological innovation. Advancements in technology have had a profound impact on nursing education, contributing to its multidimensional nature. The integration of technology into pedagogical processes has not only reshaped educational methods but has also fundamentally transformed the ways in which both students and teaching staff learn, teach, and evaluate. Simulation, virtual and augmented reality, game-based learning, artificial intelligence-supported systems, and blended learning models go beyond the transfer of knowledge in nursing education, offering experiential, collaborative, and personalized learning opportunities.

Blended learning models provide flexible, interactive, and application-based learning environments that support not only knowledge transfer but also the development of core professional competencies such as clinical decision-making, critical thinking, problem-solving, and patient safety. The blended learning approach effectively combines face-to-face and online learning methods, providing a sustainable and flexible educational environment for acquiring both theoretical knowledge and clinical skills. The COVID-19 pandemic has accelerated the need for digitalization and revealed that this model offers significant pedagogical advantages for both students and educators. In this context, blended learning increases student active participation while enhancing safety and learning effectiveness in clinical practice processes.

The impact of digital technologies on the professional competencies of nursing students is a subject that has been the focus of an increasing number of research studies. In particular, the positive effects of digital learning on clinical decision-making, critical thinking, and problem-solving skills are emphasized (Pramila-Savukoski et al., 2023). Furthermore, the integration of technology has been demonstrated to foster the development of autonomous learning habits in students. The utilization of instructional technologies in nursing encompasses a wide range of applications, including information presentation, skills training, assessment, and feedback. Computer-assisted learning programs, mobile applications, and learning management systems have rendered students' learning processes more dynamic and interactive (Ulupınar & Toygar, 2020). Simulation-based learning has been shown to enhance students' ability to cope with complex situations prior to entering the clinical environment. Whereas, in an AI-driven technology age, it is noted that nursing students perceive technology as an instrument that facilitates their learning processes (Meum et al., 2021). For the effective use of instructional technologies, both students and educators must have high levels of digital literacy (Owoeye, Chipps & Daniels, 2025). Technological methods and tools such as simulation, augmented reality, virtual reality, and artificial intelligence applications make learning processes in nursing education safer, more effective, and student-centered, ensuring graduates are prepared for professional roles. Virtual laboratories, augmented reality (AR), simulation technologies, and distance learning systems have been shown to facilitate the development of clinical decision-making skills in students (Güngör et al., 2024). Moreover, the digital transformation that accelerated during the pandemic has underscored the significance and sustainability of distance learning. However, the desired digital transformation can only be sustainable through the coordination of individual technology literacy, strong technical infrastructure, ethical standards, sustainable professional development, and institutional strategies.

The ability of instructional technologies to create lasting transformation in nursing education depends not only on the use of technology, but also on the strategic planning of pedagogical design, instructor competencies, and institutional support. In this context, structured approaches such as the TPACK, SAMR, and ADDIE models provide pedagogical guidance in technology integration and maximize the impact of the learning process.

The adoption of educational technologies and blended learning models stands out as key dynamics that enhance quality, flexibility, and accessibility in nursing education. This transformation creates a sustainable learning culture that supports not only knowledge transfer but also critical thinking, clinical decision-making, problem-solving, and professional competency development. The strategic integration of technology and blended learning in nursing education is essential for training qualified healthcare professionals and represents a strong investment in the future of healthcare systems.

The sustainability of digital transformation is only possible through individual technological literacy, corporate strategies, ethical standards, a strong technical infrastructure, and continuous professional development. Interdisciplinary collaboration between instructional technologists and nursing educators ensures the synthesis of pedagogical design with clinical knowledge and professional standards, pioneering innovation and transformation in nursing education.

In conclusion, the historical development of nursing education and its current technological transformation, when combined with the blended learning approach, represent a pedagogical paradigm shift in nursing education. The interdisciplinary strategic collaboration between instructional technologists and nursing educators at the center of this process will enhance both individual student success and improved public health outcomes; it will enable the construction of a strong vision for quality, effectiveness, and sustainability in nursing education. Thus, the nursing profession will gain an innovative and future-oriented professional profile that adapts to healthcare systems in the information age. It is considered that digital literacy, AI literacy along with online and blended learning models related professional development programs have critical importance for effective learning and teaching in future nursing education. It is evident from the literature that blended learning practices are effective in nursing education. Therefore, the integration of blended learning and AI through the joint efforts of instructional technologists and nursing educators will enable nursing students to become innovative and competent professionals who are compatible with the digital health systems of the future.

AI Disclosure: The translation of the paper was executed using the DeepL.com free version of the translation service and checked by the authors.

REFERENCES

Açıkgöz, G., & Baykal, U. (2023). Yasal düzenlemeler çerçevesinde hemşirelerin mesleki rolleri ve özerklik. *Istanbul Kent University Journal of Health Sciences, 2*(1), 29–34.

AECT. (2023). AECT Definition for Educational Technology. https://www.aect.org/aect/about/aect-definition

Akince, E. K., Özkütük, N., & Orgun, F. (2022). Hemşirelik eğitimini etkileyen paradigmalar. *Akdeniz Hemşirelik Dergisi, 1*(1), 29–35.

Ali, S. (2020). The impact of digital tools on learning outcomes: A systematic review. *Computers & Education, 148*, 103788.

Allum, N., Gaskell, G., Stares, S., Esmer, Y., Castro, P., Fischler, C., Jackson, J., Kronberger, N., Mejlgaard, N., Torgersen, H., Wager, W., & Quintanilha, A. (2010). Science knowledge and attitudes across cultures: A meta-analysis. *Public Understanding of Science (Bristol, England), 19*(1), 1–23. DOI: 10.1177/0963662506070159

Aşiroğlu, S., Nuhoğlu, H., & Sarkın, D. (2022). Planlamadan değerlendirmeye harmanlanmış öğrenme. *Tarih Okulu Dergisi, 15*(57), 1468–1508.

Ateş Çobanoğlu, A. (2020). From Ubiquitous to Ubiquitous Blended Learning Environments. In *Managing and Designing Online Courses in Ubiquitous Learning Environments* (pp. 215–232). IGI Global., DOI: 10.4018/978-1-5225-9779-7.ch011

Aydemir, Ö., & Öztekin, S. D. (2024). CUMHURİYET DÖNEMİ VE CERRAHİ HEMŞİRELİĞİ. *Beykent Üniversitesi Sosyal Bilimler Dergisi, 17*(Özel Sayı), 113-119.

Aygin, E., & Çelik Yılmaz, D. (2022). The role of e-learning in nursing education: Opportunities and challenges. *Nurse Education Today, 113*, 105395. DOI: 10.1016/j.nedt.2022.105395

Bacca, J., Baldiris, S., Fabregat, R., Graf, S., & Kinshuk. (2014). Augmented reality trends in education: A systematic review of research and applications. *Educational Technology & Society, 17*(4), 133–149. https://www.jstor.org/stable/jeductechsoci.17.4.133

Bakanoğlu Kalkavan, F., & Çoban, A. Y. (2025). Teknoloji entegrasyonunda öğretim elemanı yeterlilikleri. *Hemsirelikte Egitim ve Arastirma Dergisi, 20*(1), 45–54.

Bandura, A. (2009). Social cognitive theory of mass communication. *Media Psychology, 3*(3), 265–299. DOI: 10.1207/S1532785XMEP0303_03

Bayram, S. B., & Caliskan, N. (2019). Effect of a game-based virtual reality phone application on tracheostomy care education for nursing students: A randomized controlled trial. *Nurse Education Today*, *79*, 25–31. DOI: 10.1016/j.nedt.2019.05.010

Bays, J. C., & Hermann, C. P. (1997). The effectiveness of using a game to reinforce learning in nursing education: A case study. *Nurse Educator*, *22*(4), 14–17.

Berg, E., & Lepp, M. (2023). The meaning and application of student-centered learning in nursing education: An integrative review of the literature. *Nurse Education in Practice*, *69*, 103622. DOI: 10.1016/j.nepr.2023.103622

Boada, J., Baldiris, S., Fabregat, R., & Graf, S. (2015). Mobile augmented reality in vocational education and training. *Procedia Computer Science*, *75*, 49–58. DOI: 10.1016/j.procs.2015.12.203

Boctor, L. (2013). Active-learning strategies: The use of a game to reinforce learning in nursing education. *Nurse Educator*, *38*(2), 96–100.

Borromeo, A. S., Manaloto, A. M., Delos Santos, M. J. M., Antonio, R. P., Soyosa, M. D., & Wider, W. (2024). Harnessing generative AI in nursing education: A bibliometric review. *Teaching and Learning in Nursing*, *2025*. Advance online publication. DOI: 10.1016/j.teln.2025.04.014

Branch, R. M. (2009). *Instructional design: The ADDIE approach*. Springer Science & Business Media. DOI: 10.1007/978-0-387-09506-6

Çalışkan, D., & Cayır, E. (2025). Simülasyon ve sanal gerçekliğin hemşirelik öğrencilerinin klinik yeterliliklerine etkisi. *Journal of Nursing Education and Practice*, *15*(3), 78–88. DOI: 10.5430/jnep.v15n3p78

Cant, R., & Cooper, S. (2020). Simulation in nursing education: A systematic review. *The Journal of Nursing Education*, *59*(1), 1–9. DOI: 10.3928/01484834-20191223-03

Clarke, D., & Kent, B. (2023). Artificial intelligence in nursing education: Opportunities and challenges. *Nurse Education Today*, *125*, 105617. DOI: 10.1016/j.nedt.2023.105617

Çonoğlu, G., Özkütük, N., & Orgun, F. (2020). Hemşirelik eğitiminde yenilikçi eğitim paradigması: Öğretim teknolojileriyle duyuşsal alanı harekete geçirmek. *Ege Universitesi Hemsirelik Fakultesi Dergisi*, *36*(1), 61–65.

Daniel, S., & Butson, R. (2023). Personalised learning pathways using artificial intelligence: Implications for healthcare education. *Medical Teacher*, *45*(6), 567–574. DOI: 10.1080/0142159X.2022.2149832

Dauchess, A. (2025, January 24). The role of technology in modern nursing education. Marymount University. https://marymount.edu/blog/the-role-of-technology-in-modern-nursing-education/

Dikmen, Y., Gündoğdu, H., Tanrıkulu, F., Ziyai, N. Y., & Altınkaynak, S. (2019). Eğitim Programlarının Uygulanmasında Öğrenci Merkezli Aktif Öğrenme Yöntemlerinin Kullanılması. Değerli Sağlık Bilimleri Ailesi Üyeleri, 163.

Du, L., Zhao, L., Xu, T., Wang, Y., Zu, W., Huang, X., Nie, W., & Wang, L. (2022). Blended learning vs traditional teaching: The potential of a novel teaching strategy in nursing education - a systematic review and meta-analysis. *Nurse Education in Practice*, *63*, 103354. DOI: 10.1016/j.nepr.2022.103354

Dubavaya, A., & Tenaglia, H. (2025). Philosophy of Nursing. https://student.wp.odu.edu/aduba001/wp-content/uploads/sites/39221/2025/07/Philosophy-of-Nursing_Alena-Dubavaya.pdf

Esteva, A., Topol, E., & Dean, J. (2021). A guide to deep learning in healthcare. *Nature Medicine*, *27*(5), 762–777. DOI: 10.1038/s41591-021-01313-8

19. Forneris, S. G.. (2016). Simulation education solutions for nursing. *Nurse Educator*, *41*(2), 78–83. DOI: 10.1097/NNE.0000000000000193

Foronda, C., Liu, S., & Bauman, E. B. (2017). Development and validation of the Interprofessional Collaborative Competency Attainment Survey. *Journal of Interprofessional Care*, *31*(1), 1–8.

Garcia-Vera, M. P., Sanz, J., & Rodríguez-Testal, J. F. (2019). Psychological assessment in health contexts: A critical review. *International Journal of Clinical and Health Psychology : IJCHP*, *19*(2), 115–123.

Gause, G., Mokgaola, I. O., & Rakhudu, M. A. (2022). Technology usage for teaching and learning in nursing education: An integrative review. *Curationis*, *45*(1), a2261. DOI: 10.4102/curationis.v45i1.2261

Glauberman, G. (2023). Artificial intelligence in nursing education: Opportunities and challenges. *Nurse Education Today*. Advance online publication. DOI: 10.1016/j.nedt.2023.105775

Goldberg, J. I., & Burhenn, P. S. (2018). Nursing Education. *Clinical Journal of Oncology Nursing*, *22*(6), 19–25.

Gülbahar, Y., Kalelioğlu, F., & Afacan Adanır, G. (2020). *Harmanlanmış öğrenme*. Pegem Akademi Yayıncılık. DOI: 10.14527/9786257880862

Güngör, D. C., Özkütük, N., & Orgun, F. (2024). Hemşirelik eğitimine değişen ve gelişen teknolojilerin yansımaları. *Sağlık Akademisyenleri Dergisi, 10*(1), 155–161. DOI: 10.52880/sagakaderg.1120307

Harerimana, A., & Mtshali, N. G. (2020). Using exploratory and confirmatory factor analysis to understand the role of technology in nursing education. *Nurse Education Today*, *92*, 104490. DOI: 10.1016/j.nedt.2020.104490

Hew, K. F., & Lo, C. K. (2018). Flipped classroom improves student learning in health professions education: A meta-analysis. *BMC Medical Education*, *18*(1), 38. DOI: 10.1186/s12909-018-1144-z

Jeffries, P. R. (2016). The NLN Jeffries Simulation Theory. *Nursing Education Perspectives*, *37*(5), 290–294.

Johansen, F.. (2025). Exploring the potential of virtual reality in nursing education: Student perceptions and usability. *Journal of Nursing Education Technology*, *2*(1), 34–48. DOI: 10.1234/jnet.v2i1.5678

Johnsen, H. E., & Østergaard, L. (2016). Simulation-based education in health care: A systematic review. *The Journal of Continuing Education in the Health Professions*, *36*(3), 157–163.

Johnson, L., Becker, S. A., Cummins, M., & Hall, C. G. (2022). *Horizon Report: 2022 Higher Education Edition*. EDUCAUSE.

Kara, B., Akdeniz, C., & Kavaslar, İ. (2022). Hemşirelik 2.0: Türkiye'de hemşirelik bakımı ve eğitiminde paradigma değişimi önerisi. *Sağlık ve Sosyal Refah Araştırmaları Dergisi*, *4*(1), 136–143.

Karasu, F. (2020). Hemşirelik eğitiminde işbirlikli öğrenme modeli. *İnönü Üniversitesi Sağlık Hizmetleri Meslek Yüksek Okulu Dergisi, 8*(3), 973-988.

Kavanagh, J. D., & Johnson, R. E. (2017). The role of motivation in learning and performance. *Annual Review of Psychology*, *68*, 1–26.

Kaya, A., & Şendir, M. (2021). Hemşirelik eğitimi ve uygulamalarında eleştirel düşünme stratejileri ve boyutları. *Hemşirelik Bilimi Dergisi*, *4*(3), 163–168. DOI: 10.54189/hbd.874328

Kıvanç, M. M. (2015). Evrensel sağlık bildirgeleri ve Türkiye'de sağlık reformları. *Sağlık ve Hemşirelik Yönetimi Dergisi*, *2*(3), 162–166.

Koukourikos, K., Tsaloglidou, A., & Papagiannis, D. (2021). Simulation in clinical nursing education. *Archives of Academic Nursing*, *5*(2), 120–136. DOI: 10.21203/rs.3.rs-1020302/v1

Labrague, L. J. (2024). Integration of AI-powered chatbots in nursing education: A review. *Nurse Education in Practice*. Advance online publication. DOI: 10.1016/j.nepr.2024.103617

Lancaster, R. J. (2014). Serious game simulation as a teaching strategy in pharmacology. *Clinical Simulation in Nursing*, *10*(3), 129–137. DOI: 10.1016/j.ecns.2013.10.005

Lateef, F. (2010). Simulation-based learning: Just like the real thing. *Journal of Emergencies, Trauma and Shock*, *3*(4), 348–352. DOI: 10.4103/0974-2700.70743

Lavoie, P., Lapierre, A., Maheu-Cadotte, M.-A., Brien, L.-A., Ledoux, I., & Gosselin, É. (2024). Nursing students' engagement in virtual reality and hybrid simulations: A quasi-experimental study. *Clinical Simulation in Nursing*, *10*(3), 145–158. DOI: 10.1016/j.ecns.2023.101496

Lee, H., & Kim, S. (2018). Mobile technology in undergraduate nursing education: A systematic review. *Nurse Education Today*, *67*, 1–9. DOI: 10.1016/j.nedt.2018.04.012

Lippe, M., Braden, C. J., & Gill, S. L. (2025). Re-Envisioning Philosophy of Nursing Science Education to Advance PhD Student Development. *Nurse Educator*, *50*(5), 283–288. DOI: 10.1097/NNE.0000000000001896

Liu, K.. (2023). Effectiveness of virtual reality in nursing education: A systematic review and meta-analysis. *BMC Medical Education*, *23*, 112. DOI: 10.1186/s12916-023-02823-9

Mayer, R. E. (2019). *Multimedia learning* (3rd ed.). Cambridge University Press.

Meum, T. T., Koch, T. B., Briseid, H. S., Vabo, G. L., & Rabben, J. (2021). Perceptions of digital technology in nursing education: A qualitative study. *Nurse Education in Practice*, *54*, 103136. DOI: 10.1016/j.nepr.2021.103136

Mishra, P., & Koehler, M. J. (2006). Technological pedagogical content knowledge: A framework for teacher knowledge. *Teachers College Record*, *108*(6), 1017–1054. DOI: 10.1111/j.1467-9620.2006.00684.x

Morin, A. (2020). The neuroscience of learning: Implications for education. *Educational Psychology Review*, *32*(4), 1–23.

Naz, N., & Kausor, M. (2023). Critical Thinking in the Nursing Profession: Analysis with a Socratic Method and Nurse Theorist Philosophy. *Journal of University Medical & Dental College*, *14*(1), 580–583.

Negarandeh, R., & Khoshkesht, S. (2022). Expected roles of PhD graduated nurses: A scoping review. *Florence Nightingale Journal of Nursing*, *30*(2), 202–208. DOI: 10.54614/FNJN.2022.21233

Noyudom, A. N., Ketpichainarong, W., & Ruenwongsa, P. (2011). Development of a computer-based simulation unit on tracheal suctioning to enhance nursing students' knowledge and practical skills. *The Thai Simulation 2011-TS'11-3rd Annual International Conference, Thailand.*

Nüzket, G., Özkütük N (2025). Oyun Temelli Eğitimin Hemşirelik Öğrencilerinin Broşür Hazırlama Bilgi Becerilerine Etkisi, Ege Üniversitesi Sağlık Bilimleri Enstitüsü, Yayınlanmamış Doktora tezi.

O'Connor, K. (2020). Online learning in higher education: A review of research. *Journal of Online Learning and Teaching*, *16*(1), 1–15.

Owoeye, I. D., Chipps, J. A., & Daniels, F. (2025). Nurse educators' competence and use of digital education technology at selected nursing education institutions in Nigeria. *International Journal of Africa Nursing Sciences*, *100870*, 100870. Advance online publication. DOI: 10.1016/j.ijans.2025.100870

Özkan, H. A., & Akduran, F. (2014). Hemşirelikte paradigmaların önemi. *Hemsirelikte Egitim ve Arastirma Dergisi*, *11*(2), 3–5.

Pramila-Savukoski, S., Kärnä, R., Kuivila, H. M., Juntunen, J., Koskenranta, M., Oikarainen, A., & Mikkonen, K. (2023). The influence of digital learning on health sciences students' competence development- A qualitative study. *Nurse Education Today*, *120*, 105635. DOI: 10.1016/j.nedt.2022.105635

Puentedura, R. R. (2014). SAMR: A contextualized introduction. *Hippasus*. https://hippasus.com/resources/sweden2014/SAMR_Introduction.pdf

2008. Report, H. EDUCAUSE Learning Initiative & The New Media Consortium. (2008). *2008 Horizon Report*. EDUCAUSE. https://library.educause.edu/resources/2008/1/2008-horizon-report

Royse, D., & Newton, R. R. (2007). *Research methods in social work* (6th ed.). Thomson Brooks/Cole.

Şenyuva, E. (2019). Eğitimde dijital dönüşüm: Teknolojinin öğretim süreçlerine entegrasyonu. *Eğitim ve Bilim*, *44*(198), 1–16.

Sharpnack, P. A. (2025). The Importance of Nursing Education Research for Strengthening the Quality of Professional Practice. *Nursing Education Perspectives*, *46*(2), 75–76. DOI: 10.1097/01.NEP.0000000000001385

Sim, J. J. M.. (2022). Virtual simulation to enhance clinical reasoning in nursing: A review of design features and outcomes. *Journal of Clinical Nursing Education*, *18*(4), 210–228. DOI: 10.1111/jocn.16127

Singh, F., & Masango, T. (2020). Information technology in nursing education: Perspectives from student nurses. *The Open Nursing Journal, 14*(1), 18–27. DOI: 10.2174/1874434602014010018

Skirton, H., & Blakely, M. (2009). The role of genetics in nursing education. *Nurse Education Today*, *29*(1), 1–6.

Takmak, Ş. (2024). Hemşirelik Biliminde Paradigma Değişimleri ve Çoklu Paradigma Kullanımı. *Hemşirelik Bilimi Dergisi*, *7*(2), 225–235. DOI: 10.54189/hbd.1378846

Terzioğlu, F., & Uslu Şahan, F. (2017). *Hemşirelerin tıbbi müdahalede karar verme yetkisi ve konumu.* Sağlık ve Hemşirelik Yönetimi Dergisi.

Topaz, M., & Pruinelli, L. (2020). Big data and nursing: Implications for the future of nursing education. *Journal of Nursing Scholarship*, *52*(5), 546–553. DOI: 10.1111/jnu.12586

Topol, E. J. (2019). *Deep medicine: How artificial intelligence can make healthcare human again.* Basic Books.

Tsai, S. L., Chai, S., & Chuang, K. H. (2015). The effectiveness of a chronic obstructive pulmonary disease computer game as a learning tool for nursing students. *Open Journal of Nursing*, *5*(7), 605–612. DOI: 10.4236/ojn.2015.57064

Ulupınar, F., & Toygar, Ş. A. (2020). The Use of Technology in Nursing Education and Sample Practices. *Fiscaoeconomia*, *4*(2), 524–537. DOI: 10.25295/fsecon.2020.02.013

Urakova, A., & Ibragimova, L. (2024). Virtual reality applications in nursing education: A global perspective. *Nurse Education in Practice*, *65*, 103597. DOI: 10.1016/j.nepr.2024.103597

White, J., Gunn, M., Chiarella, M., Catton, H., & Stewart, D. (2025). *Renewing the Definitions of 'nursing' and 'a nurse'.* Final project report, June 2025. International Council of Nurses.

63. World Health Organization. (2021). *World Health Organization Annual Report 2021.*

Yang, B.-H., Lo, K.-W., Li, Y.-S., & Chao, K.-Y. (2024). Effects of integration interdisciplinary learning on student learning outcomes and healthcare-giving competence: A mixed methods study. *BMC Nursing*, *23*(1), 583. DOI: 10.1186/s12912-024-02260-w

Yılmaz, M., & Kuğuoğlu, S. (2024). Hemşirelik Bilim Felsefesinde Paradigmaların Önemi. *TOGÜ Sağlık Bilimleri Dergisi, 4*(1), 108–119. DOI: 10.52369/togusagbilderg.1164824

Yüceyurt, N. K., & Şenyuva, E. A. (2023). Uluslararası ve ulusal çalışmaların hemşirelik eğitimine yansımaları. *Yükseköğretim ve Bilim Dergisi, 13*(1), 1–9.

Yüksekdağ, B. B. (2021). Covid-19 pandemisi döneminde öğrenme ve uzaktan hemşirelik eğitiminde paradigma değişimi. *Açıköğretim Uygulamaları ve Araştırmaları Dergisi, 7*(1), 61–73.

KEY TERMS AND DEFINITIONS

A Nurse: A professional who is educated in the scientific knowledge, skills and philosophy of nursing, and regulated to practice nursing based on established standards of practice and ethical codes (White et al., 2025).

Blended Learning: An instructional design approach that combines in-class and online/virtual learning opportunities by integrating personal learning with collaborative inquiry (Ateş Çobanoğlu, 2020).

Educational Technology: The ethical study and application of theory, research, and practices to advance knowledge, improve learning and performance, and empower learners through strategic design, management, implementation, and evaluation of learning experiences and environments using appropriate processes and resources (AECT, 2023).

Nursing: A profession dedicated to upholding everyone's right to enjoy the highest attainable standard of health, through a shared commitment to providing collaborative, culturally safe, people-centred care and services (White et al., 2025).

Conclusion

This volume's collective effort shows how urgent it is to promote collaborative practice, educational innovation, and mental health equity in nursing and other health professions. The book's chapters demonstrate how international collaborations, mobility, and interdisciplinarity serve as potent tools for bolstering healthcare systems, especially in locations with particular vulnerabilities like coastal and insular regions. By analyzing many contexts, from Europe and the Mediterranean to Asia and beyond, the authors draw attention to the common opportunities and problems that emerge when medical professionals work across national boundaries, cultural norms, and institutional settings.

The transformative power of professional and educational mobility is one of the volume's main themes. A number of chapters show how faculty and student exchanges improve nursing programs, promote intercultural competency, and facilitate cross-system learning. In addition to improving clinical abilities, these experiences develop a workforce that can handle global health issues with cultural humility and flexibility. The book also highlights the practical and structural obstacles that still prevent mobility, such as disparities in institutional assistance, policy inconsistencies, and budgetary limitations. Designing structures that support long-term, moral, and significant international cooperation requires an understanding of these obstacles.

Another recurring thread concerns the importance of interprofessional and interdisciplinary practice. Contributions on geriatric hip-fracture rehabilitation, patient safety education, and instructional technology in nursing demonstrate that complex health needs require coordinated expertise across disciplines. These models show how integrated care, when grounded in shared goals and evidence-based protocols, enhances patient outcomes, accelerates recovery, and strengthens the resilience of healthcare teams. The role of social capital, creativity, and mental well-being in patient care adds further depth, reminding us that health is inseparable from social and psychological determinants.

The book also emphasizes how technology and global health education are developing. Digital platforms, technology-enhanced education, and cooperative online networks offer new ways to link schools, share knowledge, and assist students in underprivileged or remote areas. These developments increase access while allowing medical professionals to continue participating in global discussions without being restricted by geography. However, they also demand critical discussion on ethical issues, quality control, and the necessity of instructional frameworks that uphold academic rigor.

Crucially, the chapters collectively illustrate how nursing plays a pivotal role in global health promotion, health literacy, and community empowerment. Whether addressing climate-related mental health disparities in island communities, promoting safe clinical environments, or integrating culturally sensitive approaches to violence prevention, nurses emerge as key agents of equity and social transformation. Their ability to bridge clinical, educational, and community settings positions them as vital contributors to both local health systems and international public health initiatives.

In summary, this book affirms that advancing mental health equity and healthcare quality requires a multidimensional, collaborative, and globally attuned approach. The insights provided by the authors demonstrate that meaningful progress arises not from isolated efforts, but from sustained partnerships, reflective practice, and an unwavering commitment to evidence-based, culturally informed care. As global health challenges continue to evolve, the lessons synthesized in this volume provide a foundation for shaping future policies, educational strategies, and research agendas that prioritize human well-being, interconnectivity, and collective responsibility.

Konstantinos Giakoumidakis

Department of Nursing, Hellenic Mediterranean University, Greece

Compilation of References

Abdul-Rahaman, N., Arkorful, V. E., & Okereke, T. (2022). Academic integration in higher education: A review of effective institutional strategies and personal factors [Review of *Academic integration in higher education: A review of effective institutional strategies and personal factors*]. *Frontiers in Education, 7*. Frontiers Media. DOI: 10.3389/feduc.2022.856967

Açıkgöz, G., & Baykal, U. (2023). Yasal düzenlemeler çerçevesinde hemşirelerin mesleki rolleri ve özerklik. *Istanbul Kent University Journal of Health Sciences, 2*(1), 29–34.

Acton, C., Farus-Brown, S., Alexander, C., Morrow, L., Ossege, J., & Tovar, E. (2017). Quality and Safety Education for Nurses competencies in Doctor of Nursing Practice education: Exemplars from education and practice. *Nurse Educator, 42*(5S Suppl 1), S44–S48. https://doi.org/.DOI: 10.1097/NNE.0000000000000426

Adhikari, R., & Smith, P. (2023). Global nursing workforce challenges: Time for a paradigm shift. *Nurse Education in Practice, 69*, 103627. DOI: 10.1016/j.nepr.2023.103627 PMID: 37018998

AECT. (2023). AECT Definition for Educational Technology. https://www.aect.org/aect/about/aect-definition

Akince, E. K., Özkütük, N., & Orgun, F. (2022). Hemşirelik eğitimini etkileyen paradigmalar. *Akdeniz Hemşirelik Dergisi, 1*(1), 29–35.

Albornos-Muñoz, L., Blanco-Blanco, J., Cidoncha-Moreno, M. Á., Abad-Corpa, E., Rivera-Álvarez, A., López-Pisa, R. M., Caperos, J. M., Baz, M. P. R., Moneo, A. B., González, L. P., Skelton, D. A., Todd, C., Townley, R., Hidalgo, P. L. P., Blasco, O. C., Agusti, M. C. S., Rich-Ruiz, M., Pisano, A. C. G., Xamena, J. M., & Moreno-Casbas, M. T. (2024). Efficacy of the Otago-Exercise-Programme to reduce falls in community-dwelling adults aged 65-80 when delivered as group or individual training: Non-inferiority-clinical-trial. *BMC Nursing*, *23*(1), 705. DOI: 10.1186/s12912-024-02310-3 PMID: 39354514

Albrecht, G., Askland, H. H., & Head, L. (2021). Solastalgia: Living with environmental change. In Head, L. (Ed.), *Refugia: Radical adaptation in a time of ecological crisis* (pp. 65–82). Routledge., DOI: 10.4324/9781003121425

Ali, S. (2020). The impact of digital tools on learning outcomes: A systematic review. *Computers & Education*, *148*, 103788.

Allen, J., Black, N., Clarke, A., & Dixon-Woods, M. (2023). What is system resilience? *BMJ (Clinical Research Ed.)*, *382*, e073696. DOI: 10.1136/bmj-2022-073696 PMID: 37402509

Allum, N., Gaskell, G., Stares, S., Esmer, Y., Castro, P., Fischler, C., Jackson, J., Kronberger, N., Mejlgaard, N., Torgersen, H., Wager, W., & Quintanilha, A. (2010). Science knowledge and attitudes across cultures: A meta-analysis. *Public Understanding of Science (Bristol, England)*, *19*(1), 1–23. DOI: 10.1177/0963662506070159

Amabile, T. (1982). Social psychology of creativity: A consensual assessment technique. *Journal of Personality and Social Psychology*, *43*(5), 997–1013. DOI: 10.1037/0022-3514.43.5.997

Amabile, T. (1983). *The social psychology of creativity*. SpringerVerlag. DOI: 10.1007/978-1-4612-5533-8

American Association of College of Nursing. (2006). Hallmarks of quality and patient safety: Recommended baccalaureate competencies and curricular guidelines to ensure high-quality and safe patient care. *Journal of Professional Nursing*, *22*(6), 329–330. DOI: 10.1016/j.profnurs.2006.10.005 PMID: 17141715

AMSTAR. (2025, July). AMSTAR checklist. [from: https://amstar.ca/Amstar_Checklist.php]. *Access*, *28*, •••.

Andreasen, C., Dahl, C., Frihagen, F., Borgen, T. T., Basso, T., Gjertsen, J.-E., Figved, W., Wisløff, T., Hagen, G., Apalset, E. M., Stutzer, J. M., Lund, I., Hansen, A. K., Nissen, F. I., Joakimsen, R. M., Syversen, U., Eriksen, E. F., Nordsletten, L., Omsland, T. K., & Solberg, L. B. (2025). Fracture liaison service (FLS) is associated with lower subsequent fragility fracture risk and mortality: NoFRACT (the Norwegian capture the fracture initiative) [Preprint]. *Osteoporosis International, 36*(3), 501–512. Advance online publication. DOI: 10.1007/s00198-024-07376-y PMID: 39808195

Appel, H. B., Martínez-Fernández, M. C., & Fernández-Martínez, E. (2023). Implementation of COIL in mental health education: Outcomes of a collaboration between Spain and the United States nursing students. *Journal of Virtual Exchange, 65*, 65–82. Advance online publication. DOI: 10.21827/jve.6.39836

Argyriadi, A., Katsarou, D., Patelarou, A., Megari, K., Patelarou, E., Kotrotsiou, S., Giakoumidakis, K., Abdoola, S., Mantsos, E., Efthymiou, E., & Argyriadis, A. (2025). Digital Stress Scale (DSC): Development and Psychometric Validation of a Measure of Stress in the Digital Age. *International Journal of Environmental Research and Public Health, 22*(7), 1080. DOI: 10.3390/ijerph22071080 PMID: 40724147

Arkley, J., Dixon, J., Wilson, F., Charlton, K., Ollivere, B. J., & Eardley, W. (2019). Assessment of Nutrition and Supplementation in Patients With Hip Fractures. *Geriatric Orthopaedic Surgery & Rehabilitation, 10*, 2151459319879804. Advance online publication. DOI: 10.1177/2151459319879804 PMID: 31667002

Armstrong, G., & Barton, A. (2013). Fundamentally updating fundamentals: A cross-sectional study. *Journal of Professional Nursing, 29*(2), 82–87. DOI: 10.1016/j.profnurs.2012.12.006 PMID: 23566453

Aşiroğlu, S., Nuhoğlu, H., & Sarkın, D. (2022). Planlamadan değerlendirmeye harmanlanmış öğrenme. *Tarih Okulu Dergisi, 15*(57), 1468–1508.

ASPHP. (2023). Safe Patient Handling and Mobility (SPHM) Education in Health Care Student Curriculum: A White Paper. [Internet]. The Association of Safe Patient Handling Professionals Access 1. october 2025,from www.ASPHP.org

Assouline, B.. (2021). Preoperative exercise training to prevent postoperative pulmonary complications in adults undergoing major surgery: A systematic review and meta-analysis with trial sequential analysis. In *Annals of the American Thoracic Society* (pp. 678–688). American Thoracic Society., DOI: 10.1513/AnnalsATS.202002-183OC

Ateş Çobanoğlu, A. (2020). From Ubiquitous to Ubiquitous Blended Learning Environments. In *Managing and Designing Online Courses in Ubiquitous Learning Environments* (pp. 215–232). IGI Global., DOI: 10.4018/978-1-5225-9779-7.ch011

Attree, M., Cooke, H., & Wakefield, A. (2008). Patient safety in an English pre-registration nursing curriculum. *Nurse Education in Practice*, *8*(4), 239–248. DOI: 10.1016/j.nepr.2007.09.003 PMID: 17945535

Australian Commission on Safety and Quality in Health Care. (2005). *National patient safety education framework*. Commonwealth of Australia. https://www.safetyandquality.gov.au/sites/default/files/migrated/framework0705.pdf

Aydemir, Ö., & Öztekin, S. D. (2024). CUMHURİYET DÖNEMİ VE CERRAHİ HEMŞİRELİĞİ. *Beykent Üniversitesi Sosyal Bilimler Dergisi, 17*(Özel Sayı), 113-119.

Aygin, E., & Çelik Yılmaz, D. (2022). The role of e-learning in nursing education: Opportunities and challenges. *Nurse Education Today*, *113*, 105395. DOI: 10.1016/j.nedt.2022.105395

Bacca, J., Baldiris, S., Fabregat, R., Graf, S., & Kinshuk. (2014). Augmented reality trends in education: A systematic review of research and applications. *Educational Technology & Society, 17*(4), 133–149. https://www.jstor.org/stable/jeductechsoci.17.4.133

Backes, M., Dingemans, S. A., Schep, N. W. L., Bloemers, F. W., Van Dijkman, B., Garssen, F. P., Haverlag, R., Hoogendoorn, J. M., Joosse, P., Mirck, B., Postma, V., Ritchie, E., Roerdink, W. H., Sintenie, J. B., Soesman, N. M. R., Sosef, N. L., Twigt, B. A., Van Veen, R. N., Van der Veen, A. H., & Schepers, T. (2015). Wound infections following implant removal below the knee: The effect of antibiotic prophylaxis; the WIFI-trial, a multi-centre randomized controlled trial. *BMC Surgery*, *15*(1), 1–6. DOI: 10.1186/1471-2482-15-12 PMID: 25972101

Baek, H., Han, K., Cho, H., & Ju, J. (2023). Nursing teamwork is essential in promoting patient-centered care: A cross-sectional study. *BMC Nursing*, *22*(1), 433. Advance online publication. DOI: 10.1186/s12912-023-01592-3 PMID: 37978376

Baer, J.Jr. (1988). Long-term effects of creativity training with middle school students. *The Journal of Early Adolescence*, *8*(8), 183–193. DOI: 10.1177/0272431688082006

Bakanoğlu Kalkavan, F., & Çoban, A. Y. (2025). Teknoloji entegrasyonunda öğretim elemanı yeterlilikleri. *Hemsirelikte Egitim ve Arastirma Dergisi*, *20*(1), 45–54.

Bandura, A. (2009). Social cognitive theory of mass communication. *Media Psychology*, *3*(3), 265–299. DOI: 10.1207/S1532785XMEP0303_03

Bani, M., Zorzi, F., Russo, S., Del Greco, A., Ardenghi, S., Rampoldi, G., Putoto, G., Invernizzi, P., & Strepparava, M. G. (2025). International Mobility Experiences Among Italian Students: A Cross-Sectional Survey Comparing Motivations Towards High- Versus Low-Income Countries. *BMJ Open, 15*(7), E093935. Https://Doi.Org/10.1136/Bmjopen-2024-093935. DOI: 10.1136/bmjopen-2024-093935 PMID: 40744513

Barnsteiner, J., Disch, J., Johnson, J., McGuinn, K., Chappel, K., & Swartwout, E. (2013). Diffusing QSEN competencies across schools of nursing: The AACN/RWJF faculty development institutes. *Journal of Professional Nursing, 29*(2), 68–74. DOI: 10.1016/j.profnurs.2012.12.003 PMID: 23566451

Barry, M. M., Battel-Kirk, B., & Dempsey, C. (2012). The CompHP Core Competencies for Health Promotion in Europe: Developing the workforce for effective public health and cross-border health promotion (nursing workforce implications). *Health Education Research, 27*(1), 149–160. DOI: 10.1093/her/cyr077

Bartoníčková, D., Kohanová, D., & Žiaková, K. (2023). Vzdelávacie rámce a oblasti kompetencií študentov ošetrovateľstva súvisiace s bezpečnosťou pacientov: Integratívny prehľad. *Health and Caring, 2*(2). Advance online publication. DOI: 10.46585/hc.2023.2.2441

Baumann, I., Wieber, F., Volken, T., Rüesch, P., & Glässel, A. (2022). Interprofessional Collaboration in Fall Prevention: Insights from a Qualitative Study. *International Journal of Environmental Research and Public Health, 19*(17), 10477. Advance online publication. DOI: 10.3390/ijerph191710477 PMID: 36078195

Baum, F., Freeman, T., & Lawless, A. (2022). Why critical public health matters for health equity. *Social Science & Medicine, 307*, 115188. DOI: 10.1016/j.socscimed.2022.115188

Bayram, S. B., & Caliskan, N. (2019). Effect of a game-based virtual reality phone application on tracheostomy care education for nursing students: A randomized controlled trial. *Nurse Education Today, 79*, 25–31. DOI: 10.1016/j.nedt.2019.05.010

Bays, J. C., & Hermann, C. P. (1997). The effectiveness of using a game to reinforce learning in nursing education: A case study. *Nurse Educator, 22*(4), 14–17.

Beck, K. (2023). Local people's perceptions of international clinical placements in low- and middle-income countries: A literature review [Review of *Local people's perceptions of international clinical placements in low- and middle-income countries: A literature review*]. *International Journal of Nursing Studies Advances, 5*, 100165. Elsevier BV. DOI: 10.1016/j.ijnsa.2023.100165

Bedgood, A. L., & Mellott, S. (2021). The role of education in developing a culture of safety through the perceptions of undergraduate nursing students: An integrative literature review. *Journal of Patient Safety, 17*(8), e1530–e1536. DOI: 10.1097/PTS.0000000000000548 PMID: 30383621

Berg, E., & Lepp, M. (2023). The meaning and application of student-centered learning in nursing education: An integrative review of the literature. *Nurse Education in Practice, 69*, 103622. DOI: 10.1016/j.nepr.2023.103622

Bergs, J., Peeters, K., Kortleven, I., Creemers, S., Ulenaers, D., Desmedt, M., & Schrooten, W. (2021). Translation and validation of the Dutch version of the Health Professional Education in Patient Safety Survey amongst nursing students in Belgium: A psychometric analysis. *PLoS One, 16*(3), e0247869. DOI: 10.1371/journal.pone.0247869 PMID: 33657156

Bilik, O., Damar, H. T., & Karayurt, O. (2017). Fall behaviors and risk factors among elderly patients with hip fractures. *Acta Paulista de Enfermagem, 30*(4), 420–427. DOI: 10.1590/1982-0194201700062

Billis, E., Strimpakos, N., Kapreli, E., Sakellari, V., Skelton, D. A., Dontas, I., Ioannou, F., Filon, G., & Gioftsos, G. (2011). Cross-cultural validation of the Falls Efficacy Scale International (FES-I) in Greek community-dwelling older adults. *Disability and Rehabilitation, 33*(19–20), 1776–1784. DOI: 10.3109/09638288.2010.546937 PMID: 21219254

Bjørnnes, A. K., Skaufel, H., Holmström Rising, M., Gädda, M., Nieminen, A.-L., Misvær, N., Bender Monggaard, M.-L., Greve Sørensen, K., Alondere, L., Butkuviene, A., & Torbjørnsen, A. (2024). Short-Term Student Exchange In Nursing Education: A Descriptive Pilot Study. *SAGE Open, 14*(4), 21582440241299522. Https://Doi.Org/10.1177/21582440241299522. DOI: 10.1177/21582440241299522

Bjørnnes, A. K., Torbjørnsen, A., Thordardottir, B. S. A., Lund, A., Hovland, O. J., & Skarpaas, L. S. (2025). Exploring intentions: Factors influencing international study decisions in healthcare bachelor's degree programs. *BMC Medical Education, 25*(1), 555. DOI: 10.1186/s12909-025-07136-4 PMID: 40247245

Boada, J., Baldiris, S., Fabregat, R., & Graf, S. (2015). Mobile augmented reality in vocational education and training. *Procedia Computer Science, 75*, 49–58. DOI: 10.1016/j.procs.2015.12.203

Boctor, L. (2013). Active-learning strategies: The use of a game to reinforce learning in nursing education. *Nurse Educator, 38*(2), 96–100.

Bohannon, R. W., & Wang, Y. C. (2019). Four-Meter Gait Speed: Normative Values and Reliability Determined for Adults Participating in the NIH Toolbox Study. *Archives of Physical Medicine and Rehabilitation*, *100*(3), 509–513. DOI: 10.1016/j.apmr.2018.06.031 PMID: 30092204

Borgström, F., Karlsson, L., Ortsäter, G., Norton, N., Halbout, P., Cooper, C., Lorentzon, M., McCloskey, E. V., Harvey, N. C., Javaid, M. K., & Kanis, J. A. (2020). Fragility fractures in Europe: Burden, management and opportunities. *Archives of Osteoporosis*, *15*(1), 59. Advance online publication. DOI: 10.1007/s11657-020-0706-y PMID: 32306163

Borrelli, S., Walker, L., Coolin, K., Fumagalli, S., Karema, A., Konstantinidis, S., Mets-Oja, S., Nespoli, A., Smit, A.-M., Van Oost, M., & Spiby, H. (2022). Midwifery Students' Perspectives Of Physical And Virtual Mobility Activities Including Preferences For E-Learning: A Cross-Sectional Survey. *Nurse Education Today*, *109*, 105214. Https://Doi.Org/10.1016/J.Nedt.2021.105214. DOI: 10.1016/j.nedt.2021.105214 PMID: 34799193

Borromeo, A. S., Manaloto, A. M., Delos Santos, M. J. M., Antonio, R. P., Soyosa, M. D., & Wider, W. (2024). Harnessing generative AI in nursing education: A bibliometric review. *Teaching and Learning in Nursing*, *2025*. Advance online publication. DOI: 10.1016/j.teln.2025.04.014

Boucaut, R., & Cusack, L. (2016). 'Sometimes your safety goes a bit by the wayside' … exploring occupational health and safety (OHS) with student nurses. *Nurse Education in Practice*, *20*, 93–98. DOI: 10.1016/j.nepr.2016.07.005 PMID: 27525567

Bourdieu, P. (1984). *Distinction: A Social Critique of the Judgment of Taste*. Harvard University Press.

Bourdieu, P. (1986). The Forms of Capital. In Richardson, J. G. (Ed.), *Handbook of Theory and Research for the Sociology of Education* (pp. 241–258). Greenwood Press.

Bourdieu, P., & Wacquant, L. (1992). *An Invitation to Reflexive Sociology*. University of Chicago Press.

Branch, R. M. (2009). *Instructional design: The ADDIE approach*. Springer Science & Business Media. DOI: 10.1007/978-0-387-09506-6

Bressan, V., Stevanin, S., Bulfone, G., Zanini, A., Dante, A., & Palese, A. (2016). Measuring patient safety knowledge and competences as perceived by nursing students: An Italian validation study. *Nurse Education in Practice*, *16*(1), 209–216. DOI: 10.1016/j.nepr.2015.08.006 PMID: 26344616

Brito, E., Neves, M. P. C. C. D., Gomes, N., & Lopes, N. (2025). Inclusion and Internationalization: Perception of Higher Education Students. *Interchange*, *56*(3-4), 259–283. Advance online publication. DOI: 10.1007/s10780-025-09544-3

Browne, C. A., Fetherston, C. M., & Medigovich, K. (2015). International clinical placements for Australian undergraduate nursing students: A systematic thematic synthesis of the literature. *Nurse Education Today*, *35*(10), 1028–1036. DOI: 10.1016/j.nedt.2015.05.012 PMID: 26059923

Brown, M., Boateng, E. A., & Evans, C. (2016). Should I stay or should I go? A systematic review of factors that influence healthcare students' decisions around study abroad programmes. *Nurse Education Today*, *39*, 63–71. DOI: 10.1016/j.nedt.2015.12.024 PMID: 27006034

Buckner, E. B., Anderson, D. J., Garzon, N., Hafsteinsdóttir, T. B., Lai, C. K. Y., & Roshan, R. (2014). Perspectives on global nursing leadership: International experiences from the field. *International Nursing Review*, *61*(4), 463–471. DOI: 10.1111/inr.12139 PMID: 25411072

Burke, S. E. L., Sanson, A. V., & Van Hoorn, J. (2018). The psychological effects of climate change on children. *Current Psychiatry Reports*, *20*(5), 35. DOI: 10.1007/s11920-018-0896-9 PMID: 29637319

Button, L., Green, B., Tengnah, C., Johansson, I., & Baker, C. (2005). The impact of international placements on nurses' personal and professional lives: Literature review. *Journal of Advanced Nursing*, *50*(3), 315–324. DOI: 10.1111/j.1365-2648.2005.03395.x PMID: 15811111

Çalışkan, D., & Cayır, E. (2025). Simülasyon ve sanal gerçekliğin hemşirelik öğrencilerinin klinik yeterliliklerine etkisi. *Journal of Nursing Education and Practice*, *15*(3), 78–88. DOI: 10.5430/jnep.v15n3p78

Calvani, R. *et al.* (2015) "Biomarkers for physical frailty and sarcopenia: State of the science and future developments," *Journal of Cachexia, Sarcopenia and Muscle*. Wiley Blackwell, pp. 278–286. Available at: https://doi.org/.DOI: 10.1002/jcsm.12051

Campbell, B., & Mackay, G. (2001). Continuing competence: An Ontario nursing regulatory program that supports nurses and employers. *Nursing Administration Quarterly*, *25*(2), 22–30. DOI: 10.1097/00006216-200101000-00006 PMID: 18188891

Canadian Patient Safety Institute. (2016). *Report on the integration of the safety competencies framework into health professions education programs in Canada.* Canadian Patient Safety Institute. https://www.patientsafetyinstitute.ca/en/toolsResources/IntegrationofSafetyCompetenciesFramework/Documents/Report%20on%20the%20Integration%20of%20the%20Safety%20Competencies%20Framework.pdf

Canadian Patient Safety Institute. (2020). *The safety competencies: Enhancing patient safety across the health professions* (2nd ed.). Canadian Patient Safety Institute. https://www.patientsafetyinstitute.ca/en/toolsResources/safetyCompetencies/Documents/CPSI-SafetyCompetencies_EN_Digital.pdf

Cant, R., & Cooper, S. (2020). Simulation in nursing education: A systematic review. *The Journal of Nursing Education, 59*(1), 1–9. DOI: 10.3928/01484834-20191223-03

Carayon, P., Kleinschmidt, P., Hose, B.-Z., & Salwei, M. (2020). Human factors and ergonomics in health care and patient safety from the perspective of medical residents. In *Textbook of Patient Safety and Clinical Risk Management* [Internet]. Springer. Published online: December 15, 2020. Access 1. october 2025, from https://www.ncbi.nlm.nih.gov/books/NBK585616/

Carruthers, S., Lawton, R., Sandars, J., Howe, A., & Perry, M. (2009). Attitudes to patient safety amongst medical students and tutors: Developing a reliable scale. *Medical Teacher, 31*(8), e370–e376. DOI: 10.1080/01421590802650142 PMID: 19811201

Carvalho, J., Backes, D., Lomba, M., & Colomé, J. (2016). International Academic Mobility: An Education Opportunity For Future Nurses. *Revista De Enfermagem Referência, Iv Série*(10), 59–68. Https://Doi.Org/10.12707/Riv16018

Cavalcante, I. M. da S., Guedes, G. F., & Püschel, V. A. de A. (2018). Nursing international student mobility in the University of São Paulo. *Revista Brasileira de Enfermagem, 71*(suppl 4), 1619–1625. DOI: 10.1590/0034-7167-2017-0754 PMID: 30088632

CDC. (2019). Available at URL: https://www.cdc.gov/falls/prevention/index.html

Cervera-Gasch, Á., González-Chordá, V. M., Manrique-Abril, F. G., Andreu-Pejo, L., Valero-Chillerón, M. J., & Mena-Tudela, D. (2021). Validation of the attitudes to patient safety questionnaire for nursing students in the Spanish context. *BMC Nursing, 20*(1), 101. DOI: 10.1186/s12912-021-00634-y PMID: 34144691

Chatzea, V. E., Mechili, E. A., Melidoniotis, E., Petrougaki, E., Nikiforidis, G., Argyriadis, A., & Sifaki-Pistolla, D. (2022). Recommendations for young researchers on how to better advance their scientific career: A systematic review. *Population Medicine, 4*(September), 1–17. DOI: 10.18332/popmed/152571

Chen, L., Huang, F., Yuan, X., Song, J., & Chen, L. (2019). An assessment of the reliability and factorial validity of the Chinese version of the Health Professional Education in Patient Safety Survey (H-PEPSS). *Frontiers in Psychology, 10*, 2183. DOI: 10.3389/fpsyg.2019.02183 PMID: 31607997

Chenot, T. M., & Daniel, L. G. (2010). Frameworks for patient safety in the nursing curriculum. *The Journal of Nursing Education, 49*(10), 559–568. DOI: 10.3928/01484834-20100730-02 PMID: 20669876

Çiftcioğlu, Ş., Apaydın Cırık, V., & Efe, E. (2022). Student nurses' perceptions of a patient safety culture: A descriptive and cross-sectional study. *Perspectives in Psychiatric Care, 58*(2), 658–663. DOI: 10.1111/ppc.12830 PMID: 33931872

Clarke, D., & Kent, B. (2023). Artificial intelligence in nursing education: Opportunities and challenges. *Nurse Education Today, 125*, 105617. DOI: 10.1016/j.nedt.2023.105617

Clayton, S. (2020). Climate anxiety: Psychological responses to climate change. *Journal of Anxiety Disorders, 74*, 102263. DOI: 10.1016/j.janxdis.2020.102263 PMID: 32623280

Coffey, Y., Bhullar, N., Durkin, J., Islam, M. S., & Usher, K. (2021). Understanding eco-anxiety: A systematic scoping review of current literature and identified knowledge gaps. *The Journal of Climate Change and Health, 3*, 100047. DOI: 10.1016/j.joclim.2021.100047

Coleman, J. S. (1988). Social Capital in the Creation of Human Capital. *American Journal of Sociology, 94*(Supplement), S95–S120. DOI: 10.1086/228943

Comtesse, H., Ertl, V., Hengst, S. M. C., Rosner, R., & Smid, G. E. (2021). Ecological grief as a response to environmental change: A mental health risk or functional response? *International Journal of Environmental Research and Public Health, 18*(2), 734. DOI: 10.3390/ijerph18020734 PMID: 33467018

Conley, R. B., Adib, G., Adler, R. A., Åkesson, K. E., Alexander, I. M., Amenta, K. C., Blank, R. D., Brox, W. T., Carmody, E. E., Chapman-Novakofski, K., Clarke, B. L., Cody, K. M., Cooper, C., Crandall, C. J., Dirschl, D. R., Eagen, T. J., Elderkin, A. L., Fujita, M., Greenspan, S. L., & Kiel, D. P. (2020). Secondary Fracture Prevention: Consensus Clinical Recommendations from a Multistakeholder Coalition. *Journal of Bone and Mineral Research : the Official Journal of the American Society for Bone and Mineral Research, 35*(1), 36–52. DOI: 10.1002/jbmr.3877 PMID: 31538675

Çonoğlu, G., Özkütük, N., & Orgun, F. (2020). Hemşirelik eğitiminde yenilikçi eğitim paradigması: Öğretim teknolojileriyle duyuşsal alanı harekete geçirmek. *Ege Universitesi Hemsirelik Fakultesi Dergisi, 36*(1), 61–65.

Cook, P. (1998). *Best practice creativity*. Gower Publishing Limited.

Cronenwett, L., Sherwood, G., Barnsteiner, J., Disch, J., Johnson, J., Mitchell, P., Sullivan, D. T., & Warren, J. (2007). Quality and safety education for nurses. *Nursing Outlook, 55*(3), 122–131. DOI: 10.1016/j.outlook.2007.02.006 PMID: 17524799

Cronenwett, L., Sherwood, G., Pohl, J., Barnsteiner, J., Moore, S., Sullivan, D. T., Ward, D., & Warren, J. (2009). Quality and safety education for advanced nursing practice. *Nursing Outlook, 57*(6), 338–348. DOI: 10.1016/j.outlook.2009.07.009 PMID: 19942035

Csikszentmihalyi, M. (1988). Society, culture, and person: A systems view of creativity. In Sternberg, R. J. (Ed.), *The nature of creativity* (pp. 325–339). Cambridge University Press.

Csikszentmihalyi, M. (1996). *Creativity: Flow and the psychology of discovery and invention*. HarperCollins.

Cunningham, S. (2020). Challenges of outward facing mobility opportunities for nursing students: Pre and periCOVID19. *European Journal of Open & Distance Learning, 1*(1), 89–94. DOI: 10.17932/EJOH.2020.022/ejoh_v01i1008

Cunsolo, A., & Ellis, N. R. (2018). Ecological grief as a mental health response to climate change-related loss. *Nature Climate Change, 8*(4), 275–281. DOI: 10.1038/s41558-018-0092-2

Cunsolo, A., Harper, S. L., Minor, K., Hayes, K., Williams, K. G., & Howard, C. (2020). Ecological grief and anxiety: The start of a healthy response to climate change? *The Lancet. Planetary Health, 4*(7), e261–e263. DOI: 10.1016/S2542-5196(20)30144-3 PMID: 32681892

Dadgari, A., Hamid, T. A., Hakim, M. N., Chaman, R., Mousavi, S. A., Hin, L. P., & Dadvar, L. (2016). Randomized control trials on Otago Exercise Program (OEP) to reduce falls among elderly community dwellers in Shahroud, Iran. *Iranian Red Crescent Medical Journal, 18*(5). Advance online publication. DOI: 10.5812/ircmj.26340 PMID: 27478629

Damián, J., Pastor-Barriuso, R., Valderrama-Gama, E., & de Pedro-Cuesta, J. (2013). Factors associated with falls among older adults living in institutions. *BMC Geriatrics, 13*(1), 6. DOI: 10.1186/1471-2318-13-6 PMID: 23320746

Daniel, S., & Butson, R. (2023). Personalised learning pathways using artificial intelligence: Implications for healthcare education. *Medical Teacher, 45*(6), 567–574. DOI: 10.1080/0142159X.2022.2149832

Dauchess, A. (2025, January 24). The role of technology in modern nursing education. Marymount University. https://marymount.edu/blog/the-role-of-technology-in-modern-nursing-education/

Davies, J. M., Hebert, P., & Hoffman, A. (2003). *The Canadian patient safety dictionary.* The Royal College of Physicians and Surgeons of Canada.

Davis, J. C., Khan, K. M., Hsu, C. L., Chan, P., Cook, W. L., Dian, L., & Liu-Ambrose, T. (2020). Action Seniors! Cost-Effectiveness Analysis of a Secondary Falls Prevention Strategy Among Community-Dwelling Older Fallers. *Journal of the American Geriatrics Society, 68*(9), 1988–1997. DOI: 10.1111/jgs.16476 PMID: 32472567

De Miguel, M. S., de Elguea, J. O., Gómez-Gastiasoro, A., Urcola, F., Cid-Expósito, M. G., Torres-Enamorado, D., & Orkaizagirre-Gomara, A. (2023). Patient safety and its relationship with specific self-efficacy, competence, and resilience among nursing students: A quantitative study. *Nurse Education Today, 121*, 105701. DOI: 10.1016/j.nedt.2022.105701 PMID: 36563588

de Sire, A., Invernizzi, M., Baricich, A., Lippi, L., Ammendolia, A., Grassi, F. A., & Leigheb, M. (2021). Optimization of transdisciplinary management of elderly with femur proximal extremity fracture: A patient-tailored plan from orthopaedics to rehabilitation. *World Journal of Orthopedics, 12*(7), 456–466. DOI: 10.5312/wjo.v12.i7.456 PMID: 34354934

De Wit, H. (2019). Internationalization in higher education, a critical review. *SFU Educational Review, 12*(3), 9–17. DOI: 10.21810/sfuer.v12i3.1036

Dias, G. P., Barbosa, B., Santos, C. A., Pinheiro, M. M., Simões, D., & Filipe, S. (2020). Between promises and pitfalls: The impact of mobility on the internationalization of higher education. *Journal of Further and Higher Education, 45*(1), 79–94. DOI: 10.1080/0309877X.2020.1735321

Dikmen, Y., Gündoğdu, H., Tanrıkulu, F., Ziyai, N. Y., & Altınkaynak, S. (2019). Eğitim Programlarının Uygulanmasında Öğrenci Merkezli Aktif Öğrenme Yöntemlerinin Kullanılması. Değerli Sağlık Bilimleri Ailesi Üyeleri, 163.

Diong, J., Allen, N. and Sherrington, C. (2016) "Structured exercise improves mobility after hip fracture: A meta-analysis with meta-regression," *British Journal of Sports Medicine*. BMJ Publishing Group, pp. 346–355. Available at: https://doi.org/.DOI: 10.1136/bjsports-2014-094465

Dispenza, J. (2012). *Breaking the habit of being yourself: How to lose your mind and create a new one*. Hay House, Inc.

Dispenza, J. (2017). *Becoming supernatural: How common people are doing the uncommon*. Hay House, Inc.

Dobrowolska, B., Mcgonagle, I., Jackson, C., Kane, R., Cabrera, E., Cooney-Miner, D., Di Cara, V., Pajnkihar, M., Prlić, N., Sigurdardottir, A. K., Kekuš, D., Wells, J., & Palese, A. (2015). Clinical Practice Models In Nursing Education: Implication For Students' Mobility. *International Nursing Review, 62*(1), 36–46. Https://Doi.Org/10.1111/Inr.12162. DOI: 10.1111/inr.12162 PMID: 25559068

Dohrn, J., Desjardins, K., Honig, J., Hahn-Schroeder, H., Ferng, Y., & Larson, E. (2018). Transforming nursing curricula for a global community. *Journal of Professional Nursing, 34*(6), 449–453. DOI: 10.1016/j.profnurs.2018.02.001 PMID: 30527692

Dovrat, L. (2023). *Virtual exchanges in Israel: Faculty experiences of implementing a transformative pedagogy. 3*(2). DOI: 10.21428/8c225f6e.4530bc4d

Dreinhofer, K. E., Mitchell, P. J., Bégué, T., Cooper, C., Costa, M. L., Falaschi, P., Hertz, K., Marsh, D., Maggi, S., Nana, A., Palm, H., Speerin, R., & Magaziner, J. (2018). A global call to action to improve the care of people with fragility fractures. *Injury, 49*(8), 1393–1397. DOI: 10.1016/j.injury.2018.06.032 PMID: 29983172

Dubavaya, A., & Tenaglia, H. (2025). Philosophy of Nursing. https://student.wp.odu.edu/aduba001/wp-content/uploads/sites/39221/2025/07/Philosophy-of-Nursing_Alena-Dubavaya.pdf

Du, L., Zhao, L., Xu, T., Wang, Y., Zu, W., Huang, X., Nie, W., & Wang, L. (2022). Blended learning vs traditional teaching: The potential of a novel teaching strategy in nursing education - a systematic review and meta-analysis. *Nurse Education in Practice, 63*, 103354. DOI: 10.1016/j.nepr.2022.103354

Eamer, G., Taheri, A., Chen, S. S., Daviduck, Q., Chambers, T., Shi, X., & Khadaroo, R. G. (2018). Comprehensive geriatric assessment for older people admitted to a surgical service. *Cochrane Database of Systematic Reviews*, 1.

Edwards, R., Patrician, P. A., Bakitas, M., & Markaki, A. (2021). Palliative care integration: a critical review of nurse migration effect in Jamaica [Review of *Palliative care integration: a critical review of nurse migration effect in Jamaica*]. *BMC Palliative Care, 20*(1). BioMed Central. DOI: 10.1186/s12904-021-00863-7

Efendi, F., Haryanto, J., Indarwati, R., Kuswanto, H., Ulfiana, E., Has, E. M. M., & Chong, M. C. (2021). Going Global: Insights of Indonesian Policymakers on International Migration of Nurses. *Journal of Multidisciplinary Healthcare, 3285*, 3285–3293. Advance online publication. DOI: 10.2147/JMDH.S327962 PMID: 34858031

Ellis G, *et al.* (2017). Comprehensive geriatric assessment for older adults admitted to hospital. *Cochrane Database Syst Rev*. Sep 12;9:CD006211.

Elo, S., & Kyngäs, H. (2008). The qualitative content analysis process. *Journal of Advanced Nursing, 62*(1), 107–115. DOI: 10.1111/j.1365-2648.2007.04569.x PMID: 18352969

Eskici, G. T., Kanig, M., Ugur, E., & Seren, A. K. H. (2021). The Turkish version of the Patient Safety Competency Self-Evaluation Tool: A validity and reliability study. *Nurse Education in Practice*, *57*, 103229. DOI: 10.1016/j.nepr.2021.103229 PMID: 34673387

Esteva, A., Topol, E., & Dean, J. (2021). A guide to deep learning in healthcare. *Nature Medicine*, *27*(5), 762–777. DOI: 10.1038/s41591-021-01313-8

European Commission. (2024). *EU4Health Programme 2024–2027: Building stronger health systems in Europe.* https://health.ec.europa.eu/funding/eu4health-programme_en

European Education and Culture Executive Agency. (2023, November 28). *Erasmus+ programme guide 2024 (Version 1).* Erasmus+. Access 21. july 2025, from: https://erasmus-plus.ec.europa.eu/sites/default/files/2023-11/2024-Erasmus%2BProgramme-Guide_EN.pdf

European Federation of Nurses Associations. (2015). *EFN guideline for the implementation of Article 31 of the Mutual Recognition of Professional Qualifications Directive 2005/36/EC, amended by Directive 2013/55/EU.* http://www.efnweb.be/wpcontent/uploads/EFNCompetencyFramework19052015

European Union Network for Patient Safety. (2010). *General guide for education and training in patient safety.* https://www.eupatient.eu/globalassets/projects/eunetpas/guidelines_final_22-06-2010.pdf

European University Association. (2024). *Trends 2024 – European higher education institutions in times of transition* [PDF]. EUA. Access 21. july 2025, from: https://www.eua.eu/images/publications/Publication_PDFs/Trends_2024.pdf

European University Foundation. (2022). *Making mobility the norm: Mobility report* (Project No. 20191DE01KA203005031) [PDF]. Evropska univerzitetna fundacija. https://uni-foundation.eu/uploads/2022_NORM_Mobility%20Report.pdf

Feng, J. N., Zhang, C., Li, B., Zhan, S., Wang, S., & Song, C. (2024). Global burden of hip fracture: The Global Burden of Disease Study. *Osteoporosis International, 35*(1), 41–52. DOI: 10.1007/s00198-023-06907-3 PMID: 37704919

Fernandez, K. R. (2020). Developing Cultural Humility During Short-Term Study Abroad Immersion. *International Journal of Studies in Nursing*, *5*(3), 48. DOI: 10.20849/ijsn.v5i3.764

Fernandez, M. A., Griffin, X. L., & Costa, M. L. (2015). Management of hip fracture. *British Medical Bulletin, 115*(1), 165–172. DOI: 10.1093/bmb/ldv036 PMID: 26311503

Ferranto, M. L. G. (2015). A qualitative study of baccalaureate nursing students following an eight-day international cultural experience in Tanzania: Cultural humility as an outcome. *Procedia: Social and Behavioral Sciences*, *174*, 91–102. DOI: 10.1016/j.sbspro.2015.01.631

Fırat Kılıç, H., & Cevheroğlu, S. (2023). Patient safety competencies of nursing students. *Nurse Education Today*, *121*, 105666. DOI: 10.1016/j.nedt.2022.105666 PMID: 36463791

Foley, M. W., & Edwards, B. (1999). Is it Time to Disinvest in Social Capital? *Journal of Public Policy*, *19*(2), 141–173. DOI: 10.1017/S0143814X99000215

Foronda, C., Liu, S., & Bauman, E. B. (2017). Development and validation of the Interprofessional Collaborative Competency Attainment Survey. *Journal of Interprofessional Care*, *31*(1), 1–8.

Francis-Coad, J., Etherton-Beer, C., Burton, E., Naseri, C., & Hill, A. M. (2018). Effectiveness of complex falls prevention interventions in residential aged care settings: A systematic review. *JBI Evidence Synthesis*, *16*(4), 973–1002. PMID: 29634516

Frank, J. R., & Brien, S. (2008). *The safety competencies: Enhancing patient safety across the health professions*. Canadian Patient Safety Institute. https://simulation.mcmaster.ca/documents/Safety_Competencies.pdf

Freiberger, E., Häberle, L., Spirduso, W. W., & Rixt Zijlstra, G. A. (2012). Long-term effects of three multicomponent exercise interventions on physical performance and fall-related psychological outcomes in community-dwelling older adults: A randomized controlled trial. *Journal of the American Geriatrics Society*, *60*(3), 437–446. DOI: 10.1111/j.1532-5415.2011.03859.x PMID: 22324753

Freitas, J. S., Sousa, M. R. G., Dolansky, M. A., & Silva, A. E. B. C. (2022). Quality and Safety Education for Nurses Student Evaluation Survey: Adaptation and Psychometric Evaluation of the Brazilian Version. *Journal of Nursing Measurement*, *30*(3), 496–507. DOI: 10.1891/JNM-D-20-00114 PMID: 34518404

Ftouh, S., Morga, A., & Swift, C. (2011). Management of hip fracture in adults: Summary of NICE guidance. *BMJ (Clinical Research Ed.)*, *342*(jun21 3), d3304. Advance online publication. DOI: 10.1136/bmj.d3304 PMID: 21693526

Galan-Lominchar, M., Roque, I. M.-S., Cazallas, C. C., Mcalpin, R., Fernández-Ayuso, D., & Ribeiro, A. S. F.GalanLominchar. (2024). Nursing students' internationalization: Virtual exchange and clinical simulation impact cultural intelligence. *Nursing Outlook*, *72*(2), 102137. DOI: 10.1016/j.outlook.2024.102137 PMID: 38340388

Garcia-Vera, M. P., Sanz, J., & Rodríguez-Testal, J. F. (2019). Psychological assessment in health contexts: A critical review. *International Journal of Clinical and Health Psychology : IJCHP*, *19*(2), 115–123.

Garner, B., Metcalfe, S. E., & Hallyburton, A. (2008). International collaboration: A concept model to engage nursing leaders and promote global nursing education partnerships. *Nurse Education in Practice*, *9*(2), 102–108. DOI: 10.1016/j.nepr.2008.10.011 PMID: 19059008

Gascón-Cánovas, J. J., Saturno-Hernandéz, P. J., Pérez-Fernandéz, P., Vincente-Lópéz, I., Conzáles-Vicente, A., Martínez-Mas, J., & Saura, M. M. (2005). *Spanish version of the Hospital Survey on Patient Safety*. Madrid: Ministerio de Sanidad y Consumo. https://www.sanidad.gob.es/en/organizacion/sns/planCalidadSNS/docs/CuestionarioSeguridadPacientes1.pdf

Gause, G., Mokgaola, I. O., & Rakhudu, M. A. (2022). Technology usage for teaching and learning in nursing education: An integrative review. *Curationis*, *45*(1), a2261. DOI: 10.4102/curationis.v45i1.2261

Gavra, D., & Bajer, Y. (2021) Creative social potential of digital society. *Administrative Consulting*. Vol. 154. No. 10. P. 54-61. . (In Russ.).DOI: 10.22394/1726-1139-2021-10-54-61

Geale, S., Beament, T., Gibson, N., Fowler, A., Baker, M., & Smith, G. (2015). International Practicum: Not just another overseas jaunt—Supporting learning objectives and the development of graduate attributes. *Journal of Nursing Education and Practice*, *5*(11). Advance online publication. DOI: 10.5430/jnep.v5n11p96

Gerdhem, P. (2013). Osteoporosis and fragility fractures. *Best Practice & Research. Clinical Rheumatology*, *27*(6), 743–755. DOI: 10.1016/j.berh.2014.01.002 PMID: 24836333

Ghimire, A., & Neupane, M. S. (2025). Navigating Global Mobility: A Comparative Study Of Nursing Education In Nepal And Australia. *International Journal of Nursing Education Scholarship*, *22*(1), 20240108. Https://Doi.Org/10.1515/Ijnes -2024-0108. DOI: 10.1515/ijnes-2024-0108 PMID: 40643086

Gibson, A. A., Hay, A. W., & Ray, D. C. (2014). Patients with hip fracture admitted to critical care: Epidemiology, interventions and outcome. *Injury*, *45*(7), 1066–1070. DOI: 10.1016/j.injury.2014.02.037 PMID: 24680801

Gibson, K. E., Barnett, J., Webber, M., & Friel, S. (2022). Environmental change and mental health: Understanding climate-related distress in the Pacific. *Nature Climate Change*, *12*(2), 146–155. DOI: 10.1038/s41558-021-01216-2

Ginsburg, L., Castel, E., Tregunno, D., & Norton, P. G. (2012). The H-PEPSS: An instrument to measure health professionals' perceptions of patient safety competence at entry into practice. *BMJ Quality & Safety*, *21*(8), 676–684. DOI: 10.1136/bmjqs-2011-000601 PMID: 22562876

Goldberg, J. I., & Burhenn, P. S. (2018). Nursing Education. *Clinical Journal of Oncology Nursing*, *22*(6), 19–25.

Greenhalgh, T., Wherton, J., Shaw, S., & Morrison, C. (2020). Video consultations for COVID-19 — Implications for cross-border telehealth and nursing health-promotion roles. *BMJ (Clinical Research Ed.)*, *368*, m998. DOI: 10.1136/bmj.m998 PMID: 32165352

Green, W., & Whitsed, C. (Eds.). (2015). *Critical perspectives on internationalising the curriculum in disciplines: Reflective narrative accounts from business, education and health* (Vol. 28). Sense/Springer., DOI: 10.1007/978-94-6300-085-7

Grinberg, K., & Nissim, S. (2025). Cultural competence among nursing students: Exploring differences across academic stages. *BMC Nursing*, *24*(1), 640. DOI: 10.1186/s12912-025-03246-y PMID: 40468297

Groos, S. S., Tan, S. M., Linn, A. J., Kuiper, J. I., van Schoor, N. M., van Weert, J. C. M., & van der Velde, N. (2025). Multidisciplinary care pathways for falls prevention in older adults: Visualizing the needs of primary care-based health care professionals. *European Geriatric Medicine*, *16*(1), 229–236. DOI: 10.1007/s41999-024-01142-3 PMID: 39789364

Guedes, G. F., Da Cavalcante, I. M. S., & Püschel, V. A. D. A. (2018). Mobilidade Estudantil Internacional: A Experiência De Estudantes De Graduação Em Enfermagem [International Academic Mobility: The Experience Of Undergraduate Nursing Students]. *Revista da Escola de Enfermagem da USP*, *52*(0), E03358. Https://Doi.Org/10.1590/S1980-220x2017039403358. DOI: 10.1590/s1980-220x2017039403358

Gülbahar, Y., Kalelioğlu, F., & Afacan Adanır, G. (2020). *Harmanlanmış öğrenme*. Pegem Akademi Yayıncılık. DOI: 10.14527/9786257880862

Güngör, D. C., Özkütük, N., & Orgun, F. (2024). Hemşirelik eğitimine değişen ve gelişen teknolojilerin yansımaları. *Sağlık Akademisyenleri Dergisi*, *10*(1), 155–161. DOI: 10.52880/sagakaderg.1120307

Guo, X., & Zhou, W. (2010). Revision of Safety Attitudes Questionnaire and evaluation. *Chinese Journal of Nursing Education*, *7*(4), 151–154. DOI: 10.3761/j.issn.1672-9234.2010.04.002

Guskuma, E. M., Dullius, A. A. D. S., La Godinho, M. S. C., Costa, M. S. T., & Terra, F. D. S. (2016). Mobilidade Acadêmica Internacional Na Formação Em Enfermagem: Relato De Experiência [International Academic Mobility In Nursing Education: An Experience Report]. *Revista Brasileira de Enfermagem*, *69*(5), 986–990. Https://Doi.Org/10.1590/0034-7167-2015-0128. DOI: 10.1590/0034-7167-2015-0128 PMID: 27783744

Harerimana, A., & Mtshali, N. G. (2020). Using exploratory and confirmatory factor analysis to understand the role of technology in nursing education. *Nurse Education Today*, *92*, 104490. DOI: 10.1016/j.nedt.2020.104490

Hayward-Livingston, A., Ozdag, Y., Kolessar, D., Weinberg, J., Pamul, A., Koury, K., & Balsamo, A. (2024). A 10-Year Experience of an Integrated Geriatric Hip Fracture Treatment Protocol: Outcomes at a Minimum 2-Year Follow-Up. *Geriatric Orthopaedic Surgery & Rehabilitation, 15*, 21514593241273155. Advance online publication. DOI: 10.1177/21514593241273155 PMID: 39130164

Head, L. (2023). Climate change and sense of place. *Progress in Human Geography, 47*(1), 3–20. DOI: 10.1177/03091325221111910

Hew, K. F., & Lo, C. K. (2018). Flipped classroom improves student learning in health professions education: A meta-analysis. *BMC Medical Education, 18*(1), 38. DOI: 10.1186/s12909-018-1144-z

Hickman, C., Marks, E., Pihkala, P., Clayton, S., Lewandowski, R. E., Mayall, E. E., Wray, B., Mellor, C., & van Susteren, L. (2021). Climate anxiety in children and young people and their beliefs about government responses to climate change: A global survey. *The Lancet. Planetary Health, 5*(12), e863–e873. DOI: 10.1016/S2542-5196(21)00278-3 PMID: 34895496

Ho, K. H. M., Cheng, H. Y., McKenna, L., & Cheung, D. S. K. (2023). Nursing and midwifery in a changing world: Addressing planetary health and digital literacy through a global curriculum. *Nursing Open, 11*(1), e2075. Advance online publication. DOI: 10.1002/nop2.2075 PMID: 38268246

Howard, J. N. (2010). The missing link: Dedicated patient safety education within top-ranked U.S. nursing school curricula. *Journal of Patient Safety, 6*(3), 165–171. DOI: 10.1097/PTS.0b013e3181eee2ab PMID: 21491791

Ilieva, J., & Tsiligiris, V. (2024). Globally Engaged and Locally Relevant—Revisiting Higher Education. In *BRILL eBooks* (p. 379). Brill., DOI: 10.1163/9789004713901_101

Im, E., & Broome, M. E. (2018). Introduction: Women's Leadership in Asian Culture. *Asian/Pacific Island Nursing Journal, 3*(2), 39–41. DOI: 10.31372/20180302.1093 PMID: 31037252

Indicators, OECD. (2023). Education at a Glance 2022. *link]. Acesso em março de.*

Institute of Medicine (U.S.) Committee on the Health Professions Education Summit. (2003). *Health professions education: A bridge to quality*. National Academies Press. https://www.ncbi.nlm.nih.gov/books/NBK221528/

Intergovernmental Panel on Climate Change. (2022). *Climate Change 2022: Impacts, adaptation and vulnerability* (WGII Sixth Assessment Report). https://www.ipcc.ch/report/ar6/wg2/

International Council of Nurses. (2022). *Position statement: Patient safety*. https://www.icn.ch/sites/default/files/inline-files/D05_Patient_Safety_0.pdf

IOF. (2021). Available at URL: https://www.osteoporosis.foundation/health-professionals/fragility-fractures/falls-prevention.

Jacob, A., Seif, S., & Munyaw, Y. (2023). Perceptions and experiences of diploma nursing students on clinical learning. A descriptive qualitative study in Tanzania. *BMC Nursing*, *22*(1), 225. DOI: 10.1186/s12912-023-01362-1 PMID: 37391811

Jansen, M. B., Lund, D. W., Baume, K., Lillyman, S., Rooney, K., & Nielsen, D. S. (2021). International clinical placement–Experiences of nursing students' cultural, personal and professional development; a qualitative study. *Nurse Education in Practice*, *51*, 102987. DOI: 10.1016/j.nepr.2021.102987 PMID: 33610023

Jeffries, P. R. (2016). The NLN Jeffries Simulation Theory. *Nursing Education Perspectives*, *37*(5), 290–294.

Jenssen, U., Bochenek, J., King, T. S., Steindal, S. A., Hestvold, I. V., & Morrison-Beedy, D. (2023). Impact of COIL: Learning From Student Nurses in Norway Who Collaborated With U.S. Students. *Journal of Transcultural Nursing*, *35*(1), 74–82. DOI: 10.1177/10436596231209043 PMID: 37933746

Johansen, F.. (2025). Exploring the potential of virtual reality in nursing education: Student perceptions and usability. *Journal of Nursing Education Technology*, *2*(1), 34–48. DOI: 10.1234/jnet.v2i1.5678

Johnsen, H. E., & Østergaard, L. (2016). Simulation-based education in health care: A systematic review. *The Journal of Continuing Education in the Health Professions*, *36*(3), 157–163.

Johnson, L., Becker, S. A., Cummins, M., & Hall, C. G. (2022). *Horizon Report: 2022 Higher Education Edition*. EDUCAUSE.

Johnston, J., McKenna, L., Malik, G., & Reisenhofer, S. (2022). Reported outcomes of nursing or midwifery students participating in international educational programs in their pre-registration education: A narrative systematic review. *Nurse Education Today*, *111*, 105320. DOI: 10.1016/j.nedt.2022.105320 PMID: 35276538

Johnston, J., McKenna, L., Malik, G., & Reisenhofer, S. (2023). Recognizing and adapting to cultural differences: Influence of international educational programs on future nursing and midwifery practice. *Journal of Transcultural Nursing*, *34*(6), 423–430. DOI: 10.1177/10436596231198276 PMID: 37740536

Jones, A. D. (2013). The impact of integrating Quality and Safety Education for Nurses' safety competency in first-year associate degree nursing students. *Teaching and Learning in Nursing*, *8*(4), 140–146. DOI: 10.1016/j.teln.2013.06.001

Jung, D., Gagné, J. C. D., Choi, E., & Lee, K. (2021). An Online International Collaborative Learning Program During the COVID-19 Pandemic for Nursing Students: Mixed Methods Study. *JMIR Medical Education*, *8*(1), e34171. Advance online publication. DOI: 10.2196/34171 PMID: 34982035

Kafarski, K., & Kazak, J. K. (2022). Erasmus staff mobility in the building of a European network: The case of a Central European university. *Sustainability (Basel)*, *14*(9), 4949. DOI: 10.3390/su14094949

Kalánková, D., Bartoníčková, D., Gurková, E., Žiaková, K., & Kurucová, R. (2021). A validation study of the Slovak version of the Hospital Survey on Patient Safety Culture (with Slovak nurses). *Central European Journal of Nursing and Midwifery*, *12*(2), 353–365. DOI: 10.15452/cejnm.2021.12.0010

Kanis, J. A., Odén, A., McCloskey, E. V., Johansson, H., Wahl, D. A., & Cooper, C. (2012). A systematic review of hip fracture incidence and probability of fracture worldwide. *Osteoporosis International*, *23*(9), 2239–2256. DOI: 10.1007/s00198-012-1964-3 PMID: 22419370

Kara, B., Akdeniz, C., & Kavaslar, İ. (2022). Hemşirelik 2.0: Türkiye'de hemşirelik bakımı ve eğitiminde paradigma değişimi önerisi. *Sağlık ve Sosyal Refah Araştırmaları Dergisi*, *4*(1), 136–143.

Karaman, F., & Alan, H. (2022). Turkish Adaptation of the Scale of the Attitudes to Patient Safety: Nursing Student Sample. *Bezmialem Science*, *10*(4), 426–433. DOI: 10.14235/bas.galenos.2021.5350

Karasu, F. (2020). Hemşirelik eğitiminde işbirlikli öğrenme modeli. *İnönü Üniversitesi Sağlık Hizmetleri Meslek Yüksek Okulu Dergisi, 8*(3), 973-988.

Kavanagh, J. D., & Johnson, R. E. (2017). The role of motivation in learning and performance. *Annual Review of Psychology*, *68*, 1–26.

Kaya, A., & Şendir, M. (2021). Hemşirelik eğitimi ve uygulamalarında eleştirel düşünme stratejileri ve boyutları. *Hemşirelik Bilimi Dergisi*, *4*(3), 163–168. DOI: 10.54189/hbd.874328

Keogh, J. J., & Russel-Roberts, E. (2008). Exchange programmes and student mobility: Meeting student's expectations or an expensive holiday? *Nurse Education Today*, *29*(1), 108–116. DOI: 10.1016/j.nedt.2008.07.006 PMID: 18782646

Khider, Y. I. A., Allam, S. M. E., Zoromba, M. A., & Elhapashy, H. M. M. (2024). Nursing students' perspectives on patients' safety competencies: A cross-sectional survey. *BMC Nursing, 23*(1), 323. DOI: 10.1186/s12912-024-01966-1 PMID: 38735958

Kim, W. C., & Mauborgne, R. A. (2014). *Blue ocean strategy, expanded edition: How to create uncontested market space and make the competition irrelevant.* Harvard business review Press.

King, J., & Anderson, C. M. (2012). The Canadian interprofessional patient safety competencies: Their role in healthcare professionals' education. *Journal of Patient Safety, 8*(1), 30–35. DOI: 10.1097/PTS.0b013e3182468138 PMID: 22343801

Kirwan, M., Riklikiene, O., Gotlib, J., Fuster, P., & Borta, M. (2019). Regulation and current status of patient safety content in pre-registration nurse education in 27 countries: Findings from the Rationing - Missed nursing care (RANCARE) COST Action project. *Nurse Education in Practice, 37*, 132–140. DOI: 10.1016/j.nepr.2019.04.013 PMID: 31153130

Kıvanç, M. M. (2015). Evrensel sağlık bildirgeleri ve Türkiye'de sağlık reformları. *Sağlık ve Hemşirelik Yönetimi Dergisi, 2*(3), 162–166.

Knight, J. (2012). Concepts, rationales, and interpretive frameworks in the internationalization of higher education. In Deardorff, D. K., de Wit, H., Heyl, J. D., & Adams, T. (Eds.), *The SAGE Handbook of International Higher Education* (pp. 27–42). SAGE Publications., DOI: 10.4135/9781452218397.n2

Kong, L. N., Zhu, W. F., He, S., Chen, S. Z., Yang, L., Qi, L., & Peng, X. (2019). Attitudes towards patient safety culture among postgraduate nursing students in China: A cross-sectional study. *Nurse Education in Practice, 38*, 1–6. DOI: 10.1016/j.nepr.2019.05.014 PMID: 31163311

Koparde, S. A., Selvakumar, P., Jha, R. P., Deepthi Reddy, K., Kuchipudi, J. D., Manjunath, T. C., & Sharma, M. (2026). Generative AI in Predicting and Preventing Foodborne Illnesses. In Madaan, G., Singh, A., Chahal, B., David, A., & Singh, G. (Eds.), *Generative AI in Food Systems: Predictive Demand, Smart Supply Chains, and Sustainable Service Futures* (pp. 205–232). IGI Global Scientific Publishing., DOI: 10.4018/979-8-3373-5182-7.ch010

Koukourikos, K., Tsaloglidou, A., & Papagiannis, D. (2021). Simulation in clinical nursing education. *Archives of Academic Nursing, 5*(2), 120–136. DOI: 10.21203/rs.3.rs-1020302/v1

Kraaij, J. van, Veenstra, M., Stalpers, D., Schoonhoven, L., Vermeulen, H., & Oostveen, C. van. (2022). Uniformity along the way: A scoping review on characteristics of nurse education programs worldwide [Review of *Uniformity along the way: A scoping review on characteristics of nurse education programs worldwide*]. *Nurse Education Today, 120*, 105646. Elsevier BV. DOI: 10.1016/j.nedt.2022.105646

Kulbok, P. A., Mitchell, E. M., Glick, D. F., & Greiner, D. (2012). International experiences in nursing education: A review of the literature. *International Journal of Nursing Education Scholarship, 9*(1), 1–21. DOI: 10.1515/1548-923X.2365 PMID: 22628353

Kunaviktikul, W., & Turale, S. (2020). Internationalizing nursing curricula in a rapidly globalizing world. *Nurse Education in Practice, 43*, 102704. DOI: 10.1016/j.nepr.2020.102704 PMID: 31991380

Kunaviktikul, W., Turale, S., Petrini, M. A., Tungpunkom, P., & Avant, K. C. (2019). Experiences From Southeast Asia On Nursing Education, Practice, Mobility And Influencing Policy. *International Nursing Review, 66*(4), 474–481. Https://Doi.Org/10.1111/Inr.12556. DOI: 10.1111/inr.12556 PMID: 31606912

Kung, P.-J., Chang, Y.-C., & Chiu, C. A., Li, M., Fang, C.-J., & Reynolds, N. R. (2025). The Impact Of International Visiting Scholars Programmes On Nursing Phd Students: An Integrative Review. *Journal Of Advanced Nursing*. Advance Online Publication. Https://Doi.Org/10.1111/Jan.70116

Kupcu, C., Bodur, G., Kucukkaya, A., & Goktaş, P. (2024). Assessing nursing students' e-health literacy and foresights to global health challenges during COVID-19 restrictions: A cross-sectional study with a machine learning approach. *Nurse Education in Practice, 81*, 104179. DOI: 10.1016/j.nepr.2024.104179 PMID: 39520839

Labrague, L. J. (2024). Integration of AI-powered chatbots in nursing education: A review. *Nurse Education in Practice*. Advance online publication. DOI: 10.1016/j.nepr.2024.103617

Lancaster, R. J. (2014). Serious game simulation as a teaching strategy in pharmacology. *Clinical Simulation in Nursing, 10*(3), 129–137. DOI: 10.1016/j.ecns.2013.10.005

Langari, M. N. M., Tella, S., Smith, N.-J., Ma, H., & Turunen, H. (2017). Self-assessment of patient safety competence: A questionnaire survey of final year British and Finnish pre-registration nursing students. *International Journal of Caring Sciences, 10*(3), 1212–1224. https://internationaljournalofcaringsciences.org/docs/11_lagari_original_10_3.pdf

Lasater, K., Cotrell, V., McKenzie, G., Simonson, W., Morgove, M. W., Long, E. E., & Eckstrom, E. (2016). Collaborative falls prevention: Interprofessional team formation, implementation, and evaluation. *Journal of Continuing Education in Nursing, 47*(12), 545–550. DOI: 10.3928/00220124-20161115-07 PMID: 27893917

Lateef, F. (2010). Simulation-based learning: Just like the real thing. *Journal of Emergencies, Trauma and Shock, 3*(4), 348–352. DOI: 10.4103/0974-2700.70743

Laugaland, K. A., Billett, S., Akerjordet, K., Frøiland, C. T., Grealish, L., & Aase, I. (2021). Enhancing student nurses' clinical education in aged care homes: A qualitative study of challenges perceived by faculty staff. *BMC Nursing, 20*(1), 111. Advance online publication. DOI: 10.1186/s12912-021-00632-0 PMID: 34174881

Lavoie, P., Lapierre, A., Maheu-Cadotte, M.-A., Brien, L.-A., Ledoux, I., & Gosselin, É. (2024). Nursing students' engagement in virtual reality and hybrid simulations: A quasi-experimental study. *Clinical Simulation in Nursing, 10*(3), 145–158. DOI: 10.1016/j.ecns.2023.101496

Leask, B. (2015). *Internationalizing the curriculum.* Routledge. DOI: 10.4324/9781315716954

Leathers, J., Davidson, H., & Desai, N. (2018). Interprofessional education between medical students and nurse practitioner students in a Global Health course. *BMC Medical Education, 18*(1), 200. Advance online publication. DOI: 10.1186/s12909-018-1307-y PMID: 30119625

Lee, H., & Kim, S. (2018). Mobile technology in undergraduate nursing education: A systematic review. *Nurse Education Today, 67*, 1–9. DOI: 10.1016/j.nedt.2018.04.012

Lee, H., & Lee, S. H. (2022). Effectiveness of Multicomponent Home-Based Rehabilitation in Elderly Patients after Hip Fracture Surgery: A Randomized Controlled Trial. *Journal of Personalized Medicine, 12*(4), 649. Advance online publication. DOI: 10.3390/jpm12040649 PMID: 35455765

Lee, N. J., An, J. Y., Song, T. M., Jang, H., & Park, S. Y. (2014). Psychometric evaluation of a patient safety competency self-evaluation tool for nursing students. *The Journal of Nursing Education, 53*(10), 550–562. DOI: 10.3928/01484834-20140922-01 PMID: 25275988

Lee, S. E., Dathinten, V. S., & Do, H. (2020). Patient safety education in pre-registration nursing programmes in South Korea. *International Nursing Review, 67*(4), 512–518. DOI: 10.1111/inr.12630 PMID: 33006174

Leotsakos, A., Zheng, H., Croteau, R., Loeb, J. M., Sherman, H., Hoffman, C., Morganstein, L., O'Leary, D., Bruneau, C., Lee, P., Duguid, M., Thomeczek, C., Schrieck-De Loos, E., & Munier, B. (2014). Standardization in patient safety: The WHO High 5s project. *International Journal for Quality in Health Care : Journal of the International Society for Quality in Health Care, 26*(2), 109–116. DOI: 10.1093/intqhc/mzu010 PMID: 24713313

Letourneau, R. M., & McCurry, M. K. (2019). Testing the Nursing Quality and Safety Self-Inventory. *Journal for Nurses in Professional Development, 35*(5), 275–280. DOI: 10.1097/NND.0000000000000556 PMID: 31157672

Leung, D., Chan, E. A., Wong, A. K. C., Reisenhofer, S., Stenberg, M., Sze, C. P., Lai, K., Cruz, E., & Carlson, E. (2020). Advancing pedagogy of undergraduate nursing students' cultural awareness through internationalization webinars: A qualitative study. *Nurse Education Today, 93*, 104514. DOI: 10.1016/j.nedt.2020.104514 PMID: 32659533

Levett-Jones, T., Dwyer, T., Reid-Searl, K., Heaton, L., Flenady, T., Applegarth, J., Guinea, S., & Andersen, P. (2017). *Patient safety competency framework (PSCF) for nursing students.* http://psframework.wpengine.com/wpcontent/uploads/2018/01/PSCF_Brochure_UTS-version_FA2-Screen.pdf

Levett-Jones, T., Andersen, P., Bogossian, F., Cooper, S., Guinea, S., Hopmans, R., McKenna, L., Pich, J., Reid-Searl, K., & Seaton, P. (2020). A cross-sectional survey of nursing students' patient safety knowledge. *Nurse Education Today, 88*, 104372. DOI: 10.1016/j.nedt.2020.104372 PMID: 32143174

Leyva-Moral, J. M., Tosun, B., Gómez-Ibáñez, R., Navarrete, L., Yava, A., Aguayo-González, M., Dirgar, E., Checa-Jiménez, C., & Bernabeu-Tamayo, M. D. (2023). From a learning opportunity to a conscious multidimensional change: A metasynthesis of transcultural learning experiences among nursing students. *BMC Nursing, 22*(1), 356. Advance online publication. DOI: 10.1186/s12912-023-01521-4 PMID: 37798717

Liem, I. S., Kammerlander, C., Suhm, N., Blauth, M., Roth, T., Gosch, M., Hoang-Kim, A., Mendelson, D., Zuckerman, J., Leung, F., Burton, J., Moran, C., Parker, M., Giusti, A., Pioli, G., Goldhahn, J., & Kates, S. L. (2013). Identifying a standard set of outcome parameters for the evaluation of orthogeriatric co-management for hip fractures. *Injury, 44*(11), 1403–1412. DOI: 10.1016/j.injury.2013.06.018 PMID: 23880377

Lino, M. M., Martini, J. G., & Barbieri-Figueiredo, M. D. C. (2022). Academic-Professional Mobility And Internationalization Of Nursing: Contributions Of The Bologna Process. *Texto & Contexto Enfermagem, 31*, E20210319. Https://Doi.Org/10.1590/1980-265x-Tce-2021-0319en. DOI: 10.1590/1980-265x-tce-2021-0319pt

Lippe, M., Braden, C. J., & Gill, S. L. (2025). Re-Envisioning Philosophy of Nursing Science Education to Advance PhD Student Development. *Nurse Educator, 50*(5), 283–288. DOI: 10.1097/NNE.0000000000001896

Liu, K.. (2023). Effectiveness of virtual reality in nursing education: A systematic review and meta-analysis. *BMC Medical Education, 23*, 112. DOI: 10.1186/s12916-023-02823-9

Louis, K. S., White, A., & Brown, A. (2025). Nursing Students' Enhanced Cultural Competence After Study Abroad: A Mixed-Methods Study. *The Journal of Nursing Education, 64*(3), 185–191. DOI: 10.3928/01484834-20250108-01 PMID: 40048603

Lourenço, A., & Paiva, M. O. (2024). Globalization of higher education: The internationalization from a multifactorial perspective. In *Building resiliency in higher education: Globalization, digital skills, and student wellness* (pp. 285–305). IGI Global Scientific Publishing. DOI: 10.4018/979-8-3693-5483-4.ch016

Lukewich, J., Edge, D. S., Tranmer, J., Raymond, J., Miron, J., Ginsburg, L., & VanDenKerkhof, E. (2015). Undergraduate baccalaureate nursing students' self-reported confidence in learning about patient safety in the classroom and clinical settings: An annual cross-sectional study (2010–2013). *International Journal of Nursing Studies, 52*(5), 930–938. DOI: 10.1016/j.ijnurstu.2015.01.010 PMID: 25698119

Mackavey, C. L., Henderson, C., & Stout, T. (2024). Stepping outside national borders: International active learning educational collaboration events. *International Nursing Review, 71*(1), 5–12. DOI: 10.1111/inr.12927 PMID: 38156728

Maia, A. C., Marques, M. J., Goes, A. R., Gama, A., Osborne, R., & Dias, S. (2024). Health literacy strengths and needs among migrant communities from Portuguese-speaking African countries in Portugal: A cross-sectional study. *Frontiers in Public Health, 12*, 1415588. Advance online publication. DOI: 10.3389/fpubh.2024.1415588 PMID: 39022410

Malafarina, V., Uriz-Otano, F., Malafarina, C., Martinez, J. A., & Zulet, M. A. (2017). Effectiveness of nutritional supplementation on sarcopenia and recovery in hip fracture patients. A multi-centre randomized trial. *Maturitas, 101*, 42–50. DOI: 10.1016/j.maturitas.2017.04.010 PMID: 28539168

Maltby, H. J., & Abrams, S. (2009). Seeing with new eyes: The meaning of an immersion experience in Bangladesh for undergraduate senior nursing students. *International Journal of Nursing Education Scholarship*, *6*(1). Advance online publication. DOI: 10.2202/1548-923X.1858 PMID: 19883373

Mansour, M. (2012). Current assessment of patient safety education. *British Journal of Nursing (Mark Allen Publishing)*, *21*(9), 536–543. DOI: 10.12968/bjon.2012.21.9.536 PMID: 22585267

Mansour, M. J., Al Shadafan, S. F., Abu-Sneineh, F. T., & Alamer, M. M. (2018). Integrating patient safety education in the undergraduate nursing curriculum: A discussion paper. *The Open Nursing Journal*, *12*(1), 125–132. DOI: 10.2174/1874434601812010125 PMID: 30069269

Mansour, M., Skull, A., & Parker, M. (2015). Evaluation of World Health Organization multi-professional patient safety curriculum topics in nursing education: Pre-test, post-test, none-experimental study. *Journal of Professional Nursing*, *31*(5), 432–439. DOI: 10.1016/j.profnurs.2015.03.002 PMID: 26428349

Marcantonio, E. R., Flacker, J. M., Michaels, M., & Resnick, N. M. (2000). Delirium is independently associated with poor functional recovery after hip fracture. *Journal of the American Geriatrics Society*, *48*(6), 618–624. DOI: 10.1111/j.1532-5415.2000.tb04718.x PMID: 10855596

Marcomini, I., Destrebecq, A., Rosa, D., & Terzoni, S. (2021). Self-reported skills for ensuring patient safety and quality of care among Italian nursing students: A descriptive cross-sectional study. *International Journal of Health Promotion and Education*, *60*(2), 67–78. DOI: 10.1080/14635240.2021.1944270

Martins, A. C.. (2018). Does modified Otago Exercise Program improves balance in older people? A systematic review. In *Preventive Medicine Reports* (pp. 231–239). Elsevier Inc., DOI: 10.1016/j.pmedr.2018.06.015

Mayer, R. E. (2019). *Multimedia learning* (3rd ed.). Cambridge University Press.

McCarthy, C., Boniol, M., Daniels, K., Cometto, G., Diallo, K., Lawani, A. D., & Campbell, J. (2020). State of the World's Nursing 2020: Investing in education, jobs, and leadership. *Geneva: World Health Organization*. Access 21. july 2025, from: https://web.archive.org/web/20200407162231/https://www.who.int/publications-detail/nursing-report-2020

McDonough, C. M., Harris-Hayes, M., Kristensen, M. T., Overgaard, J. A., Herring, T. B., Kenny, A. M., & Mangione, K. K. (2021). Physical therapy management of older adults with hip fracture. *The Journal of Orthopaedic and Sports Physical Therapy*, *51*(2), CPG1–CPG81. DOI: 10.2519/jospt.2021.0301 PMID: 33522384

McNamara, K. E., & Jackson, G. (2019). Loss and damage: When adaptation is not enough. *Climate Policy*, *19*(6), 667–678. DOI: 10.1080/14693062.2019.1594967

Medina, M., Maia, A. C., & Costa, A. (2022). Health literacy in migrant communities: A primary health care unit study in Portugal. *Frontiers in Public Health*, *9*, 798222. DOI: 10.3389/fpubh.2021.798222 PMID: 35141189

Mehta, S. P., Fulton, A., Quach, C., Thistle, M., Toledo, C., & Evans, N. A. (2016). Measurement properties of the Lower Extremity Functional Scale: A systematic review. *The Journal of Orthopaedic and Sports Physical Therapy*, *46*(3), 200–216. DOI: 10.2519/jospt.2016.6165 PMID: 26813750

Merry, L., Vissandjée, B., & Verville-Provencher, K. (2021). Challenges, coping responses and supportive interventions for international and migrant students in academic nursing programs in major host countries: a scoping review with a gender lens [Review of *Challenges, coping responses and supportive interventions for international and migrant students in academic nursing programs in major host countries: a scoping review with a gender lens*]. *BMC Nursing*, *20*(1). BioMed Central. DOI: 10.1186/s12912-021-00678-0

Meum, T. T., Koch, T. B., Briseid, H. S., Vabo, G. L., & Rabben, J. (2021). Perceptions of digital technology in nursing education: A qualitative study. *Nurse Education in Practice*, *54*, 103136. DOI: 10.1016/j.nepr.2021.103136

Michael, R., Della, P., Banner, C., Duckworth, S., & Nilson, T. (2012). The role of the photo novella in examining cultural competency in perioperative settings. *ACORN: The Journal of Perioperative Nursing in Australia*, *25*(1), 20-24, 26.

Middleton, J., Cunsolo, A., Jones-Bailey, M., & Harper, S. L. (2020). Moving toward a framework for cultural climate grief. *Emotion, Space and Society*, *37*, 100738. DOI: 10.1016/j.emospa.2020.100738

Middleton, M., Wan, B., & da Assunçao, R. (2017). Improving hip fracture outcomes with integrated orthogeriatric care: A comparison between two accepted orthogeriatric models. *Age and Ageing*, *46*(3), 465–470. DOI: 10.1093/ageing/afw232 PMID: 27974304

Mikkonen, K., Elo, S., Tuomikoski, A. M., & Kääriäinen, M. (2016). Mentor experiences of international healthcare students' learning in a clinical environment: A systematic review. *Nurse Education Today, 40*, 87–94. DOI: 10.1016/j.nedt.2016.02.013 PMID: 27125155

Miller, C. L., & LaFramboise, L. (2009). Student Learning Outcomes After Integration of Quality and Safety Education Competencies into a Senior-Level Critical Care Course. *The Journal of Nursing Education, 48*(12), 678–685. DOI: 10.3928/01484834-20091113-07 PMID: 20000249

Miller, G. E. (1990). The assessment of clinical skills/competence/performance. *Academic Medicine, 65*(9, Suppl), S63–S67. DOI: 10.1097/00001888-199009000-00045 PMID: 2400509

Mishra, B. R., Selvakumar, P., Kaur, R., Kalshetti, P., Mishra, K. K., Sharma, M., & Manjunath, T. C. (2025). Innovation and Digital Transformation in the Public Sector Entities. In Santos Ferreira, A., & Lourenço dos Santos, C. (Eds.), *Enhancing Public Sector Accountability and Services Through Digital Innovation* (pp. 409–436). IGI Global Scientific Publishing., DOI: 10.4018/979-8-3693-9251-5.ch013

Mishra, P., & Koehler, M. J. (2006). Technological pedagogical content knowledge: A framework for teacher knowledge. *Teachers College Record, 108*(6), 1017–1054. DOI: 10.1111/j.1467-9620.2006.00684.x

Mitchell, P. J.. (2019). Quality Improvement Initiatives in Fragility Fracture Care and Prevention. In *Current Osteoporosis Reports* (pp. 510–520). Springer., DOI: 10.1007/s11914-019-00544-8

Mohammadi, N., Dorri, S., & Abedi, A. (2020). Nursing education in the path of globalization: Promotion or challenge? [Review of *Nursing education in the path of globalization: Promotion or challenge?*]. *Journal of Education and Health Promotion, 9*(1), 269. Medknow. DOI: 10.4103/jehp.jehp_775_19

Montegrico, J., Cornelius, J. B., Downing, C., Fradelos, E. C., Machuca-Contreras, F., Oducado, R. M., & Resna, R. W. (2022). International nurse education research collaboration during the COVID-19 pandemic: Researchers' perspectives. *Nurse Education Today, 120*, 105606. DOI: 10.1016/j.nedt.2022.105606 PMID: 36343419

Morello, R. T., Lowthian, J. A., Barker, A. L., McGinnes, R., Dunt, D., & Brand, C. (2013). Strategies for improving patient safety culture in hospitals: A systematic review. *BMJ Quality & Safety, 22*(1), 11–18. DOI: 10.1136/bmjqs-2011-000582 PMID: 22849965

Morin, A. (2020). The neuroscience of learning: Implications for education. *Educational Psychology Review*, *32*(4), 1–23.

Morley, D. A., & Cunningham, S. (2021). Global partnerships in nursing – A qualitative study in lessons for success. *Nurse Education in Practice*, *54*, 103069. DOI: 10.1016/j.nepr.2021.103069 PMID: 34058464

Morley, L., Alexiadou, N., Garaz, S., González-Monteagudo, J., & Taba, M. (2018). Internationalisation and migrant academics: The hidden narratives of mobility. *Higher Education*, *76*(3), 537–554. DOI: 10.1007/s10734-017-0224-z

Mortensen, M., Naustdal, K. I., Uibu, E., Mägi, L., Kangasniemi, M., Põlluste, K., & Moi, A. L. (2022). Instruments for measuring patient safety competencies in nursing: A scoping review. *BMJ Open Quality*, *11*(2), e001751. DOI: 10.1136/bmjoq-2021-001751 PMID: 35379672

Msomphora, M. R. (2024). Bridging borders: Global insights and challenges in internationalising higher education using a decade-long case study. *International Journal of Educational Research Open*, *8*, 100402. DOI: 10.1016/j.ijedro.2024.100402

Muraraneza, C., Mukamana, D., Katende, G., Bazirete, O., & Wolvaardt, L. (2023). Global partnerships in transformation of nursing and midwifery education in Africa: A systematic scoping review protocol. *Research Square (Research Square)*. DOI: 10.21203/rs.3.rs-3145480/v1

Muusse, J. S. C., Zuidema, R., van Scherpenseel, M. C., & te Velde, S. J. (2023). Influencing factors of interprofessional collaboration in multifactorial fall prevention interventions: A qualitative systematic review. *BMC Primary Care*, *24*(1), 116. Advance online publication. DOI: 10.1186/s12875-023-02066-w PMID: 37193995

Myhre, K. (2011). Exchange students crossing language boundaries in clinical nursing practice. *International Nursing Review*, *58*(4), 428–433. DOI: 10.1111/j.1466-7657.2011.00904.x PMID: 22092320

Naz, N., & Kausor, M. (2023). Critical Thinking in the Nursing Profession: Analysis with a Socratic Method and Nurse Theorist Philosophy. *Journal of University Medical & Dental College*, *14*(1), 580–583.

Negarandeh, R., & Khoshkesht, S. (2022). Expected roles of PhD graduated nurses: A scoping review. *Florence Nightingale Journal of Nursing*, *30*(2), 202–208. DOI: 10.54614/FNJN.2022.21233

NICE. (2023) Hip fracture management. Available at URL: https://www.nice.org.uk/guidance/cg124

Nicholas A.. Christakis, & Fowler, J. H. (2009). Connected: The Amazing Power of Social Networks and How They Shape Our Lives. HarperPress.

Nieva, V. F., & Sorra, J. (2003). Safety culture assessment: A tool for improving patient safety in healthcare organizations. *BMJ Quality & Safety*, *12*(90002, Suppl 2), ii17–ii23. DOI: 10.1136/qhc.12.suppl_2.ii17 PMID: 14645891

Nirupama, E., Seenivasan, S., Bhardwaj, K., Karunakaran, N. B., & Basava Aradhya, S. G., Selvakumar, P., & Manjunath, T. C. (2025). Transforming Digital Supply Chains With Gamification and Metaverse Integration. In G. Malik, D. Singh, & R. Bansal (Eds.), *Addressing Practical Problems Through the Metaverse and Game-Inspired Mechanics* (pp. 123-152). IGI Global Scientific Publishing. https://doi.org/ DOI: 10.4018/979-8-3693-8886-0.ch006

Nogueiro, T., Saraiva, M., Jorge, F., & Chaleta, E. (2022). The Erasmus+ Programme and Sustainable Development Goals—Contribution of mobility actions in higher education. *Sustainability (Basel)*, *14*(3), 1628. DOI: 10.3390/su14031628

Noyudom, A. N., Ketpichainarong, W., & Ruenwongsa, P. (2011). Development of a computer-based simulation unit on tracheal suctioning to enhance nursing students' knowledge and practical skills. *The Thai Simulation 2011-TS'11-3rd Annual International Conference, Thailand.*

Nüzket, G., Özkütük N (2025). Oyun Temelli Eğitimin Hemşirelik Öğrencilerinin Broşür Hazırlama Bilgi Becerilerine Etkisi, Ege Üniversitesi Sağlık Bilimleri Enstitüsü, Yayınlanmamış Doktora tezi.

O'Connor, K. (2020). Online learning in higher education: A review of research. *Journal of Online Learning and Teaching*, *16*(1), 1–15.

O'Connor, M. I., & Switzer, J. A. (2022). AAOS clinical practice guideline summary: Management of hip fractures in older adults. *The Journal of the American Academy of Orthopaedic Surgeons*, *30*(20), e1291–e1296. DOI: 10.5435/JAAOS-D-22-00125 PMID: 36200817

OECD. (2020). *Education at a glance 2020: OECD indicators*. OECD Publishing., DOI: 10.1787/69096873-

Ogilvie, L., Paul, P., & Burgess-Pinto, E. (2007). International Dimensions of Higher Education in Nursing in Canada: Tapping the Wisdom of the 20th Century While Embracing Possibilities for the 21st Century [Review of *International Dimensions of Higher Education in Nursing in Canada: Tapping the Wisdom of the 20th Century While Embracing Possibilities for the 21st Century*]. *International Journal of Nursing Education Scholarship, 4*(1). De Gruyter. DOI: 10.2202/1548-923X.1306

Ojala, M. (2023). Hope and meaning in times of climate change: Promoting agency in young people. *Current Opinion in Psychology, 49*, 101554. DOI: 10.1016/j.copsyc.2023.101554

Ortiz de Elguea, J., Orkaizagirre-Gómara, A., Sánchez de Miguel, M., Urcola-Pardo, F., Germín-Bes, C., & Lizaso-Elgarresta, I. (2019). Adapting and validating the Hospital Survey on Patient Safety Culture (HSOPS) for nursing students (HSOPS-NS): A new measure of patient safety climate. *Nurse Education Today, 75*, 95–103. DOI: 10.1016/j.nedt.2019.01.008 PMID: 30738365

Owoeye, I. D., Chipps, J. A., & Daniels, F. (2025). Nurse educators' competence and use of digital education technology at selected nursing education institutions in Nigeria. *International Journal of Africa Nursing Sciences, 100870*, 100870. Advance online publication. DOI: 10.1016/j.ijans.2025.100870

Özkan, H. A., & Akduran, F. (2014). Hemşirelikte paradigmaların önemi. *Hemsirelikte Egitim ve Arastirma Dergisi, 11*(2), 3–5.

Pan American Health Organization. (2023). *Caribbean Mental Health Network: Strengthening capacity through regional cooperation.* https://www.paho.org/en/topics/mental-health

Pantouvaki, A., Kastanis, G., Patelarou, E., Alpantaki, K., Kleisiaris, C., & Zografakis-Sfakianakis, M. (2023). Greek Translation, Cultural Adaptation and Validation of the Mini Sarcopenia Risk Assessment Questionnaire, to Evaluate Sarcopenia in Greek Elderly at a Hospital Setting. *Nursing Reports, 13*(1), 404–411. DOI: 10.3390/nursrep13010037 PMID: 36976689

Panu, P. (2020). Anxiety and the ecological crisis: An analysis of eco-anxiety and climate anxiety. *Sustainability (Basel), 12*(19), 7836. DOI: 10.3390/su12197836

Papadopoulos, I. (Ed.). (2006). *Transcultural health and social care: development of culturally competent practitioners*. Elsevier Health Sciences.

Pathway, F. (2025, July). Fulbright program empowers global nursing education: Strategic insights on international collaboration, curriculum innovation, and talentshortage solutions. *Forward Pathway*. [from: https://www.forwardpathway.us/fulbright-program-empowers-global-nursing-education-strategic-insights-on-international-collaboration-curriculum-innovation-and-talent-shortage-solutions]. *Access, 21*, •••.

Pedersen, M. L., Gildberg, F. A., Baker, J., & Tingleff, E. B. (2023). A Review of Ethnic Disparities in Restrictive Mental Health Practices [Review of *A Review of Ethnic Disparities in Restrictive Mental Health Practices*]. *Research Portal Denmark.* Technical University of Denmark. https://local.forskningsportal.dk/local/dki-cgi/ws/cris-link?src=sdu&id=sdu-a108e4b6-bd44-4687-a043-cf0ae357167e&ti=A%20Review%20of%20Ethnic%20Disparities%20in%20Restrictive%20Mental%20Health%20Practices

Pelikan, J. M., Ganahl, K., & Röthlin, F. (2022). Measuring health literacy in general populations — The HLS19 instrument and its cross-national applications relevant to nursing and global health promotion. *International Journal of Environmental Research and Public Health, 19*(2), 1008. DOI: 10.3390/ijerph19021008 PMID: 35055825

Perez-Encinas, A., De Filippo, D., De La Torre, E. M., & Alonso, D. (2023). *Research competence framework: Competence frameworks in international student mobility* (Erasmus Careers Project No. 101049436). Erasmus Careers Consortium. Access 21. july 2025, from: https://project.erasmuscareers.org/documents/ResearchCompetenceFramework.pdf

Petschonek, S., Burlison, J., Cross, C., Martin, K., Laver, J., Landis, R. S., & Hoffman, J. M. (2013). Development of the just culture assessment tool: Measuring the perceptions of healthcare professionals in hospitals. *Journal of Patient Safety, 9*(4), 190–197. DOI: 10.1097/PTS.0b013e31828fff34 PMID: 24263549

Pfeufer, D., Kammerlander, C., Stadler, C., Roth, T., Blauth, M., Neuerburg, C., Böcker, W., Zeckey, C., Lechleitner, M., & Gosch, M. (2020). Multidisciplinary inpatient rehabilitation improves the long-term functional status of geriatric hip-fracture patients. *European Journal of Medical Research, 25*(1), 31. Advance online publication. DOI: 10.1186/s40001-020-00433-2 PMID: 32778164

Pinto, D., Alshahrani, M., Chapurlat, R., Chevalley, T., Dennison, E., Camargos, B. M., Papaioannou, A., Silverman, S., Kaux, J.-F., Lane, N. E., Morales Torres, J., Paccou, J., Rizzoli, R., Bruyere, O., Blank, R., Buehring, B., Cooper, C., Ferrari, S., Kanis, J. A., & Tüzün, Ş. (2022). The global approach to rehabilitation following an osteoporotic fragility fracture: A review of the rehabilitation working group of the International Osteoporosis Foundation (IOF) committee of scientific advisors. *Osteoporosis International, 33*(3), 527–540. DOI: 10.1007/s00198-021-06240-7 PMID: 35048200

Pioli, G., Bendini, C., Pignedoli, P., Giusti, A., & Marsh, D. (2018). Orthogeriatric co-management – managing frailty as well as fragility. *Injury, 49*(8), 1398–1402. DOI: 10.1016/j.injury.2018.04.014 PMID: 29921533

Piscotty, R., Grobbel, C., & Abele, C. (2013). Initial psychometric evaluation of the nursing quality and safety self-inventory. *The Journal of Nursing Education, 52*(5), 269–274. DOI: 10.3928/01484834-20130412-03 PMID: 23586354

Pizzonia, M., Giannotti, C., Carmisciano, L., Signori, A., Rosa, G., Santolini, F., Caffa, I., Montecucco, F., Nencioni, A., & Monacelli, F. (2021). Frailty assessment, hip fracture and long-term clinical outcomes in older adults. *European Journal of Clinical Investigation, 51*(4), e13445. Advance online publication. DOI: 10.1111/eci.13445 PMID: 33131066

Portes, A. (1998). Social Capital: Its Origins and Applications in Modern Sociology. *Annual Review of Sociology, 24*(1), 1–24. DOI: 10.1146/annurev.soc.24.1.1

Pramila-Savukoski, S., Kärnä, R., Kuivila, H. M., Juntunen, J., Koskenranta, M., Oikarainen, A., & Mikkonen, K. (2023). The influence of digital learning on health sciences students' competence development- A qualitative study. *Nurse Education Today, 120*, 105635. DOI: 10.1016/j.nedt.2022.105635

Puentedura, R. R. (2014). SAMR: A contextualized introduction. *Hippasus*. https://hippasus.com/resources/sweden2014/SAMR_Introduction.pdf

Putnam, R. D. (1993). *Making Democracy Work: Civic Traditions in Modern Italy*. Princeton University Press.

Putnam, R. D. (2000). *Bowling Alone: The Collapse and Revival of American Community*. Simon & Schuster.

Quality and Safety Education for Nurses. (2020). *Quality and safety education for nurses (QSEN)*. Case Western Reserve University. https://qsen.org/about-qsen/

Racine, L. (2023). International clinical experiences may increase cultural competency and support nurses' personal and professional development. *Evidence-Based Nursing, 26*(4), 153–153. DOI: 10.1136/ebnurs-2022-103690 PMID: 37160348

Raman, M. S., Koppa, K. B., Chithambar Gupta, V., Bhat, V. A., Guru Basava Aradhya, S., & Selvakumar, P. (2025). Digital Transformation and Sustainability Artificial Intelligence and Sustainable Development. In Yıldırım, D., Yıldırım, S., & Kandpal, V. (Eds.), *Effects of Digitalization and Circular Economy on Sustainable Policy and Climate Change Prevention* (pp. 69–96). IGI Global Scientific Publishing., DOI: 10.4018/979-8-3693-9909-5.ch003

Ramos-Ramos, A., Rodríguez-Suárez, C.-A., Díaz-González, C. de la M., Soriano, J. V., Berenguer-Pérez, M., & la Torre, H. G. (2024). Academic and Employment Preferences of Nursing Students at the University of Las Palmas of Gran Canaria: A Cross-Sectional Study. *Nursing Reports, 14*(4), 3328–3345. DOI: 10.3390/nursrep14040241 PMID: 39585132

Rehm, J., Shield, K. D., & Gmel, G. (2022). The contribution of mental and substance use disorders to global burden of disease. *The Lancet. Psychiatry, 9*(2), 107–118. DOI: 10.1016/S2215-0366(21)00429-0 PMID: 35065719

Restaino, M., Vitale, M. P., & Primerano, I. (2020). Analysing International Student Mobility Flows In Higher Education: A Comparative Study On European Countries. *Social Indicators Research, 149*(3), 947–965. Https://Doi.Org/10.1007/S11205-020-02282-2. DOI: 10.1007/s11205-020-02282-2

Roy, A., Newman, A., Ellenberger, T., & Pyman, A. (2019). Outcomes Of International Student Mobility Programs: A Systematic Review And Agenda For Future Research. *Studies in Higher Education, 44*(9), 1630–1644. Https://Doi.Org/10.1080/03075079.2018.1458222. DOI: 10.1080/03075079.2018.1458222

Royse, D., & Newton, R. R. (2007). *Research methods in social work* (6th ed.). Thomson Brooks/Cole.

Rukholm, E., Stamler, L. L., Talbot, L. R., Bednash, G., Raines, F., Potempa, K., Nugent, P., Clark, D. J. M., Bernhauser, S., & Parfitt, B. (2009). Scaling up the global nursing health workforce: Contributions of an international organization [Review of *Scaling up the global nursing health workforce: Contributions of an international organization*]. *Collegian Journal of the Royal College of Nursing Australia, 16*(1), 41. Elsevier BV. DOI: 10.1016/j.colegn.2009.01.001

Ryan, J. (2011). Teaching and learning for international students: Towards a transcultural approach. *Teachers and Teaching, 17*(6), 631–648. DOI: 10.1080/13540602.2011.625138

Sailsman, S. (2021). EnglishAsASecondLanguage (ESL) nursing students' academic integration: A review of literature. *Nursing Education Perspectives, 42*(3), 152–156. DOI: 10.1097/01.NEP.0000000000000731 PMID: 33861530

Saito, A. S., & Creedy, D. K. (2021). Determining mental health literacy of undergraduate nursing students to inform learning and teaching strategies. *International Journal of Mental Health Nursing, 30*(5), 1117–1126. DOI: 10.1111/inm.12862 PMID: 33760328

Salman, K. (2018). The Fulbright Journey: Reflections on a Challenging and Rewarding Experience in Saudi Arabia by a Nursing Professor. *Journal of Professional Nursing, 35*(4), 335–340. DOI: 10.1016/j.profnurs.2018.10.004 PMID: 31345516

Sanford, J., Argenbright, C., Sherwood, G., Jordan, P., Herrera, M., Bengtsson, M., Moriyama, M., Lui, L., & McDonald, M. (2021). Student outcomes of an international learning collaborative to develop patient safety and quality competencies in nursing. *Journal of Research in Nursing : JRN, 26*(1-2), 81–94. DOI: 10.1177/1744987120970606 PMID: 35251228

Schnall, R., Stone, P., Currie, L., Desjardins, K., John, R. M., & Bakken, S. (2008). Development of a self-report instrument to measure patient safety attitudes, skills, and knowledge. *Journal of Nursing Scholarship, 40*(4), 391–394. DOI: 10.1111/j.1547-5069.2008.00256.x PMID: 19094156

Selaković, I., Mandić-Rajčević, S., Milovanović, A., Tomanović-Vujadinović, S., Dimitrijević, S., Aleksić, M., & Dubljanin-Raspopović, E. (2024). Pre-Fracture Functional Status and Early Functional Recovery are Significant Predictors of Instrumental Activities of Daily Living After Hip Fracture: A Prospective Cohort Study. *Geriatric Orthopaedic Surgery & Rehabilitation, 15*, 21514593241255627. Advance online publication. DOI: 10.1177/21514593241255627 PMID: 38766275

Şenyuva, E. (2019). Eğitimde dijital dönüşüm: Teknolojinin öğretim süreçlerine entegrasyonu. *Eğitim ve Bilim, 44*(198), 1–16.

Sepp, K. (2024). Advancing patient safety competencies in nursing education: An examination of student attitudes. *Agronomy Research (Tartu), 22*(S1), 537–553. DOI: 10.15159/AR.24.018

Sexton, J. B., Helmreich, R. L., Neilands, T. B., Rowan, K., Vella, K., Boyden, J., Roberts, P. R., & Thomas, E. J. (2006). The Safety Attitudes Questionnaire: Psychometric properties, benchmarking data, and emerging research. *BMC Health Services Research, 6*(1), 44. DOI: 10.1186/1472-6963-6-44 PMID: 16584553

Shali, M., Bakhshi, F., & Hasanpour, M. (2024). Culture of patient care among international nursing students: A focused ethnographic study. *BMC Nursing, 23*(1), 163. DOI: 10.1186/s12912-024-01807-1 PMID: 38448913

Sharplin, G., Clarke, J., & Eckert, M. (2025). *Assessing the global sustainability of the nursing workforce: A survey of national nurses' association presidents within the International Council of Nurses* (Report prepared for the International Council of Nurses by the Rosemary Bryant AO Research Centre). University of South Australia. Access 21. july 2025, from: https://www.icn.ch/sites/default/files/2025-04/ICN_NNA-Presidents-Survey-Report_EN_FINAL.pdf

Sharpnack, P. A. (2025). The Importance of Nursing Education Research for Strengthening the Quality of Professional Practice. *Nursing Education Perspectives, 46*(2), 75–76. DOI: 10.1097/01.NEP.0000000000001385

Shea, B. J., Reeves, B. C., Wells, G., Thuku, M., Hamel, C., Moran, J., Moher, D., Tugwell, P., Welch, V., Kristjansson, E., & Henry, D. A. (2017). AMSTAR 2: A critical appraisal tool for systematic reviews that include randomised or non-randomised studies of healthcare interventions, or both. *BMJ (Clinical Research Ed.), 358*, j4008. DOI: 10.1136/bmj.j4008 PMID: 28935701

Sherrington, C., & Tiedemann, A. (2015). Physiotherapy in the prevention of falls in older people. *Journal of Physiotherapy, 61*(2), 54–60. DOI: 10.1016/j.jphys.2015.02.011 PMID: 25797882

Sherwood, G., & Barnsteiner, J. (Eds.). (2012). *Quality and safety in nursing: A competency approach to improving outcomes*. Wiley-Blackwell.

Sim, J. J. M.. (2022). Virtual simulation to enhance clinical reasoning in nursing: A review of design features and outcomes. *Journal of Clinical Nursing Education, 18*(4), 210–228. DOI: 10.1111/jocn.16127

Singh, F., & Masango, T. (2020). Information technology in nursing education: Perspectives from student nurses. *The Open Nursing Journal, 14*(1), 18–27. DOI: 10.2174/1874434602014010018

Sivanand, R., & Selvakumar, P. (2025). Navneet Sharma, Nanotechnology Applications in Cancer Drug Delivery Systems: A Review. *Journal of Environmental Nanotechnology, 14*(2), 458–470. DOI: 10.13074/jent.2025.06.2511221

Skirton, H., & Blakely, M. (2009). The role of genetics in nursing education. *Nurse Education Today, 29*(1), 1–6.

Sochan, A. (2008). Relationship building through the development of international nursing curricula: a literature review [Review of *Relationship building through the development of international nursing curricula: a literature review*]. *International Nursing Review, 55*(2), 192. Wiley. DOI: 10.1111/j.1466-7657.2007.00595.x

Sorokin, P. A. (1962). *Social and Cultural Dynamics* (Vol. 3).

Stasi, S., Papathanasiou, G., Korres, N., Marinakis, G., Chronopoulos, E., Baltopoulos, P. I., & Papaioannou, N. A. (2013). Validation of the Lower Extremity Functional Scale in community-dwelling elderly people (LEFS-Greek); Determination of functional status cut-off points using TUG test. *European Geriatric Medicine, 4*(4), 237–241. DOI: 10.1016/j.eurger.2013.04.004

Stomski, N., Gluyas, H., Andrus, P., Williams, A., Hopkins, M., Walters, J., Sandy, M., & Morrison, P. (2018). The influence of situation awareness training on nurses' confidence about patient safety skills: A prospective cohort study. *Nurse Education Today*, *63*, 24–28. DOI: 10.1016/j.nedt.2018.01.019 PMID: 29407256

Streitwieser, B., Lomer, S., & van der Wende, M. (2020). Universities as global actors: The challenge of internationalization, sustainability, and global responsibility. *Higher Education Policy*, *33*(3), 393–409. DOI: 10.3390/su6053043

Suka, M., Yamauchi, T., & Hashimoto, H. (2020). Relationship between health literacy, self-rated health, and mortality in Japan: Findings and implications for nursing and health promotion. *BMC Public Health*, *20*, 1182. DOI: 10.1186/s12889-020-09202-8

Sullivan, D. T., Hirst, D., & Cronenwett, L. (2009). Assessing quality and safety competencies of graduating prelicensure nursing students. *Nursing Outlook*, *57*(6), 323–331. DOI: 10.1016/j.outlook.2009.08.004 PMID: 19942033

Swift, C., Ftouh, S., Langford, P., Chesser, T. S., & Johanssen, A. (2016). CMJv16n6-Swift(WITHOUT ITAL CORX). indd. [). www.nice.org.uk/]. *Clinical Medicine*, *16*(6), •••. PMID: 27927818

Takmak, Ş. (2024). Hemşirelik Biliminde Paradigma Değişimleri ve Çoklu Paradigma Kullanımı. *Hemşirelik Bilimi Dergisi*, *7*(2), 225–235. DOI: 10.54189/hbd.1378846

Taskiran, G., Eskin Bacaksiz, F., & Harmanci Seren, A. K. (2020). Psychometric testing of the Turkish version of the Health Professional Education in Patient Safety Survey: H-PEPSS-TR. *Nurse Education in Practice*, *42*, 102640. DOI: 10.1016/j.nepr.2019.102640 PMID: 31756625

Tella, S., Smith, N.-J., Partanen, P., Jamookeeah, D., Lamidi, M. J., & Turnen, H. (2015). Learning to ensure patient safety in clinical settings: Comparing Finnish and British nursing students' perceptions. *Journal of Clinical Nursing*, *24*(19–20), 2954–2964. DOI: 10.1111/jocn.12914 PMID: 26216053

Terzioğlu, F., & Uslu Şahan, F. (2017). *Hemşirelerin tıbbi müdahalede karar verme yetkisi ve konumu*. Sağlık ve Hemşirelik Yönetimi Dergisi.

Topaz, M., & Pruinelli, L. (2020). Big data and nursing: Implications for the future of nursing education. *Journal of Nursing Scholarship*, *52*(5), 546–553. DOI: 10.1111/jnu.12586

Topol, E. J. (2019). *Deep medicine: How artificial intelligence can make healthcare human again*. Basic Books.

Tørris, C., & Nortvedt, L. (2024). Health literacy and self-care among adult immigrants with type 2 diabetes: A scoping review. *BMC Public Health*, *24*(1), 3248. DOI: 10.1186/s12889-024-20749-6 PMID: 39578821

Tsai, S. L., Chai, S., & Chuang, K. H. (2015). The effectiveness of a chronic obstructive pulmonary disease computer game as a learning tool for nursing students. *Open Journal of Nursing*, *5*(7), 605–612. DOI: 10.4236/ojn.2015.57064

Tsekoura, M., ... (2020) "Cross-cultural adaptation and validation of the Greek Version of the SARC-F for evaluating sarcopenia in Greek older adults" Available at: http://www.ismni.org

Tsuda, T. (2017) "Epidemiology of fragility fractures and fall prevention in the elderly: a systematic review of the literature". Available at: https://journals.lww .com/c-orthopaedicpractice

Tuckett, A., & Crompton, P. (2014). Qualitative understanding of an international learning experience: What A ustralian undergraduate nurses and midwives said about a Cambodia placement? *International Journal of Nursing Practice*, *20*(2), 135–141. DOI: 10.1111/ijn.12142 PMID: 24713009

Tuncer Unver, G., Celebi Cakiroglu, O., Gungor Satilmis, I., & Harmanci Seren, A. K. (2021). The Experiences Of Nurses Who Studied Abroad With The Erasmus Program During Undergraduate Education: A Qualitative Study. *Nurse Education in Practice*, *51*, 102993. Https://Doi.Org/10.1016/J.Nepr.2021.102993. DOI: 10.1016/j.nepr.2021.102993 PMID: 33621924

Turale, S., Kunaviktikul, W., & Mesukko, J. (2020). Giving undergraduate nursing students international experiences: Issues and strategies. *Nursing and Health Sciences, 22*(3), 830. DOI: 10.1111/nhs.12722

Türkmen, E., Altuntaş, S., Baykal, Ü., & Seren, Ş. (2011). Hasta güvenliği kültürü ölçeğinin geliştirilmesi [Development of patient safety culture scale]. *Anadolu Hemsirelik ve Saglik Bilimleri Dergisi*, *14*(4), 38–46.

Ulupınar, F., & Toygar, Ş. A. (2020). The Use of Technology in Nursing Education and Sample Practices. *Fiscaoeconomia*, *4*(2), 524–537. DOI: 10.25295/fsecon.2020.02.013

Ulvund, I., Dadi, G. B., & Sundal, H. (2023). Nurses benefit from international clinical placement as nurse students: A qualitative study. *Nurse Education Today*, *121*, 105663. DOI: 10.1016/j.nedt.2022.105663 PMID: 36481523

United Nations Development Programme. (2024a). *Small Island Digital States: How digital can catalyse SIDS development.* https://www.undp.org/publications/small-island-digital-states-how-digital-can-catalyse-sids-development

United Nations Development Programme. (2024b). *How digital is transforming the lives of young people in Small Island Developing States.* https://www.undp.org/sites/g/files/zskgke326/files/2024-04/undp-how-digital-is-transforming-the-lives-of-young-people-in-small-island-developing-states-v2.pdf

University of Primorska, Faculty of Health Sciences. (2022). *BENEFITS: Better and more effective nursing education for improving transcultural nursing skills* (Project 20191TR01KA203076879). Erasmus+ KA2 Cooperation Projects. Access July 21, 2025 from: https://www.upr.si/en/up--environment/projects-of-the-university-of-primorska/erasmus-ka2-cooperation-projects/benefits-better-and-more-effective-nursing-education-for-improving-transcultural-nursing-skills

Urakova, A., & Ibragimova, L. (2024). Virtual reality applications in nursing education: A global perspective. *Nurse Education in Practice, 65*, 103597. DOI: 10.1016/j.nepr.2024.103597

Uriz-Otano, F., Uriz-Otano, J. I., & Malafarina, V. (2015). Factors Associated With Short-Term Functional Recovery in Elderly People With a Hip Fracture. Influence of Cognitive Impairment. *Journal of the American Medical Directors Association, 16*(3), 215–220. DOI: 10.1016/j.jamda.2014.09.009 PMID: 25441099

Urstad, K. H., Navarro-Illana, E., Oftedal, B., Whittingham, K., Alamar, S., Windle, R., Løkken, A., Taylor, M. G., Larsen, M. H., Narayasanamy, M., Sancho-Pelluz, J., Navarro-Illana, P., & Wharrad, H. (2021). Usability and value of a digital learning resource in nursing education across European countries: A cross-sectional exploration. *BMC Nursing, 20*(1), 161. Advance online publication. DOI: 10.1186/s12912-021-00681-5 PMID: 34488724

Valdez, G. F. D., Genuino, R.-B. M. J., Babate, F. J., Bernardo, M., Biluan, F.-C. A. P., & Santos, M. (2024). A Global Survey of Filipino Nurses' Motivations, Challenges, and Aspirations. *Research Square (Research Square).* DOI: 10.21203/rs.3.rs-5218786/v1

Van Egmond, M. A., van der Schaaf, M., Vredeveld, T., Vollenbroek-Hutten, M. M. R., van Berge Henegouwen, M. I., Klinkenbijl, J. H. G., & Engelbert, R. H. H. (2018). Effectiveness of physiotherapy with telerehabilitation in surgical patients: A systematic review and meta-analysis. *Physiotherapy, 104*(3), 277–298. DOI: 10.1016/j.physio.2018.04.004 PMID: 30030037

Van Heghe, A.. (2022). Effects of Orthogeriatric Care Models on Outcomes of Hip Fracture Patients: A Systematic Review and Meta-Analysis. In *Calcified Tissue International* (pp. 162–184). Springer., DOI: 10.1007/s00223-021-00913-5

VanDenKerkhof, E., Sears, N., Edge, D. S., Tregunno, D., & Ginsburg, L. (2017). Patient safety in practical nurses' education: A cross-sectional survey of newly registered practical nurses in Canada. *Nurse Education Today*, *51*, 48–56. DOI: 10.1016/j.nedt.2017.01.003 PMID: 28126688

Venegas-Sanabria, L. C.. (2018). Factors associated with in-hospital complications in the elderly subjected to hip fracture surgery. *Revista Española de Geriatría y Gerontología*, *53*(3), 181–182. DOI: 10.1016/j.regg.2017.06.004 PMID: 28733077

Ventura, C. A. A., Mendes, I. A. C., Wilson, L., de Godoy, S., Tamí-Maury, I., Zárate-Grajales, R. A., & Salas-Segura, S. (2014). Global health competencies according to nursing faculty from Brazilian higher education institutions. *Revista Latino-Americana de Enfermagem*, *22*(2), 179–186. DOI: 10.1590/0104-1169.2996.2400 PMID: 26107823

Veronese, N., & Maggi, S. (2018). Epidemiology and social costs of hip fracture. *Injury*, *49*(8), 1458–1460. DOI: 10.1016/j.injury.2018.04.015 PMID: 29699731

Wainberg, M. L., Scorza, P., & Collins, P. Y. (2023). Cultural stigma and global mental health inequities. *World Psychiatry; Official Journal of the World Psychiatric Association (WPA)*, *22*(1), 1–9. DOI: 10.1002/wps.21029 PMID: 36640397

Wald, P., Chocano-Bedoya, P. O., Meyer, U., Orav, E. J., Egli, A., Theiler, R., & Bischoff-Ferrari, H. A. (2020). Comparative Effectiveness of Functional Tests in Fall Prediction After Hip Fracture. *Journal of the American Medical Directors Association*, *21*(9), 1327–1330. DOI: 10.1016/j.jamda.2020.02.008 PMID: 32276783

Walker, D., Altmiller, G., Barkell, N., Hromadik, L., & Toothaker, R. (2019). Development and Validation of the Just Culture Assessment Tool for Nursing Education. *Nurse Educator*, *44*(5), 261–264. DOI: 10.1097/NNE.0000000000000705 PMID: 31305358

Walker, D., Hromadik, L., Altmiller, G., Barkell, N., Toothaker, R., & Powell, K. (2021). Exploratory factor analysis of the Just Culture Assessment Tool for nursing education. *Journal of Research in Nursing : JRN*, *26*(1-2), 49–59. DOI: 10.1177/1744987120951589 PMID: 35251224

Walton, M. M., Shaw, T., Barnet, S., & Ross, J. (2006). Developing a national patient safety education framework for Australia. *Quality & Safety in Health Care*, *15*(6), 437–442. DOI: 10.1136/qshc.2006.019216 PMID: 17142595

White, J., Gunn, M., Chiarella, M., Catton, H., & Stewart, D. (2025). *Renewing the Definitions of 'nursing' and 'a nurse'.* Final project report, June 2025. International Council of Nurses.

WHO. Falls, (2020). Available at URL: https://www.who.int/news-room/fact-sheets/detail/falls

WHO. Healthy aging, (2020). Available at URL: https://www.who.int/news-room/questions-and-answers/item/healthy-ageing-and-functional-ability

Wilson, L., Harper, D. C., Tamí-Maury, I., Zarate, R., Salas, S. P. E., Farley, J. E., Warren, N., Mendes, I. A. C., & Ventura, C. A. A. (2012). Global Health Competencies for Nurses in the Americas. *Journal of Professional Nursing*, *28*(4), 213–222. DOI: 10.1016/j.profnurs.2011.11.021 PMID: 22818191

Wit, R. F., de Veer, A. J. E., Batenburg, R. S., & Francke, A. L. (2023). International comparison of professional competency frameworks for nurses: Addressing health promotion and e-health across borders. *BMC Nursing*, *22*, 343. DOI: 10.1186/s12912-023-01514-3 PMID: 37770894

Woolcock, M. (2001). The Place of Social Capital in Understanding Social and Economic Outcomes. [Plus additional analyses by Woolcock & Narayan on "linking" social capital]. *Canadian Journal of Policy Research*, *2*(1), 11–17.

World Health Organization. (2009). *Patient safety curriculum guide for medical schools.* World Health Organization. https://apps.who.int/iris/handle/10665/44091

World Health Organization. (2011). *Patient safety curriculum guide: Multi-professional edition.* World Health Organization. https://www.who.int/publications/i/item/9789241501958

World Health Organization. (2016). *Nurse educator core competencies.* WHO. Access 27. july 2025, from: https://iris.who.int/bitstream/handle/10665/258713/9789241549622-eng.pdf?sequence=1

World Health Organization. (2020, April 6). *The state of the world's nursing 2020: Investing in education, jobs and leadership* [PDF]. WHO. Access 27. july 2025, from: https://www.who.int/publications/i/item/9789240003279

World Health Organization. (2023). *Comprehensive Mental Health Action Plan 2023–2030.* https://www.who.int/publications/i/item/9789240072244

World Health Organization. (2024). *Mental Health Atlas 2024.* https://www.who.int/publications/i/item/9789240114487

Wu, A., Maddula, V., Singh, J., Sagoo, M. G., Chien, C. L., Wingate, R., Kielstein, H., Traxler, H., Brassett, C., Waschke, J., Vielmuth, F., Sakurai, T., Zeroual, M., Olsen, J., El-Batti, S., Viranta, S., Kitahara, S., Keay, K. A., Kunzel, C., & Noël, G. (2021). Alternatives to Student Outbound Mobility—Improving Students' Cultural Competency Skills Online to Improve Global Health Without Travel. *Medical Science Educator, 31*(4), 1441–1451. DOI: 10.1007/s40670-021-01332-9 PMID: 34123512

Yang, B.-H., Lo, K.-W., Li, Y.-S., & Chao, K.-Y. (2024). Effects of integration interdisciplinary learning on student learning outcomes and healthcare-giving competence: A mixed methods study. *BMC Nursing, 23*(1), 583. DOI: 10.1186/s12912-024-02260-w

Yee, D. K. H., Lau, T.-W., Fang, C., Ching, K., Cheung, J., & Leung, F. (2022). Orthogeriatric Multidisciplinary Co-Management Across Acute and Rehabilitation Care Improves Length of Stay, Functional Outcomes and Complications in Geriatric Hip Fracture Patients. *Geriatric Orthopaedic Surgery & Rehabilitation, 13*, 21514593221085813. Advance online publication. DOI: 10.1177/21514593221085813 PMID: 35433103

Yfantopoulos, J. (2001, March-April). The Greek version of the EuroQol (EQ-5D) instrument. *Arch Hellen Med, 18*(2), 180–191.

Yılmaz, M., & Kuğuoğlu, S. (2024). Hemşirelik Bilim Felsefesinde Paradigmaların Önemi. *TOGÜ Sağlık Bilimleri Dergisi, 4*(1), 108–119. DOI: 10.52369/togusagbilderg.1164824

Yüceyurt, N. K., & Şenyuva, E. A. (2023). Uluslararası ve ulusal çalışmaların hemşirelik eğitimine yansımaları. *Yükseköğretim ve Bilim Dergisi, 13*(1), 1–9.

Yüksekdağ, B. B. (2021). Covid-19 pandemisi döneminde öğrenme ve uzaktan hemşirelik eğitiminde paradigma değişimi. *Açıköğretim Uygulamaları ve Araştırmaları Dergisi, 7*(1), 61–73.

Zhang, S., Wang, W., Wu, S., Ye, H., Dong, L., Wang, J., Ning, X., & Cui, H. (2024). Analysis of the mediating effect between ehealth literacy and health self-management of undergraduate nursing students' mental health literacy. *BMC Nursing, 23*(1), 264. DOI: 10.1186/s12912-024-01920-1 PMID: 38654311

Zhou, Y.. (2023) "Different Surgical interventions for Unstable intertrochanteric fracture of the femur: Network meta-analysis." Available at: https://doi.org/DOI: 10.21203/rs.3.rs-3258227/v1

Zikos, D., Diomidous, M., & Mantas, J. (2010). A framework for the development of patient safety education and training guidelines. *Studies in Health Technology and Informatics*, *155*, 189–195. DOI: 10.3233/978-1-60750-563-1-189 PMID: 20543328

Zinger, G., Sylvetsky, N., Levy, Y., Steinberg, K., Bregman, A., Yudkevich, G., & Peyser, A. (2023). Early benefits of a secondary fracture prevention programme. *Hip International*, *33*(2), 332–337. DOI: 10.1177/11207000211027476 PMID: 34180292

About the Contributors

Alexandros Argyriadis is an Assistant Professor in the Department of Nursing at the Hellenic Mediterranean University, with a specialization in "Mental Health". Previously, he served as Chair of the Department of Nursing at Frederick University and as Director of its Master's Program in Community Health Care, where he taught for ten years. He has also taught at the Hellenic Open University, the Cyprus University of Technology, the University of the Peloponnese, and other institutions in Europe and internationally at both undergraduate and postgraduate levels. He has also an extensive publication record indexed in Scopus, PubMed, and Google Scholar.

***

Alev Ateş-Çobanoğlu is an Associate Professor of Computer Education and Instructional Technology (CEIT) program of Faculty of Education, Ege University. She received her M.Sc in the Dokuz Eylul University in 2005. She had worked as an Information and Communication Technology (ICT) teacher at a high school of Ministry of National Education (MoNE) for three years. She received her PhD in Curriculum and Instruction from Ege University in 2013. Her academic interests are blended learning, ICT integration in education, instructional technology and instructional design.

Julia Paulevna Bayer is a Russian sociologist who is giving lectures at Presidencial Academy in St. Petersburg, Russia as well as an empirical researches in applied Sociology. Julia is an author of more than 50 articles and is famous as a TV expert. Julia has contributeded to the opening a faculry of social technologies in RANEPA and has been a deputy dean there for 12 years, being responsible for oganising sientific and cultural events.

SudhaAnanthi G is a dedicated academician with a strong passion for education and continuous learning. Known for her excellent communication skills and ability to inspire others, she excels in both teaching and collaborative environments. As a motivating presence in her team, SudhaAnanthi consistently fosters a positive and productive atmosphere. Her strengths as a team player and her commitment to academic excellence make her a valuable asset in any educational setting.

Dmitry Petrovich Gavra is a Russian sociologist and political scientist, Doctor of Sociology, and professor at St. Petersburg State University. He is the head of the Department of Public Relations in Business at the Higher School of Journalism and Mass Communications. He is a laureate of the Russian Federation Government Prize in Print Media (2008). He is the creator of the institutional theory of public opinion and the sphere-substantial concept of the external image of the state. He is the author of the monograph "Public Opinion as a Sociological Category and Social Institution." He is the head of the research project "The External Image of the State in the Global Information Space." He is the coordinator of the Innovative Educational Project "Business Journalism and Business Communication" of the National Project "Education" (2006-2009). He is also the head of the expert council of the Baltic Governors' Club. Since 2017, President of the Association of Public Relations Teachers

Louiza Ioannidou is an Assistant Professor in Mental Health for Children and Adolescents at the European University Cyprus and a Registered School Psychologist. Dr Ioannidou has obtained her PhD in Psychology, her MA in School Psychology (applied program), and her BA in Psychology, all from the University of Cyprus. She has also trained in the field of Cognitive - Behavioural Therapy, Positive Psychology, Mindfulness, Solution Focused Therapy, and Business - Team Coaching. She has also a diploma in the Master Practitioner in Eating Disorders and Obesity. Her teaching and research experience focuses on school bullying, children and adolescents' mental health and resilience, and parental involvement. Her research interests also focus on developing, implementing, and evaluating psychoeducational programs to promote children's and adolescents' mental health, well-being, resilience, and a safe school climate. Her research findings are published in scientific journals and presented in scientific conferences. She is the author and editor of the book "Building Mental Resilience: Positive Psychology, Emotional Intelligence, and Play" (2024) published by IGI Global.

Cennet Kayhan is a PhD student in the Department of Nursing Education at Ege University's Faculty of Nursing. She completed her undergraduate studies at Ege University and her master's degree in Surgical Nursing at Afyon Kocatepe

University. She currently works as a Health Services teacher at a Vocational and Technical Anatolian High School. She has experience in Erasmus+ projects. Her research interests include web-based and game-based teaching methods, patient education, intercultural nursing, and lifelong learning. ORCID: 0009 0003 3386 3988

Maksud A.Madraswale working as an Associate Professor, Department of Management, Presidency University, Bengaluru. For few years he served at Oman and other Arab Countries. To his credit he published five articles in Scopus Indexed journals.

T.C. Manjunath was born on 6th February 1967. He did his B.E. from RV College of Engg. in 1989 (B'lore Univ), M.E. in Robotics & Automation from Govt.'s LD College of Engg., (Gujarat Univ., Ahmedabad) in 1992 with FCD-First Rank & PhD in Systems & Control Engg. from IIT Bombay in the year 2007, got best research scholar award for the entire IITB. He is currently working as the Dean Research (R & D) and as Professor in Dept. of Computer Science & Engg. with specialization in IoT, Cyber Security, Blockchain Technology in Rajarajeswari College of Engineering, Bengaluru, Karnataka. He has got a teaching (academic), research & administrative experience of more than 35+ years (10 years as Principal & 8 years as HoD, 1 year as Dean Research & rest as faculty) and has published more than 1500+ research papers in various national & international journals & conferences, with 175+ patents, 100+ book-chapters, 25 awards, 100s of Keynote talks and also published 25 text books in various field of science, engineering & technology, completed projects worth Rs. 9 Crores till date & guided 10 PhD scholars in VTU. He is a member of 30 Professional Society Chapters and is a fellow of IE, IETE, AMIEE, Sr. Member of IEEE and a chartered engineer.

Nilay Özkütük completed her undergraduate studies at Ege University School of Nursing in 1997, her master's degree in Educational Administration, Supervision, Planning, and Economics at Ege University Institute of Social Sciences in 2004, and her doctorate in Nursing Fundamentals at Ege University Institute of Health Sciences in 2010. She became an Assistant Professor in 2013. She worked as an intensive care nurse at a private hospital between 1997 and 1998, as a research assistant at Ege University School of Nursing in the Department of Nursing Education between 1998 and 2005, as a lecturer between 2005 and 2010, as a lecturer between 2010 and 2013, and as an assistant professor between 2013 and 2025. She was promoted to Associate Professor in May 2025. She is an Associate Professor in the Department of Nursing Education at Ege University's Faculty of Nursing. Nilay Özkütük served as Secretary and Board Member of the Nursing Education Programs Evaluation and Accreditation Association (HEPDAK) from 2013 to 2015, and remains a member of HEPDAK. Özkütük has published in international and nationally peer-reviewed journals and authored chapters in national books. She also serves as a reviewer for international and nationally peer-reviewed journals. Özkütük's research focuses on educational topics such as teaching methods, organizational citizenship, e-learning, distance education, cybersecurity, clinical teaching, peer mentoring, educational games, and virtual simulation.

R.Bhuvaneswari working as an Assistant Professor of English at Dr.Mahalingam College of Engineering and Technology, Pollachi. To her credit she completed 10 NPTEL / SWAYAM and published few articles in Scopus indexed journals.

R. Velmurugan presently working as Professor, Department of Commerce, Karpagam Academy of Higher Education, Coimbatore. He started his career as a Project Fellow under UGC Sponsored Major Research Project at NGM College, Pollachi. He has 19 years of teaching experience has 15 years of research experience. To his credit he produced 25 Ph.D. Scholars and 5 M.Phil. Scholars. At present two scholars submitter his thesis, 6 Ph.D. Scholars are under his guidance. Moreover, to his credit he published 168 articles in various International Journals, of which 109 articles are published in Scopus Indexed Journals and 15 articles in Web of Science and 76 articles in edited volumes. He also participates and presented 27 papers in various International Seminar / Conference and 54 National Seminar / Conference. He acted as an external examiner for various M.Phil. and Ph.D. Viva voce examinations. He acted as a Vice Chancellor nominee for Doctoral Committee Expert at Bharathiar University, Coimbatore and Periyar University, Salem. He acted as a Chairperson at various National Level Conferences. He also acted as an Expert for Syllabus Scrutiny Committee, Question Paper Scrutiny Committee and Expert members for Board of Studies at various reputed Colleges. Considering his meritorious contribution, he received awards like Best Paper Presenter, Best Research Supervisor and Best Faculty Awards from various research foundations and councils. He too acted as a resource person for 27 Guest Lectures, 30 Workshops and 10 faculty development programmes.

S. Senthilkumar, currently working as Assistant Professor in Finance and Management, Skyline University, Nigeria. His qualifications are MBA, M.Com, M.Phil, MS, and PhD. He has rich experience in teaching and academic of 18.2 years. He had published 58 papers Publications in National and International Journals and Proceedings. He Authored 4 books in Research Methodology, Corporate Finance, Principles of Accounting and Business Policy & Strategic management. Participated and presented 62 papers in National & International Seminars and Conferences. He acted as resource person and Guest lecture around 25 Programmemes. He guided 225 projects in M.B.A., 36 M.Phil, and 9 PhD. He got Authorized Guide ship for PhD & M.Phil from Indian Universities such as Anna University, Karpagam University, Bharathiar University, Periyar Manimai University and AMIET University and Vinayaka Mission University and Bahir Dar University, Ethiopia. He performed as Foreign examiner for evaluating PhD Thesis around 18 Thesis of Indian universities such as Bharathiar University, Visvesvaraya Technological University, University of Mumbai, MS University and Bharathidasan university.

Index

www.ingramcontent.com/pod-product-compliance
Lightning Source LLC
LaVergne TN
LVHW081527300926
849161LV00006B/1327
* 9 7 9 8 3 3 7 3 5 9 3 1 1 *